MORE 4U!

P9-CCM-955

the**clinics**.com

This Clinics series is available online.

ere's what
ou get:

- Full text of EVERY issue from 2002 to NOW

- Figures, tables, drawings, references and more

- Searchable: find what you need fast

  Search [All Clinics ▼] for [   ] [GO]

- Linked to MEDLINE and Elsevier journals

- E-alerts

NDIVIDUAL
UBSCRIBERS

lick __Register__
nd follow
nstructions

ou'll need an
ccount number

LOG ON TODAY. IT'S FAST AND EASY.

Your subscriber
account number ——→
is on your mailing
label

This is your copy of:

THE CLINICS OF NORTH AMERICA

CXXX   **2296532-2**   2   Mar 05

J.H. DOE, MD
531 MAIN STREET
CENTER CITY, NY 10001-001

BOUGHT A SINGLE ISSUE? Sorry, you won't be able to access full text online. Please subscribe today to get complete content by contacting customer service at 800 645 2552 (US and Canada) or 407 345 4000 (outside US and Canada) or via email at elsols@elsevier.com.

NEW!

Now also available for INSTITUTIONS

Works/Integrates with MD Consult

Available in a variety of packages: Collections containing 14, 31 or 50 Clinics titles

Or Collection upgrade for existing MD Consult customers

Call today! 877-857-1047 or e-mail: mdc.groupinfo@elsevier.com

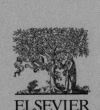

ELSEVIER

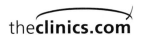

CLINICS IN CHEST MEDICINE

The Lung in Extreme Environments

GUEST EDITORS
Stephen Ruoss, MD, and
Robert B. Schoene, MD

September 2005 • Volume 26 • Number 3

SAUNDERS

An Imprint of Elsevier, Inc.
PHILADELPHIA   LONDON   TORONTO   MONTREAL   SYDNEY   TOKYO

W.B. SAUNDERS COMPANY
A Division of Elsevier Inc.

Elsevier, Inc. • 1600 John F. Kennedy Boulevard • Suite 1800 • Philadelphia, Pennsylvania 19103-2899

http://www.chestmed.theclinics.com

CLINICS IN CHEST MEDICINE	**Volume 26, Number 3**
September 2005	**ISSN 0272-5231**
Editor: Sarah E. Barth	**ISBN 1-4160-2812-9**

Reprints: For copies of 100 or more, of articles in this publication, please contact the Commercial Reprints Department, Elsevier Inc., 360 Park Avenue South, New York, New York 10010-1710. Tel. (212) 633-3813 Fax: (212) 462-1935 e-mail: reprints@elsevier.com.

The ideas and opinions expressed in *Clinics in Chest Medicine* do not necessarily reflect those of the Publisher. The Publisher does not assume any responsibility for any injury and/or damage to persons or property arising out of or related to any use of the material contained in this periodical. The reader is advised to check the appropriate medical literature and the product information currently provided by the manufacturer of each drug to be administered to verify the dosage, the method and duration of administration, or contraindications. It is the responsibility of the treating physician or other health care professional, relying on independent experience and knowledge of the patient, to determine drug dosages and the best treatment for the patient. Mention of any product in this issue should not be construed as endorsement by the contributors, editors, or the Publisher of the product or manufacturers' claims.

Clinics in Chest Medicine (ISSN 0272-5231) is published quarterly by W.B. Saunders Company. Corporate and editorial offices: Elsevier, Inc., 1600 John F. Kennedy Boulevard, Suite 1800, Philadelphia, PA 19103-2899. Accounting and circulation offices: 6277 Sea Harbor Drive, Orlando, FL 32887-4800. Periodicals postage paid at Orlando, FL 32887, and additional mailing offices. Subscription price is $185.00 per year (US individuals), $285.00 per year (US institutions), $206.00 per year (Canadian individuals), $340.00 per year (Canadian institutions), $240.00 per year (international individuals), and $340.00 per year (international institutions). International air speed delivery is included in all *Clinics* subscription prices. All prices are subject to change without notice. POSTMASTER: Send address changes to *Clinics in Chest Medicine* (ISSN 0272-5231), W.B. Saunders Company, Periodicals Fulfillment, Orlando, FL 32887-4800. **Customer Service: 1-800-654-2452 (US). From outside of the US, call 1-407-345-4000.**

Clinics in Chest Medicine is covered in *Index Medicus, Current Contents/Clinical Medicine, EMBASE/Excerpta Medica, Science Citation Index*, and *ISI/BIOMED*.

Printed in the United States of America.

GUEST EDITORS

STEPHEN RUOSS, MD, Associate Professor of Medicine, Division of Pulmonary and Critical Care Medicine, Stanford University School of Medicine, Stanford, California

ROBERT B. SCHOENE, MD, Professor of Medicine, Division of Pulmonary and Critical Care Medicine, University of California—San Diego, School of Medicine, San Diego, California

CONTRIBUTORS

ULRICH BROECKEL, MD, Associate Professor, Division of Cardiovascular Medicine, Human and Molecular Genetics Center, Medical College of Wisconsin, Milwaukee, Wisconsin

THOMAS A. DILLARD, MD, Professor of Medicine, Division of Pulmonary/Critical Care, Medical College of Georgia, Augusta, Georgia

ULRICH EHRMANN, MD, Resident in Anesthesia, Sektion Anaesthesiologische Pathophysiologie und Verfahrensentwicklung, Universitaetsklinikum, Ulm, Germany

MARLOWE W. ELDRIDGE, MD, Medical Director, The John Rankin Laboratory of Pulmonary Medicine, Department of Population Health Sciences, University of Wisconsin at Madison; and Assistant Professor, Department of Pediatrics, Critical Care Medicine, and Biomedical Engineering, University of Wisconsin School of Medicine, Madison, Wisconsin

FRANK W. EWALD, Jr, MD, Assistant Professor of Medicine, Veteran's Administration Medical Center, Augusta, Georgia

HANS C. HAVERKAMP, PhD, Postdoctoral Fellow, Vermont Lung Center, University of Vermont, Burlington, Vermont

SUSAN R. HOPKINS, MD, PhD, Associate Professor, Division of Physiology, Department of Medicine; and Department of Radiology, University of California—San Diego, La Jolla, California

JEAN-PAUL JANSSENS, MD, Head of Outpatient Section of the Division of Pulmonary Diseases, Geneva University Hospital, Geneva, Switzerland

M. ASIF KALEEM, MBBS, Senior Fellow, Division of Pulmonary/Critical Care, Medical College of Georgia, Augusta, Georgia

SEEMA KHOSLA, MD, Senior Fellow, Division of Pulmonary/Critical Care, Medical College of Georgia, Augusta, Georgia

ANDREW T. LOVERING, PhD, Postdoctoral Fellow, The John Rankin Laboratory of Pulmonary Medicine, Department of Population Health Sciences, University of Wisconsin at Madison, Madison, Wisconsin

JAMES P. MALONEY, MD, Associate Professor, Division of Pulmonary and Critical Medicine, University of Colorado Health Sciences Center, Denver, Colorado

CLAUS-MARTIN MUTH, MD, Assistant Professor of Anesthesiology, Sektion Anaesthesiologische Pathophysiologie und Verfahrensentwicklung, Universitaetsklinikum, Ulm, Germany

G. KIM PRISK, PhD, DSc, Professor, Division of Physiology, Department of Medicine, University of California—San Diego, La Jolla, California

PETER RADERMACHER, MD, Professor of Anesthesiology, Sektion Anaesthesiologische Pathophysiologie und Verfahrensentwicklung, Universitaetsklinikum, Ulm, Germany

ROBERT B. SCHOENE, MD, Professor of Medicine, Division of Pulmonary and Critical Care Medicine, University of California—San Diego, School of Medicine, San Diego, California

KAY TETZLAFF, MD, Associate Professor, Department of Sports Medicine, Medical Clinic and Polyclinic, University of Tübingen, Tübingen, Germany

EINAR THORSEN, MD, PhD, Professor, Department of Hyperbaric Medicine, Haukeland University Hospital, University of Bergen, Bergen, Norway

CONTRIBUTORS

CONTENTS

Preface   ix
Stephen Ruoss and Robert B. Schoene

**Breathing at Depth: Physiologic and Clinical Aspects of Diving while
Breathing Compressed Gas**   355
Kay Tetzlaff and Einar Thorsen

> When diving, human beings are exposed to hazards that are unique to the hyperbaric
> underwater environment and the physical behavior of gases at higher ambient pressure.
> Hypercapnia, hyperoxia, carbon monoxide intoxication, inert gas (predominantly nitro-
> gen) narcosis, and decompression illness all may lead to impaired consciousness, with a
> high risk of drowning in this nonrespirable environment. Proper physiologic function and
> adaptation of the respiratory system are of the utmost importance to minimize the risks
> associated with compressed gas diving. This article provides an introduction to the diving
> techniques, the physics, and the pertinent human physiology and pathophysiology asso-
> ciated with this extreme environment. The causes of the major medical problems encoun-
> tered in diving are described, with an emphasis on the underlying respiratory physiology.

Physiological and Clinical Aspects of Apnea Diving   381
Claus-Martin Muth, Ulrich Ehrmann, and Peter Radermacher

> Apnea diving is a fascinating example of applied physiology. The record for apnea div-
> ing as an extreme sport is 171 meters, 8:58 minutes. The short time beneath the surface
> induces profound cardiovascular and respiratory effects. Variations of blood-gas tensions
> result from the interaction of metabolism and the rapid sequence of compression and
> decompression. Decompression sickness is possible. Apnea divers can reach depths
> beyond the theoretic physiologic limit by using the lung-packing maneuver. Apnea
> divers exhibit a fall in heart rate, which can be trained and is an oxygen-conserving
> effect, but increases the incidence of ventricular arrhythmia.

**Epidemiology, Risk Factors, and Genetics of High-Altitude–Related
Pulmonary Disease**   395
James P. Maloney and Ulrich Broeckel

> High-altitude–related pulmonary disease is a spectrum of acute and chronic illnesses
> with a well-described epidemiology. The risk for these illnesses is related to well-known
> environmental risk factors and lesser-known but important genetic factors. Prevention
> of acute high-altitude illness is possible in most visitors from lower elevations. Chronic
> high-altitude illnesses have an important worldwide impact.

Limits of Respiration at High Altitude 405
Robert B. Schoene

Under most conditions, the lungs compensate for the stresses of illness to ensure adequate acquisition of oxygen. Even with exposure to high altitude, the lungs' adaptations ensure that this process takes place. This process is challenged by global hypoxia, especially if there is impairment in the three processes needed for adequate tissue oxygenation: (1) intact ventilatory drive to breathe; (2) sufficient increase in alveolar ventilation, which is stimulated by that drive; and (3) intact gas exchange at the alveolar-capillary interface. This article reviews the mechanisms that make the study of high altitude relevant to patients who have heart or lung disease at low altitude.

The Lung in Space 415
G. Kim Prisk

The lung is exquisitely sensitive to gravity, which induces gradients in ventilation, blood flow, and gas exchange. Studies of lungs in microgravity provide a means of elucidating the effects of gravity. They suggest a mechanism by which gravity serves to match ventilation to perfusion, making for a more efficient lung than anticipated. Despite predictions, lungs do not become edematous, and there is no disruption to gas exchange in microgravity. Sleep disturbances in microgravity are not a result of respiratory-related events; obstructive sleep apnea is caused principally by the gravitational effects on the upper airways. In microgravity, lungs may be at greater risk to the effects of inhaled aerosols.

Responses and Limitations of the Respiratory System to Exercise 439
Andrew T. Lovering, Hans C. Haverkamp, and Marlowe W. Eldridge

During maximal exercise, the gas exchange function of the lung is challenged because of the major cardiopulmonary changes that must occur to meet the increased metabolic demands imposed by exercise. In healthy untrained young adults, the respiratory system is able to meet these demands imposed on it during maximal exercise by implementing several key mechanisms. Nonetheless, there are several exceptional cases in which the lung is unable to accommodate the demands of exercise because of vascular or airway limitations.

The Lung at Maximal Exercise: Insights from Comparative Physiology 459
Susan R. Hopkins

Horses are bred selectively for aerobic performance and have extraordinarily high maximal oxygen consumption, approximately double the mass-specific value for human athletes. Pulmonary limitations to exercise performance are well described in these animals, including exercise-induced arterial hypoxemia and exercise-induced pulmonary hemorrhage. In human athletes, pulmonary limitations are recognized increasingly as affecting athletic performance. Potential pulmonary limitations during maximal exercise are compared in human and equine athletes.

Aging of the Respiratory System: Impact on Pulmonary Function Tests and Adaptation to Exertion 469
Jean-Paul Janssens

Normal aging of the respiratory system is associated with a decrease in static elastic recoil of the lung, in respiratory muscle performance, and in compliance of the chest wall and respiratory system, resulting in increased work of breathing compared with younger subjects and a diminished respiratory reserve in cases of acute illness, such as heart failure, infection, or airway obstruction. In spite of these changes, the respiratory system remains capable of maintaining adequate gas exchange at rest and during exertion during the entire lifespan, with only a slight decrease in PaO_2 and no significant change in $PaCO_2$.

Pulmonary Function Testing and Extreme Environments   485
Thomas A. Dillard, Seema Khosla, Frank W. Ewald, Jr, and M. Asif Kaleem

Millions of people worldwide engage in leisure or occupational activities in extreme environments. These environments entail health risks even for normal subjects. The presence of lung disease, or other conditions, further predisposes to illness or injury. Patients who have lung conditions should, but often do not, consult with their pulmonary clinicians before traveling. Normal subjects, including elderly or deconditioned adults, may be referred to pulmonologists for evaluation of risk prior to exposure. Other patients may present for consultations after complications occur. Pulmonary function testing before or after exposure can assist physicians counseling patients about the likelihood of complications.

Index   509

FORTHCOMING ISSUES

December 2005

Pulmonary Considerations in Organ and Hematopoietic Stem Cell Transplantation
Robert M. Kotloff, MD, and
Vivek N. Ahya, MD, *Guest Editors*

March 2006

Asthma
Monica Kraft, MD, *Guest Editor*

June 2006

Pleural Diseases
Steven A. Sahn, MD, *Guest Editor*

RECENT ISSUES

June 2005

Tuberculosis
Neil W. Schluger, MD, *Guest Editor*

March 2005

Pneumonia in the Hospital Setting
Marin H. Kollef, MD, *Guest Editor*

December 2004

Interstitial Lung Disease: Idiopathic Interstitial Pneumonia
Ganesh Raghu, MD, *Guest Editor*

ELSEVIER
SAUNDERS

CLINICS
IN CHEST
MEDICINE

Clin Chest Med 26 (2005) ix – x

Preface

The Lung in Extreme Environments

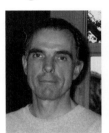 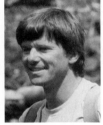

Stephen Ruoss, MD   Robert B. Schoene, MD
Guest Editors

Humans evolved in a temperate, low-altitude environment, but early continental migration, more recent commerce, and modern recreation have exposed humans to environments in which the physiologic stresses are beyond our genetic capabilities. Unlike other species that have adapted, each in their own way, to the extremes of temperature and altitude, humans cannot survive for long periods in these environments. On the other hand, human physiology is resourceful in its acute and chronic adaptations to intentional or accidental environmental extremes, and a better understanding of human health and disease can be gleaned from knowing more about the response to the extremes to which we are exposed. Furthermore, we can also learn from more "niche-specific" species whose abilities to survive seem phenomenal. Through expanded technologic capabilities and continued exploration of unusual environments, humans are exposed to physiologic extremes that not too long ago would have been considered unthinkable or unachievable.

The lung is the first barrier between the body and its surrounding atmosphere, yet it is one of the more resilient in its immediate and long-term responses to environmental extremes. This issue of the *Clinics in Chest Medicine* explores important aspects of pulmonary physiology and medicine in a broad range of extreme environments. Multiple aspects of diving physiology are covered in the first

two articles. These include discussions of the physiology and medical problems encountered while diving with compressed gases for breathing, and also the fascinating circumstances and physiology of breath-hold diving to extreme depths. The issue then addresses the world of hypobaric hypoxia encountered at extreme altitudes. An article discussing the epidemiology and genetics of high-altitude pulmonary diseases in humans is followed by a review of gas exchange at extreme altitude. The truly otherworldly physiology of life in the weightless, zero gravity environment of space is the next subject. The final series of articles addresses the extreme of physiologic performance, rather than that necessarily produced solely by survival in an unnatural environment. The function and limits of pulmonary physiology during exercise is examined in two nicely paired articles. The first principally explores the responses and limitations in humans, while the second provides a wonderful insight into the extremes of lung physiologic tolerance during exercise, though this is undertaken as a comparison of human and equine physiology. We want to note in particular that multiple contributing authors in this issue took the opportunity to compare human and relevant animal physiology in these "niche" extreme environments. This provides an added insight into the adaptive range of some animals, and the relatively narrow adaptive range for our species by comparison. We have also chosen to address the very important extreme of age in this issue. This is a particularly important subject, especially as we are living increasingly active lives to greater ages. Concluding this issue is a very necessary and practical review of the relevant and appropriate evaluation considerations and testing methods for evaluation of individuals who are to explore these environmental extremes.

Befitting our focus on the world of extreme pulmonary physiology and medicine, we have been very fortunate to be able to include in this issue the excellent work from a world-class as well as geographically diverse group of contributing authors. Notwithstanding the rather "environmentally unchallenging" California locations of the Guest Editors, our contributing authors span a wonderful geographic diversity and bring to this project their respective impressive backgrounds in these various disciplines. To them we owe a great debt of gratitude for their willingness to participate, and for the entertaining and educational articles they have contributed to this issue.

Stephen Ruoss, MD
Division of Pulmonary and Critical Care Medicine
H3149
Stanford University School of Medicine
Stanford University Medical Center
300 Pasteur Drive
Stanford, CA 94305, USA
E-mail address: ruoss@stanford.edu

Robert B. Schoene, MD
Division of Pulmonary and Critical Care Medicine
University of California—San Diego
School of Medicine
200 West Arbor Drive
San Diego, CA 92103, USA
E-mail address: rschoene@ucsd.edu

ELSEVIER
SAUNDERS

Clin Chest Med 26 (2005) 355 – 380

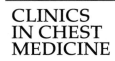

CLINICS
IN CHEST
MEDICINE

Breathing at Depth: Physiologic and Clinical Aspects of Diving while Breathing Compressed Gas

Kay Tetzlaff, MD[a],*, Einar Thorsen, MD, PhD[b]

[a]Department of Sports Medicine, Medical Clinic and Polyclinic, University of Tübingen, Silcherstrasse 5,
72076 Tübingen, Germany
[b]Department of Hyperbaric Medicine, Haukeland University Hospital, University of Bergen, 5021 Bergen, Norway

When diving, human beings are exposed to hazards that are unique to the hyperbaric underwater environment and the physical behavior of gases at higher ambient pressure. Hypercapnia, hyperoxia, carbon monoxide intoxication, inert gas (predominantly nitrogen) narcosis, and decompression illness (DCI) all may lead to impaired consciousness, with a high risk of drowning in this nonrespirable environment. Proper physiologic function and adaptation of the respiratory system are of the utmost importance to minimize the risks associated with compressed gas diving. This article provides an introduction to the diving techniques, the physics, and the pertinent human physiology and pathophysiology associated with this extreme environment. The causes of the major medical problems encountered in diving are described, with an emphasis on the underlying respiratory physiology.

Methods of diving

Diving has become a popular recreational activity and is no longer restricted to military and commercial underwater operations. Although the number of recreational divers is still increasing, the number of professional divers has been more or less the same over the last few decades. It was estimated by the American National Sporting Goods Association [1]

that recreational diving ranks third among the fastest growing outdoor activities and that approximately 2.1 million Americans were engaged in this activity in 2001.

Several methods of underwater diving exist. Diving from submerged air-filled diving bells and diving with air supplied from the surface via an umbilical cord allowing a free flow of gas into a diving helmet have been in use from the early nineteenth century. Problems encountered with diving, including decompression sickness (DCS) and barotrauma, were well known early in the twentieth century. The breakthrough for underwater exploration was the development of the open-circuit breathing apparatus by Cousteau and Gagnan in the French Navy in 1943. This self-contained underwater breathing apparatus (scuba) allowed the diver to breathe air supplied from a high-pressure tank carried by the diver and delivered through a pressure regulator that accommodated the changing ambient pressure of the diving environment. This system provided divers with previously unknown freedom and mobility under water.

With bounce diving (where the diver starts the dive from the surface using scuba equipment, spending a limited time at depth before returning to the surface), the exposure to bottom pressure is limited to minimize decompression stress and the risk of DCI. When breathing air, the practical limit is at a pressure corresponding to a depth of 50–60 m of sea water (msw). The narcotic effects of nitrogen, the high gas density, and the decompression stress all contribute to adverse effects on the body beyond that depth range. Some of these effects can be reduced by changing the breathing gas mixture. Mixtures enriched with oxy-

* Corresponding author.
E-mail address: Kay.Tetzlaff@bc.boehringer-ingelheim.com (K. Tetzlaff).

gen reduce the uptake of inert gas and thereby reduce the risks of decompression, whereas mixtures using added helium reduce the gas density. Increasing the oxygen faction in the gas mixture increases the risk of toxic oxygen effects. Most dangerous is the risk of cerebral oxygen toxicity with sudden unconsciousness, and seizures can occur with exposure to partial pressures of oxygen higher than 150 kPa. Because of the risk of hyperoxic cerebral toxicity, military combat divers who are diving using pure oxygen in a closed-circuit breathing apparatus usually restrict their diving depth range to 0–10 msw.

For diving operations of long duration and deeper than 50–60 msw, the technique of saturation diving was developed in the period from 1960 to 1980. The divers undergo compression in hyperbaric chambers to a pressure equivalent to the diving depth, and they are transferred to the work site in a diving bell. Their body tissues are allowed to become saturated with the gas mixture, which usually is a mixture of helium and oxygen, with a partial pressure of oxygen in the range of 35–70 kPa. Theoretically, they can stay under pressure for an infinite length of time. Most commonly, periods up to 2 weeks are used in diving operations on the offshore oil and gas fields. The divers' effective working time at the work site is not limited by the time constraints of bounce diving. Routine saturation diving operations are typically restricted to depths of 100–150 msw, although an experimental saturation dive to a maximal depth of 701 msw has been performed. In the depth range deeper than 250 msw, there may arise problems, with the pressure effect causing high-pressure nervous syndrome.

The decompression procedures with saturation dives must take into account that body tissues are saturated with the inert gases and the rate of decompression is limited to 25–30 m/d, meaning that some saturation diving operations require that divers stay and live in the hyperbaric chambers for periods up to 30 days or more. Most of the time, the diver is in a dry environment in the hyperbaric chamber, and some operations, such as welding in dry habitats, can be undertaken without the diver having been submerged at all when the diver is transferred from the diving bell to the habitat directly.

Physical and physiologic factors affecting lung function during diving

Diving exposure

Diving is associated with exposure to higher than normal ambient pressure. A dive is typically charac-

terized by compression, isobaric, and decompression phases. The major difference between the diving described in this article and breath-hold diving is that a gas mixture is breathed at increased ambient pressure freely in the atmosphere of a diving bell or a hyperbaric chamber or supplied by an underwater breathing apparatus. Diving usually takes place submerged in water, but some diving operations can be done in a dry environment in a hyperbaric chamber or underwater habitat.

Normal atmospheric pressure or one atmosphere absolute is equivalent to the pressure of a column of 760 mm Hg or 101.3 kPa. One bar corresponds to a pressure of 750 mm Hg, 100 kPa, or 10 msw. For example, at a depth of 30 msw, the diver is exposed to a pressure of 4 bars, and at 100 msw, the diver is exposed to a pressure equivalent of 11 bars.

The fractional concentrations of each gas in a mixture of ideal gases remain the same independent of pressure, and the partial pressure of each component gas is dependent on its fractional concentration and total pressure. The fractional concentration of oxygen in air is 0.21, and at normal atmospheric pressure, the partial pressure of oxygen is 21 kPa. At an ambient pressure of 4 bars or a depth of 30 msw, the fractional concentration of oxygen is still 0.21 but the partial pressure is 84 kPa.

Gases dissolve in fluids proportionately with their partial pressures in the gas phase, which means that the volume of dissolved gases in blood and tissues increases until equilibrium with the gas phase is achieved. The fluid is then saturated with the gas. During the compression and decompression phases of a dive, this process follows first-order exponential functions, with each tissue having its characteristic time constant.

Exposure to factors associated with pressure and gas mixture, such as hyperoxia, decompression stress, and gas density, are known to have acute effects on pulmonary function that may limit ventilatory capacity and exercise tolerance. The effects of hyperoxia and decompression stress may even be toxic or harmful, resulting in acute inflammatory reactions and disease, and possibly long-term residual effects. Other factors associated with the equipment used and the environment in which the diving takes place may impose additional physiologic limitations of the divers' performance.

Hyperoxia

The toxic effects of oxygen on the lung are well known and the dose-response relation and pulmonary tolerance limits have been settled as far as changes in vital capacity (VC) are concerned [2]. Above a threshold of 50 kPa, there is a reduction in VC dependent on the pressure of oxygen and exposure time. The asymptotic threshold was found to be somewhat lower than 50 kPa [3], and the threshold is definitely lower for changes in lung function variables other than VC. After some saturation dives in which the partial pressure of oxygen has been at or lower than 50 kPa for periods of up to 4 weeks [4,5] and after exposures in which no changes in VC were predicted or demonstrated, there have been reductions in transfer factor for carbon monoxide (Tl_{CO}) and maximal expiratory flow rates at low lung volumes as well as an increase in the slope of phase III of the single breath nitrogen washout test [6].

The toxic effects of oxygen are mediated by reactive oxygen species, and inflammatory changes in the lung parenchyma are induced [7]. First, this process gives rise to symptoms of nonproductive coughing and a retrosternal burning sensation before a reduction in VC takes place. The recovery of VC reductions as large as 20%–30% is usually complete within 1 or 2 weeks.

The toxic effects of oxygen must be accounted for in practical diving and hyperbaric treatment procedures. The unit pulmonary toxic dose (UPTD) is the toxic effect equivalent to the exposure to oxygen at 101 kPa for 1 minute [2]. For a given reduction in VC to take place, there is a hyperbolic relation between the exposure time and partial pressure of oxygen. A dose of 615 UPTDs results in an average 2% decrease in VC, and a dose of 1425 UPTDs results in a 10% decrease. For operational diving activity, a 2% decrease in VC is generally considered acceptable, and for recompression and hyperbaric oxygen therapy for DCI and arterial gas embolism (AGE), a 10% or even larger decrease in VC may be accepted.

Decompression stress and venous gas microembolism

In the decompression phase, blood and tissues are supersaturated with the inert gas of the atmosphere. This provides the pressure gradient for diffusion of gas out of the fluid, but supersaturated fluids are inherently unstable and there is a risk of free gas evolving in gas bubbles. Gas bubbles can form interstitially in the tissues or, probably more commonly, intravascularly in venous blood. Because of the unloading of inert gas in the lung during the decompression phase, bubbles do not form and grow in the arterial circulation. Bubbles can, however, obtain access to the arterial circulation if the pulmonary capillary bed in which the venous bubbles lodge is bypassed. These right-to-left shunts can occur as

intracardiac shunts or as intrapulmonary arteriovenous malformations and can contribute to AGE (discussed elsewhere in this article).

By controlled infusion of gas bubbles in the venous circulation in sheep, there is an immediate increase in pulmonary arterial pressure and disturbances in gas exchange function consistent with the mechanical effects of microembolization [8]. Some hours later, there is increased fluid transport across the capillaries, with increased protein content in the lymphatic fluid indicating damage to the capillary endothelium [9]. Inflammatory processes mediated by activated leukocytes contribute to this endothelial damage [10]. A large increase in pulmonary arterial pressure, which can be a result of a large shower of venous gas microemboli (VGM), may facilitate spillover of gas bubbles to the pulmonary veins [11].

VGM are frequently detected by Doppler ultrasound monitoring. They are commonly observed with generally accepted decompression procedures but do not necessarily cause clinical DCS.

Immediately after air bounce dives [12,13] and saturation dives in which VGM were demonstrated during and after the decompression phase, reductions in Tl_{CO} and maximal oxygen uptake correlating with the cumulative load of VGM have been demonstrated.

Gas density and respiratory mechanical loading

For a given gas mixture, density increases proportionately with pressure. Airway resistance is proportional to density with turbulent flow characteristics, and maximal expiratory flow rate is inversely proportional to the square root gas density, which has been shown experimentally for maximal voluntary ventilation and forced expiratory volume in 1 second (FEV_1) as well [14]. When breathing air at a pressure of 4 bars, corresponding to a depth of 30 msw, the gas density is four times normal and maximum voluntary volume (MVV) and FEV_1 are reduced by 50% of normal. The ventilatory capacity is then limiting exercise performance. Because of the increased partial pressure of oxygen in the breathing gas and some carbon dioxide retention, however, tolerated peak oxygen uptake is not significantly reduced in healthy fit subjects.

To reduce the internal resistance of breathing gas mixtures, helium is usually used instead of air when diving deeper than 50–60 msw when saturation diving techniques are preferred. Even hydrogen has been used experimentally but is associated with problems because of its narcotic effects and the danger of fire.

Gas transport in alveoli is by diffusion. The helium and oxygen mixture breathed in deep experimental saturation dives to pressures corresponding to depths of 500–700 msw has a fractional concentration of oxygen of less than 2%, with the rest being helium and, sometimes, some nitrogen. The density can be as high as 8–10 times that of air at atmospheric pressure. There is some alveolar-capillary diffusion limitation of oxygen in this low fraction of inspired oxygen (FIO_2) environment contributing to pulmonary gas exchange limitation in deep diving [15]. Within the depths accessible with today's diving techniques, however, this effect is small and is estimated to depress alveolar oxygen pressure by a few kilopascal only.

Resistance to breathing is further increased by an external breathing apparatus and the effects of static lung loading attributable to submersion. The combination of increased internal and external breathing resistances and static lung loading may facilitate the development of lung edema associated with diving and swimming, particularly in a cold environment and with high exercise intensity [16,17].

Respiratory heat and water loss

Inhaled gas is heated and humidified during its passage through the airways. The energy required to heat the gas is dependent on the physical characteristics of the gas mixture, including temperature, density, and specific heat as well as the physiologic requirement for ventilation. Some of the energy used for heating the inspired gas is recovered in the upper airways during exhalation. The mean temperature of exhaled gas is normally lower than body temperature but higher than ambient temperature. The energy required to humidify the gas is assumed to be independent of pressure, but gas mixtures used for diving are dry so as to prevent icing in the gas supply lines. The specific heat capacity for helium is five times greater than for nitrogen, 5.19 and 1.04 $J/g^{-1}/K^{-1}$, but density is only 0.18 g/L^{-1} for helium and 1.25 g/L^{-1} for nitrogen. Therefore, the respiratory heat loss when diving with air remains higher compared with diving with helium-oxygen mixtures, because it is the product of density and specific heat capacity that determines heat loss. The respiratory heat loss when diving is always larger than at normal atmospheric pressure whatever the gas mixture is, however, and the heat loss as well as the water loss for gas humidification may induce a bronchomotor response [18–20].

The thermal problems related to saturation diving with helium and oxygen gas mixtures are mainly attributable to the increased heat loss over the skin surface in the dry helium oxygen environment, which is a function of heat conductance rather than heat capacity. Heat conductance for helium is 1.51 $W/m^{-1}/K^{-1}$, and for nitrogen, it is 0.26 $W/m^{-1}/K^{-1}$. The range of comfortable temperatures in this environment is usually 27°C–29°C compared with 20°C–22°C in air at atmospheric pressure.

Respiratory effects of single dives

Immediately after dives, changes in pulmonary function can be demonstrated that are the combined effects of all the specific exposure factors associated with the dive. After deep saturation dives to depths of 300 m or more, a reduction in Tl_{CO} of 10%–15% and reduced maximal oxygen uptake have been consistently demonstrated in several studies [21–23]. Exposures to hyperoxia and VGM have been shown to contribute to these effects [4,5,12,13]. Any reduction in VC as a result of oxygen toxicity has, however, not been demonstrated. On the contrary, a small increase in VC has been seen after some dives. This could be caused by the opposing effects of hyperoxia and respiratory muscle training attributable to the effects of increased gas density. The recovery time for the changes in Tl_{CO} is 4–6 weeks.

After short air bounce dives, small reductions in Tl_{CO} and VC as well as a decrease in airway conductance have also been demonstrated [24,25], but the recovery time after these dives of a short duration (ie, hours) compared with days in saturation is much shorter, only 1–2 days. In these dives, the effects of submergence and static lung loading as well as the effects of respiratory heat and water loss are believed to contribute significantly to the changes in lung function.

Clinical problems

The important clinical problems encountered in diving medicine are listed in Box 1, and are described and discussed here.

Pulmonary barotrauma

Although the lung can withstand considerably high absolute ambient pressures without harm, exposure to abrupt changes in pressure may severely affect the lung at even small pressure differences. The term "pulmonary barotraumas" (PBTs) refers to lung injury that is induced by a change in intrapulmonary pressure relative to ambient pressure. Astronauts, aviators, compressed air workers, and divers are inherently exposed to rapid changes in ambient pressure and are thus at risk of PBT. The following section focuses on diving-related PBTs, which is a feared complication of compressed gas diving and consistently ranks second among all causes for scuba diving fatalities after drowning [26].

Definition and mechanisms

Diving-related PBT may occur during the descent of a breath-hold dive when intrathoracic gas volume falls short of residual volume and intrathoracic pressure becomes negative relative to hydrostatic pressure. This complication, also known as lung squeeze, is rare [27].

PBT during the ascent from a scuba dive, however, is defined as lung rupture that occurs during decompression when ambient pressure decreases [28]. According to Boyle's law, the volume of an enclosed gas expands with decreasing pressure. Expanding intrapulmonary gas during the ascent from a scuba dive eventually must be exhaled properly. If the rate of decrease in pressure during the ascent exceeds the rate at which the expanding gas can escape through the airways, overdistension of the alveoli and bronchi may cause lung rupture. Closure of the upper airways by, for example, breath-holding, airway obstruction attributable to pulmonary pathologic

changes, or both, may precipitate this pathophysiology [28]. Unprotected dogs with a closed trachea that were rapidly decompressed from ambient pressures of 306.3 or 612.6 kPa, equivalent to depths of approximately 31 and 62 msw, developed PBT when the intratracheal pressure reached a critical level of approximately 10.7 kPa (80 mm Hg) [29]. This could be prevented by the application of thoracoabdominal binders, despite a rise in intratracheal pressure to levels of 24 kPa (180 mm Hg). Accordingly, experiments with fresh unchilled human cadavers showed that lung barotrauma occurred at intrapulmonary pressures of approximately 9.7–10.7 kPa (73–80 mm Hg) [30]. Binding of the chest and abdomen required much higher pressures of 17.7–25.3 kPa (133–190 mm Hg). It was further observed that rupture of the visceral pleura occurred when basal pleural adhesions were present. Thus, the transpulmonary pressure (ie, the difference between intratracheal and intrapleural pressure) is the critical factor for the development of PBT rather than the absolute level of the intratracheal pressure.

Intrapulmonary air trapping during ascent may occur in any particular region of the lung. Localized overdistension of the lung then results in rising local transpulmonary pressure with subsequent rupture of the alveolar wall [31]. Once rupture occurs, gas is sucked into the peribronchial space and causes pulmonary interstitial emphysema [29]. Gas may track into the tissues by the mechanics of breathing and cause pneumomediastinum with emphysema of the neck. Alternatively, it may dissect toward the lung periphery, rupturing via subpleural blebs into the pleural space, causing pneumothorax, or mediastinal gas may rupture the mediastinal pleura and enter the pleural space. The latter mechanism is supported by observations from experimental animal studies showing that the mediastinum contained dissecting gas in all cases in which there was pneumothorax [29]. Moreover, extra-alveolar gas may pass the diaphragm through the esophageal hiatus into the peritoneal cavity and cause pneumoperitoneum [32,33].

Gas may also track along the perivascular sheaths of the pulmonary arteries and erupt into such an artery or move toward the hilum on expiration and dissect into the thin-walled pulmonary veins. In consequence, the gas may then rapidly enter the systemic circulation and cause AGE, a clinical condition that is associated with high morbidity and mortality [34]. A pressure gradient between the air passages and the left atrium in excess of 8 kPa (60 mm Hg) has been found to enable the transfer of gas into the vasculature [29]. If gas has entered the left side of the heart via the pulmonary veins, it may be distributed into

Table 1
Systematic studies that reported clinical and radiologic evidence of pulmonary barotraumas in case series of divers/submarine escape trainees suffering from PBT with or without arterial gas embolism

First author, year [reference]	No. of subjects	PBT	AGE	Combined PBT/AGE
Elliott, 1978 [71][a]	88	N/A	9	79
Kizer, 1987 [58][b]	42	N/A	1	41
Leitch, 1986 [60]	140	23	59	58
Harker, 1993 [64][b]	31	N/A	15	16
Tetzlaff, 1997 [59]	15	2	10	3

Abbreviation: N/A, not applicable.
[a] Only submarine escape trainees included.
[b] Only divers with clinical diagnosis of AGE included.

nearly all organs, causing embolic occlusion of end arteries. Head position during ascent in relation to the torso, buoyancy of the gas bubbles, and blood flow dynamics favors the distribution of gas bubbles to the brain. Because of the extremely short hypoxia tolerance of the central nervous system, critical injury may occur depending on the absolute quantity of gas and the areas affected. Small gas bubbles may rapidly be absorbed and only briefly interrupt blood flow. Larger gas bubbles, however, may cause severe harm by ischemic cell injury and disruption of the blood-brain barrier. Immediate pathologic changes are characterized by a rise in cerebrospinal fluid pressure, systemic hypertension, cessation of neuronal activity, and changes in vascular permeability [35]. Cellular and humoral responses induced by the effects of gas-blood as well as gas-endothelial interfaces contribute to inflammation that is maintained even after absorption of the gas [34].

In contrast to PBT induced by mechanical ventilation [36], AGE is the most frequent sequel to diving-related PBT (Table 1). The direction and amount of transpulmonary pressure generated by rapid decompression during diving may account for this distinct feature. Often, AGE is combined with pneumomediastinum (Fig. 1), and severe cases of PBT have been reported in which the gas had tracked into the vasculature causing AGE into pleural spaces and the mediastinum [37,38]. In fatal cases of PBT, death may result from obstruction of the heart (pneumocardium) and central circulation after massive AGE [39–41]. The detailed pathophysiologic changes causing death in human beings, however, are not yet entirely understood [40].

PBT may also occur with the use of breathing gases other than air. There are two case reports of PBT with and without AGE in divers using a closed-circuit oxygen rebreathing diving apparatus. Remarkably, the highly elevated oxygen fraction may have accelerated the resorption of extra-alveolar gas in

these cases, where symptoms were reported to have resolved rapidly [42,43].

Because of the common misapprehension that diving accidents do not occur in shallow water, it is worth mentioning that the risk for PBT is greatest just below the surface, because the ambient pressure doubles between 0 and 10 msw and the relative change in volume is maximal at that depth range. Accordingly, cases of severe AGE have been reported that occurred during shallow water dives of less than 5 msw and even during swimming [44–46].

Decompression-related PBT is not restricted to scuba diving only. It may occur during the ascent of a commercial airplane when the passenger cabin pressure decreases by approximately 26.7 kPa (200 mm Hg) [47] or during hypobaric chamber training performed for military aircrew members throughout the world [48–50]. Cerebral AGE after PBT has been reported in ground maintenance crew members after cabin pressure tests to approximately 55 kPa (413 mm Hg) [51,52]. Few cases have occurred during hyperbaric oxygen therapy in a hyper-

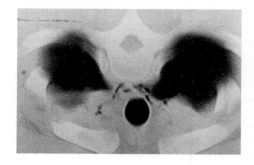

Fig. 1. CT scan of a 23-year-old Navy scuba diver who developed chest pain and nausea while performing free ascent training from a depth of 11 msw. The scan was taken after the first recompression treatment. The chest radiograph was unremarkble. MRI of the neurocranium revealed a large cerebellar infarction.

baric chamber [53–55]. All these exposures have in common the fact that the pressure change during the ascent is of minor magnitude and occurs more slowly when compared with scuba diving ascents. Thus, PBT is infrequent in these occupations. Remarkably, pre-existing lung pathologic findings have been described more often in these cases [47,49,53–55], supporting the concept that air-trapping pulmonary lesions increase the risk of PBT.

Clinical presentation of pulmonary barotrauma

The clinical presentation of diving-related PBT largely depends on feature and localization of injury. Pulmonary symptoms alone may be present in cases with pneumothorax or mediastinal emphysema without concurrent gas embolism. Pneumomediastinum has been detected by chest radiographs in even asymptomatic subjects after buoyant ascents [56]. Hoarseness only or a strange voice with mild chest pain should prompt the physician to consider PBT in the differential diagnosis after scuba dives [43,57]. More prominent pulmonary symptoms reported from larger case series comprised chest discomfort, chest pain or tightness, dyspnea or apnea, and hemoptyses [58–60]. Among these, chest pain and dyspnea were the most frequent and accounted for approximately 25% and 13% of all cases of combined PBT and AGE, respectively.

In most cases, however, neurologic symptoms are present as a consequence of AGE (Table 2). A stroke-like syndrome with unilateral neurologic symptoms has been considered typical for diving-related AGE [28,61]. A less typical presentation with bilateral symptoms may also be seen [62,63]; therefore, AGE is not excluded. Cognitive symptoms and unconsciousness are most frequently present, whereas seizures, focal motor deficits, visual disturbances, vertigo, and sensory changes are also common (see Table 2) [58–60,64,65]. Most importantly, these symptoms appear on or shortly after surfacing within

Table 2
Most frequent symptoms of arterial gas embolism and pulmonary barotrauma

Symptom	Range (%)
Unconsciousness	17–81
Paraesthesias and/or paralyses	23–77
Dizziness	10–43
Nausea and/or vertigo	9–39
Visual disturbances	13–26
Convulsions	0–31
Headache	0–26

Data from five larger case series published in peer-reviewed literature: Refs. [58–60,64,65].

5 minutes (>90% of cases) [26,59,60]. However, time to onset of symptoms may take longer than 10 minutes [65], and there are case reports with delayed onset after hours up to several days [66,67]. Symptoms generally progress rapidly when not treated, but spontaneous recovery may occur and has been reported even following resuscitation after initial apnea and pulselessness [68]. A small, but important number (approximately 4%) of patients present fatally with immediate unconsciousness and cardiopulmonary arrest [69]. Postmortem radiography in fatal AGE revealed massive gas in cardiac chambers and large thoracic vessels in these cases [39–41,70]. Some fatalities, however, may simply be attributable to drowning subsequent to loss of consciousness under water; thus, the actual incidence of PBT and/or AGE may be underestimated.

Risk factors for pulmonary barotrauma

Incident statistics show that the technique of ascent (ie, the decompression procedure that the body is exposed to) is a major risk factor. At depth, the diver inhales gas from the scuba equipment at normal lung volumes. When surfacing from depth during a free ascent (ie, without breathing from the scuba equipment), the expanding gas must be exhaled continuously. Thus, certain diving techniques, such as out-of-air emergency training, buddy-breathing during ascent, or buoyant ascents during submarine escape tank training, pose significantly increased risks to the subjects. Accordingly, reported incidences per number of dives are 0.04%–0.06% for buoyant ascent training [71,72] and 0.005% for military scuba dives [60,73].

Among individual factors contributing to the risk of PBT, conditions that predispose to intrapulmonary air trapping play a major role. An autopsy study on 13 diving fatalities revealed that in the cases with fatal pneumothorax occurring during ascent from depths between 10 and 40 msw, the site of rupture was related to pleural adhesions and lung bullae [74]. Such adhesions were also present in 26% of investigated lungs that were not involved in PBT, however. Poorly ventilated intrapulmonary structures, such as lung bullae or air cysts, may hinder the expanding gas from being exhaled properly or simply be a locus minor resistentiae. Accordingly, flap-valve mechanisms have been described from emphysematous lesions that may support air trapping during expiration [31]. There are case reports of PBT in which plain film radiography revealed evidence of pre-existing large lung cysts [71,75,76] that were considered to be causally related to the injury. Indeed, in one case report of fatal AGE occurring after the descent of a commercial flight, the rupture of a large pre-existing intrapulmonary air cyst was confirmed by autopsy [47]. More recent studies using CT of the chest [43,77–81] have frequently detected bullae and cysts that had escaped detection by chest radiographs and thus support the hypothesis that in cases of diving-related PBT with normal plain chest radiographs, subtle pre-existing pulmonary lesions may still be potentially implicated in the injury (Fig. 2). Some doubt remains as to whether these bullae detected by postinjury radiology were pre-existing. Their persistence over long-term follow-up may support this assumption [43,62,77].

An analysis of the database of the Royal Navy Institute of Naval Medicine revealed a series of 140 cases of PBT with and without AGE, of which 8% were recurrent incidents [82]. In these cases as well as in another reported case [83], there were no identifiable predisposing findings. A chest CT scan was only available in the latter case, however. We are aware of a 26-year old female diver who asked for consultation after she had suffered twice from unilateral neurologic limb symptoms and nausea after emergency ascents from open water scuba dives within 2 years. Only after the second incident was chest CT was performed, which revealed a subpleural bulla in the right lower lobe [84].

Some studies investigated the idea that PBT might be predictable by means of pulmonary function testing. In a controlled study of 14 divers who had suffered from PBT that was established clinically or by chest radiography, pulmonary conductance and static recoil pressure were measured, on average, 0.8 years after the injury [85]. It was found that a derived index of lung distensibility was significantly decreased in the PBT group compared with 10 healthy divers and 34 healthy controls. The authors postulated that stresses in peribronchial alveolar tissue would be magnified near total lung capacity if bronchi are relatively stiffer. Limitations to that study

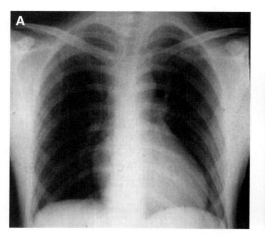

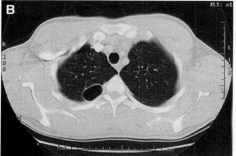

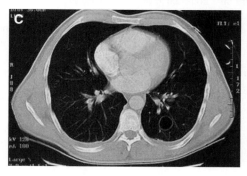

Fig. 2. (*A*) Chest radiograph of a 38-year-old sport scuba diver who complained of sudden leg paralysis and right-sided chest tightness after an uneventful 25-m dive with 20 minutes of bottom time in the Red Sea. The radiograph was taken after the initial treatment for decompression illness and repatriation. Chest CT scan of the same diver shows bilateral lung bullae in the right upper lobe (*B*) and in the left lower lobe (*C*). (Courtesy of Armin Kemmer, MD, Murnau, Germany.)

were the finding of a significant difference in the index of lung distensibility between the control divers and healthy nonsmokers in measurements spanning over a time range of more than 10 years. In a retrospective review of a large series of submarine escape training tank incidents that occurred in the Royal Navy during a 22-year period, there were only six cases in which there was radiologic or clinical evidence of extra-alveolar gas and four additional cases that were considered to be related to PBT for other reasons [86]. Standardized residuals were calculated for FEV_1 and forced vital capacity (FVC) as well as for the quotient of FEV_1/FVC. The authors found significant associations between values of FVC and FEV_1 below those predicted and PBT ($P < .01$ and $P < .05$, respectively) but not for FEV_1/FVC. Surprisingly, these studies revealed some correlation between restrictive lung indices and risk of PBT rather than indices of obstruction. Thus, individuals with small and stiff lungs may be at increased risk of PBT. In another retrospective study of 15 scuba divers who had consecutively suffered from PBT with or without AGE, however, expiratory flows at low lung volumes were found to be less than predicted and significantly less than those values of a control group of divers who had experienced diving injuries other than PBT [59]. Thus, peripheral airflow limitation may have indicated obstructive lung disease in some of these cases. The issue with these latter studies is that the differences from the control populations were rather small (ie, within two times the standard deviation); in fact, there are a large number of subjects diving safely with spirometric indices within that range. In conclusion, there are as yet no convincing data indicating pulmonary function to be predictive for detecting those divers who are at risk of PBT, mostly because of the small samples investigated.

Decompression illness

General features of pathophysiology

Severe injury from scuba diving is predominantly caused by decompression-related pathophysiology. The term "decompression illness" has been introduced to encompass those distinct disease entities that may result from tissue damage by excess intracorporeal gas during and after decompression [87]. Included under the broader definition of DCI are AGE, which occurs as a consequence of PBT, and DCS, a multiorgan system disorder that results from micro- or macroscopic nitrogen bubble formation when ambient pressure decreases on surfacing.

As outlined in the section on diving exposure, body tissues become saturated at depth with inert gas molecules as a function of time, the partial pressure of the gas in the breathing mix, and a constant depending on the type of tissue [88]. On ascent from a scuba dive, the sum of tissue gas tensions and vapor pressure may exceed ambient pressure (ie, the body tissues become supersaturated). Dissolved inert gas in the tissue and blood forms a free gas phase to equalize the pressures. Current theories favor the hypothesis that bubbles are predominantly formed by small pre-existing gas nuclei that are commonly contained in body tissues. Spontaneous bubble formation may contribute to this process. Once nucleated, gas bubbles are subject to tissue diffusion and perfusion. The pressure gradient for the partial pressure of the inert gas toward alveolar gas eventually forces the inert gas to leave the tissues. Excess inert gas physiologically reaches the lungs by venous return, where it is trapped in the lung microvasculature and removed by diffusion into the alveolar space [89].

With the introduction of Doppler ultrasound methodology, intravascular gas bubbles have been frequently been observed with decompression. Exposure to even mild hyperbaria of 138 kPa ambient pressure (3.8 msw) for 48 hours revealed detectable venous gas emboli a few hours after direct ascent in 20% of asymptomatic subjects, and bubbles were even detectable after 12 hours in subjects who ascended from 4.8 msw [90]. Intravascular gas bubbles are often present in the absence of symptoms after scuba dives [90–93]. These bubbles may elicit acute respiratory responses, such as a decrease in the Tl_{CO} [12,13]. In animal models, intravascular air bubbles have been shown to exert diverse pathophysiologic effects. Hemodynamic changes after venous gas embolism comprised a rise in pulmonary artery pressure and pulmonary vascular resistance and a decrease in arterial oxygen tension [94–96]. Humoral and cellular changes in general concern the activation of the complement system and leukocytes [97,98]. These effects induce proinflammatory cascades that result in hemocentration and leakage of the vascular endothelium [9,99]. The magnitude of these changes depends on the amount of venous gas emboli, and smaller bubble numbers are less likely to produce gross hemodynamic or fluid abnormalities. Whether these so-called "silent bubbles" cause any long-term effects on the organism is not yet known. Moreover, the factors that determine whether bubble formation becomes pathologic remain to be elucidated.

Clinical features of decompression sickness

The term "decompression sickness" refers to a multiorgan system disorder that results from micro- or macroscopic nitrogen bubble formation when ambient pressure decreases on surfacing. Thus, the presence of these pathologic bubbles per se does not predict the clinical manifestations of DCS but is pivotal for its pathologic diagnosis.

One major clinical presentation of DCS is limited to musculoskeletal or cutaneous symptoms only and is also known commonly by the lay term "the bends." The pathophysiologic basis for these manifestations, which have historically been classified as type I DCS, is still under investigation. It is believed that tendon sheaths or joint capsules may be irritated mechanically by gas bubbles that form within these inhomogeneously perfused tissue compartments. Bubbles may also grow within the bone marrow, causing a rise in intermedullary pressure, or may be delivered by the blood toward these sites. This mechanistic hypothesis is supported by the observation that limb, joint, or muscle pain is immediately responsive to recompression in most cases. The cutaneous manifestation of DCS presents as cutis marmorata with skin itching and rash. In swine, it was shown that the violaceous color of the lesions was presumably attributable to congestion of deeper vessels in the dermis and subcutis, and vascular inflammation was apparent on electron microscopy [100].

More severe DCS historically has been classified as type II and is characterized by neurologic, audiovestibular, or respiratory manifestations. The particular nitrogen saturation and elimination kinetics of neural tissues and their minimal ischemia tolerance favor the development of neurologic symptoms in the presentation of DCS. Neurologic injury is presumed to be attributable to the thrombogenetic effect of venous gas bubbles in the epidural venous plexus surrounding the spinal cord, causing venous stasis and spinal cord ischemia in the thoracic region. There may also be evidence for the in situ generation of so-called "autochthonous bubbles" within the tissue of the spinal cord because of its high solubility for inert gas [101,102]. More recently, however, it was shown in decompressed goats that autochthonous bubbles arise as an artifact and that the nature of the lesion in the spinal cord is a focal infarct or necrosis after events that occurred in local vessels [103]. In swine that underwent a hyperbaric exposure to 612.6 kPa, equivalent to 50 msw, for 24 minutes, 67.2% of animals developed neurologic DCS or died [104]. Histologic examination revealed an association between the hemorrhage within the spinal cord gray matter and increasing disease severity [105]. Brain lesions were present in 23% of pigs, whereas cord lesions, mostly thoracic, were evident in 63% of pigs and in 23% of those clinically unaffected. Using the

same animal model for neurologic DCS, another study revealed high rates of microembolic Doppler ultrasound signals in animals that died within 1 hour after a dive [106]. Chest CT performed 20 minutes after a dive showed massive amounts of ectopic gas in the right side of the heart, probably causing death by mechanical outflow obstruction in some of these animals (Fig. 3). In conclusion, these animal experiments confirmed observations from human beings that there is a considerable interindividual range of DCS severity associated with the same decompression stress.

Neurologic DCS may cover a gamut of signs and symptoms depending on localization, the amount of bubbles, and the type of affected tissue. Sensory symptoms, including numbness, tingling, paresthesias, and abnormal sensation, are far more common than more severe neurologic symptoms [26]. Typically, these symptoms develop progressively, beginning with mild paresthesia, followed by regional numbness, weakness, and, occasionally, paresis of the affected limbs. Symptoms usually occur within hours after decompression, but in severe cases, they may present immediately [26]. Thus, a clinical diagnosis of DCS may be difficult to establish, and clinical symptoms may overlap with those of AGE. Furthermore, cases of combined DCS and AGE have been reported [107].

The risk of DCS is considered to be negligible at shallow water depths of 0–10 msw, because the limited gas supply from the scuba equipment prevents the body from a significant inert gas uptake. Beyond that depth, however, the risk proportionally increases with pressure and the time spent at that pressure. The time needed for desaturation on ascent increases accordingly. It has been shown in human beings after

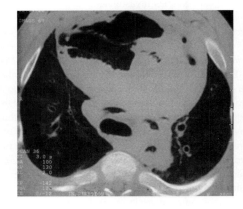

Fig. 3. CT scan of a pig that had been exposed to a hyperbaric chamber depth of 50 msw for 24 minutes. Large amounts of ectopic gas can be seen in the right ventricle.

scuba dives that the presence of intravascular bubbles is correlated with the rate of ascent [91]. In a pig model of DCS, the use of nonlinear ascent profiles with a combined fast/slow ascent was associated with a 30% reduction of the DCS rate [108]. To minimize the risk of DCS, decompression tables and schedules have been established that outline certain gradual decompression profiles. Modern dive computers use algorithms that consider different tissue desaturation kinetics and calculate surface intervals that must be kept before the next dive. Nevertheless, DCS may occur unpredictably even when strictly following decompression requirements. An incidence of 0.003% of "undeserved" DCS (ie, scuba dives with no obvious risk profile) has been reported [73].

There are environmental and individual factors that may place the subject at increased risk. Temperature and exercise influence tissue perfusion and thus may affect the probability of bubble formation. An analysis of accident records of the Royal Navy Institute of Naval Medicine revealed a significant association between the exposure to cold and the occurrence of DCS [109]. Increased pulmonary gas exchange during exercise at depth may be detrimental, because tissues equilibrate more rapidly with increased blood flow. It was recently shown in subjects who performed arm or leg exercise during graded decompression beginning at 9 msw after a 30-minute wet chamber dive at 450 kPa that there were significantly less venous gas bubbles detectable by Doppler ultrasound compared with sedentary control divers [110]. Moreover, in animal models, exercise before diving has been shown to have beneficial effects. In swine, predive exercise conditioning of approximately 20 sessions on a treadmill reduced the rate of DCS by 31% versus that in control animals [111]. Recent data in rats indicate that it is not the aerobic capacity per se but the acute effect of predive exercising that contributes to the risk reduction. Rats that performed a single bout of exercise lasting for 1.5 hours, with 20 hours of rest before the dive, were protected from bubble formation, as were those who had trained regularly for 2 weeks [112]. This effect was recently confirmed in human subjects who underwent two experimental chamber dives to 280 kPa for 80 minutes in a cross-over fashion while performing a single interval exercise 24 hours before one of the dives. There were significantly fewer bubbles and decreased maximum bubble grades detectable after the dives with predive exercise compared with the dives without predive exercise [113]. The reasons for the beneficial effect of a single predive exercise in the rate of diving-related DCS remain speculative. An interesting theory is that the population of gas micronuclei may be depleted by exercise, thus diminishing the chance for gas bubbles to nucleate [114].

Individual factors also contribute to the risk of bubble formation and DCS. Observational studies from diving populations revealed that obesity may be contributory to the occurrence of DCS [115]. In fact, Doppler ultrasound investigations of divers confirmed a significant relation between detected postdive bubble grades and body weight [116]. Moreover, general physical fitness, as indicated by maximal oxygen uptake, does seem to prevent bubble formation in human beings [91]. Age and sex have historically been considered risk factors for DCS [117], but conflicting data have arisen more recently. In a field study monitoring venous gas emboli after recreational open water dives, male and older divers had a higher incidence of high bubble grades by Doppler ultrasound [118]. The investigated divers, however, had a relatively high mean age, and divers were only monitored once. In a retrospective cohort study of recreational diving instructors in Sweden, the incidence of self-reported DCS symptoms among younger divers 18–24 years of age equaled that among those older than 25 years of age [119]. In a survey among recreational divers in the United Kingdom, the physician-confirmed rate of DCS was 0.026% in woman versus 0.016% in men, suggesting a 1.67-fold greater DCS rate in women [120]. When adjusting these rates by diving experience, however, the sex difference became insignificant. The overall DCS rate across male and female divers was 0.02%, which is within the range reported from other sources [26,73,119]. Recent diving accident statistics show a bell-shaped distribution over the complete age range, peaking at the age of 38 years, and the sex distribution of injured divers exactly mirrors the distribution among the total diving population [26]. It is thus less likely that age and sex grossly influence the risk of diving-related DCS.

Remarkably, approximately one quarter of injured divers indicate that they have been exposed to altitude after diving [26], confirming the theoretic concept that further decompression from sea level pressure aggravates bubble formation. A case-control study using recreational dive profiles found that the relative odds of DCS increased with decreased preflight surface intervals [121]. In most divers who developed DCS symptoms during or after the flight, the preflight surface interval was less than 12 hours [26]. This mechanism also applies to those who expose themselves to altitude while driving across mountains after diving. Thus, to be on the safe side, a minimum interval of 24 hours is recommended before flying when the dive profile did not require decompression stops; otherwise, it should even be longer [122].

Respiratory decompression illness

The respiratory effects of gas bubbles have been well characterized in different animal species. In anesthetized dogs that were decompressed from a 17-minute hyperbaric exposure at 90 msw, pulmonary hypertension, systemic hypotension, hemoconcentration, and hypoxia occurred [123]. Moreover, a decrease in pulmonary compliance but unchanged resistance was measured. Pathologic findings revealed the regular occurrence of pulmonary edema without an elevation of left ventricular end-diastolic pressure. The authors postulated that microvascular permeability was altered by venous bubble emboli formed during decompression. In anesthetized dogs ventilated with oxygen and nitrogen (30%:70% ratio), it was shown that venous gas emboli could remain in the pulmonary vasculature as discrete bubbles for periods lasting up to 43 ± 11 minutes after air infusion at a rate of 0.25 mL/kg^{-1}/min^{-1} and that infused air doses were correlated with bubble residence times [124]. In sheep, it has been shown that the amount of lung microvascular injury could be controlled by the rate of venous gas embolism and was reversible within $1-2$ days [99]. In another sheep model of experimental respiratory DCS, animals were exposed to compressed air at 230 kPa for 22 hours, followed by simulated altitude at 76 kPa (570 mm Hg) [125]. In that study, clinical findings were found to be correlated to pathophysiologic changes; an increased mean pulmonary artery pressure after the detection of high precordial bubble grades corresponded with the onset of restlessness, respiratory difficulty, and collapse. Radiography revealed interstitial pulmonary edema in five animals and patchy infiltrates as well as pleural effusions in two. It was concluded that massive embolization of the pulmonary capillary bed precipitates respiratory DCS. These changes are accompanied by impaired endothelial function [126,127] that may be prevented by administration of antibodies to complement factors, such as C5a in rabbits [128].

In diving, however, respiratory DCS is rare, probably because common scuba dive profiles do not exert the significant decompression stress to the lung that is needed for pulmonary manifestations. Clinical symptoms are characterized by increased breathing frequency, cough, cyanosis, and thoracic discomfort or pain. This symptomatology has also been called "the chokes." There is one case report of a 40-year old previously healthy woman who became dyspneic and coughed frothy white sputum immedi-ately after she had made her third dive on the same day [129]. Chest radiography showed bilateral lower lobe airspace consolidation that completely resolved 5 hours after treatment. In contrast to diving, however, incidence of the chokes in altitude DCS has been reported to achieve a rate of 6% [130].

Paradoxic gas embolism

Paradoxic gas embolism may occur when gas that has entered the venous side of the circulation gains access to the systemic arterial circulation. Routes for the transpulmonary passage of venous gas bubbles include the pulmonary capillaries and intra- or extra-pulmonary right-to-left shunts.

The lung serves as an excellent filter for microbubbles in the healthy state. Its capacity to effectively filter gas bubbles depends on the size, location, and amount of bubbles trapped in the pulmonary circulation and may be impaired by administration of pulmonary vasodilators, such as aminophylline [131]. The overload threshold of the pulmonary vasculature in dogs could be determined at an infusion rate of 0.3 mL/kg^{-1}/min^{-1} [131]. Higher infusion doses of 0.35 mL/kg^{-1}/min^{-1} resulted in arterial bubbles as detected by Doppler sonography in more than 50% of the dogs. An elevation in pulmonary artery pressure was required before the spillover of venous gas bubbles occurred, with a pressure gradient between pulmonary artery pressure and left atrial pressure of approximately 52 mm Hg [11]. In swine, the breakthrough of bubbles was already apparent at 0.1 mL/kg^{-1}/min^{-1} and occurred in pigs experiencing a substantial reduction in mean arterial pressure and pulmonary artery pressure that had returned to normal at the time of spillover [132]. The time course of changes in mean pulmonary artery pressure in swine after rapid decompression from a 30-minute exposure to 500 kPa was related to the Doppler sonography bubble counts in the pulmonary artery, with a great variation in the degree of bubble formation [133]. In conclusion, these animal models showed that a significant decompression stress is associated with an increased risk of a spillover of venous gas bubbles into the arterial side of the circulation, and the occurrence of arterial gas bubbles seemed to follow the same time course as the venous bubble count in pigs [106,134].

Extrapulmonary right-to-left shunts represent another pathway for paradoxic gas embolism. A patent foramen ovale, as the most common right-to-left shunt, has been demonstrated to be related to otherwise unexplained DCI in divers [135–137]. Normally, the fossa ovalis, a persisting remnant of a physiologic communication between the venous and arterial sides of the fetal circulation, closes at birth by the postnatal increase in left atrial pressure and fuses within the first 2 years of life. In approximately one third of the population, fusion does not occur, which is not of significance in normal life, because the high left atrial pressure forces the interseptal valve against the septum. In divers, however, the Valsalva maneuver or other procedures that raise intra-abdominal pressure during and after diving lead to a concomitant increase in right atrial pressure and eventually enable the passage of gas bubbles through the foramen ovale. Accordingly, a shunt of venous bubbles could be shown by transcranial Doppler ultrasound in divers with a patent foramen ovale who had developed venous gas emboli after two experimental chamber dives [138]. In a field study investigating recreational divers after scuba dives, arterial micro-embolic signals were detected by transcranial Doppler ultrasound in 6 of 40 asymptomatic divers who also had significant venous bubbles [93]. In contrast, in another field study using transcranial Doppler ultrasound, no evidence of AGE was detected after multiple dives in commercial divers with a patent foramen ovale [139]. The authors concluded that strict adherence to decompression procedures prevented the divers from significant intravascular bubble formation. The latter studies clearly revealed that it is not the patency of the foramen ovale but the presence of inert gas bubbles that drives the pathologic finding of right-to-left shunts in diving. This concept is supported by the overall incidence of AGE by right-to-left shunting: the prevalence of a patent foramen ovale among the diving population equals that of the total population [93,137,139]. A meta-analysis of three studies that reported incidences for DCI and the echocardiographic presence of a patent foramen ovale in different diving populations revealed a 2.6-fold increase in the risk for DCS, however [140]. The incidence of DCI in that population averaged 0.02%; thus, the absolute increase of risk in the presence of a patent foramen ovale remained small.

Management of decompression illness

As outlined previously, DCI resembles a pattern of diseases that differ fundamentally in their pathophysiology but share, to some extent, the pathologic changes induced by excess intracorporeal gas. There may be a considerable overlap in symptomatology between them [26,141], thus complicating diagnosis.

Evidence has arisen from experimental animal data and experience in human beings that the same treatment algorithms apply for DCI independent of the way in which the excess gas entered the body

[142–144]. This is particularly helpful in view of the facts that delay to treatment is inversely related to outcome [26] and time-consuming diagnostic procedures must be postponed until treatment has been initiated.

Diagnosis of DCI mainly relies on careful examination and a detailed medical history, including data on the dive profiles preceding the accident. Other diseases that may mimic DCI, such as cardiovascular or cerebrovascular events, must be considered in view of the present findings. Laboratory and radiographic evaluation should only be applied initially if readily available. Laboratory investigations are useful to assess hemoconcentration and dehydration [145], and an elevated serum creatine kinase level has been shown to be related to the size and severity of AGE [146]. A chest radiograph may be helpful in evaluating the presence of pneumothorax, which must be treated before any recompression therapy is initiated [28]. Costly radiography, such as CT or MRI, may be applied after initial treatment. MRI has been proven useful in further evaluation of neurologic DCI but may be insensitive in some cases [147,148]. For the assessment of further fitness to dive after DCI, it is mandatory to evaluate pulmonary conditions that increase the risk of barotrauma (eg, by chest CT and pulmonary function testing) as well as cardial conditions that predispose to right-to-left shunting.

Effective treatment of tissue damage caused by excess gas includes the fast elimination of the gas phase and the correction of tissue hypoxia. This is best achieved by the application of oxygen at increased ambient pressure, that is, hyperbaric oxygen therapy [149]. It accelerates the elimination of the gas phase by raising the ambient pressure and by creating systemic hyperoxia. Current treatment schedules involve placement of the patient in an environment pressurized at two to three times the sea level pressure while breathing 100% oxygen, which results in arterial oxygen tensions in excess of 2000 mm Hg (267 kPa). The most commonly used treatment algorithm for DCI is the US Navy Table 6, with cycles of oxygen breathing at 18 msw for approximately 75 minutes and at 9 msw for approximately 3 hours, with air pauses in between to minimize adverse oxygen effects [61]. Approximately 40% of injured divers show complete resolution after the first treatment, and only 20% need more than three treatments [26]. If hyperbaric oxygen therapy is not immediately available (eg, at remote locations), early administration of 100% oxygen has been shown to improve clinical outcome significantly [26].

As with any medical emergency, however, cardiopulmonary resuscitation and adjunctive therapies may be necessary, and transportation of the patient with DCI requires certain prerequisites. A more detailed review on the treatment of DCI exceeds the scope of this article and may be found elsewhere [144,150].

Pulmonary edema

Pulmonary edema has only recently been recognized as a diving-related clinical problem [17,151], probably attributable to the fact that an affected individual may recover spontaneously; therefore, it is largely underreported in scuba diving. Moreover, cases of pulmonary edema may have been misinterpreted as DCI previously [129,152,153].

The first observation was on 11 divers who had developed pulmonary edema while scuba diving in cold British waters. It was assumed that an abnormal increase in vascular resistance to cold exposure may have precipitated edema by raising preload and afterload, because healthy controls did not show the same degree of increase in forearm vascular resistance to experimental cold exposure [17]. Increased oxygen partial pressure at depth might have been contributory, but in 2 divers, episodes of pulmonary edema had occurred even during surface swimming. During follow-up of the divers, most of them had become hypertensive, thus indicating that an abnormal vascular reactivity may be predictive for developing hypertension. A subsequent study reported on four subjects who had developed pulmonary edema while scuba diving or swimming [151]. By distribution of a questionnaire addressing possible symptoms of pulmonary edema, one additional subject (0.22%) of 460 responders was identified as having a positive history of edema. All these subjects who had no history of cardiac or pulmonary disease exhibited no abnormal vascular reactivity when compared with healthy controls. It was thus speculated that a combination of factors, such as immersion and cold exposure, together with an increase in cardiac output, might lead to an excessive increase in pulmonary capillary pressure. Simultaneously, another study reported on a group of eight military subjects who developed hemoptysis and cough while engaged in an open sea swimming competition in warm (23°C) water [154]. The authors suggested that a combination of immersion, exercise, and overhydration had increased pulmonary capillary pressure and eventually caused edema. Subsequently, more cases were reported that occurred during diving in warm waters [155–157], thus diminishing the cold water hypothesis. In Israeli military trainees participating in a 2-month fitness

program with distance swims of 2.4 and 3.6 km, there were 29 events of pulmonary edema in 21 individuals (ie, 60% of the study group) [158]. The authors postulated that stress failure of the pulmonary capillary during strenuous swimming precipitated the events and that immersion contributed to this mechanism significantly. In fact, immersion elicits diverse cardiovascular and ventilatory effects that may increase capillary transmural pressure (eg, blood displacement into the lungs, increase in preload, ventilation-perfusion mismatch). The human blood-gas barrier is extremely thin to allow adequate gas exchange to occur by passive diffusion, and its strength to resist higher capillary pressures is mainly provided by the extracellular matrix [159]. It is the type IV collagen matrix that allows intracellular disruptions of the capillary endothelial and alveolar epithelial cells to occur, which are reversible on stress reduction. Pulmonary edema is extremely rare in healthy athletes in a dry environment, albeit there is evidence from animal species that capillary breakage with alveolar bleeding occurs routinely at a high level of exercise. In elite competition cyclists, it could, in fact, be shown that the blood-gas barrier was altered by maximal exercise, whereas it was not changed when exercising at 77% of their maximal oxygen consumption [160,161]. Thus, exhaustive exercise elicits subtle changes to the blood-gas barrier that may become aggravated in the wet environment. Recently, it was reported from the US Naval Medical Center at San Diego that there are more than 20 cases of swimming-induced pulmonary edema annually [162], underlining the high incidence of swimming-induced pulmonary edema during strenuous in-water exercise. Dyspnea and cough are complained of most often and may be accompanied by hemoptyses, hypoxemia, increased breathing frequency, and crackles [163,164]. Radiographic findings, such as Kerley-B lines and airspace consolidation (Fig. 4), usually normalize within 48 hours. Clinical symptoms often improve simply by removal from water and with supportive treatment, so that diuretics are mostly superfluous [163]. Remarkably, in combat swimmers who primarily swim in the lateral decubitus position to allow constant eye contact with the partner and to maintain a low surface profile, it was the dependent submersed lung that was more often affected on chest radiographs [162]. Pulmonary edema has recently been described in an Israeli combat swimmer using a closed-circuit oxygen breathing apparatus [164]. In that case, oxygen may have contributed to the development of edema by its vasoconstrictive effects.

In conclusion, a large variety of different factors may precipitate pulmonary edema during scuba

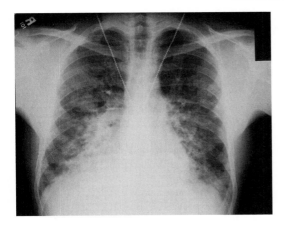

Fig. 4. Chest radiograph of a 28-year-old US Marine who complained of cough and hemoptysis after a 1000-m swim with a wetsuit and fins in the cold (14.4°C [58°F]) Pacific Ocean. (Courtesy of Richard T. Mahon, MD, San Diego, CA.)

diving or swimming, and there is yet no evidence of a single common risk factor. Exertion in the immersed state may be a major causative factor in swimming-induced pulmonary edema, whereas strenuous exercise was only rarely reported in published cases of pulmonary edema during scuba diving [17,151, 155–157,165,166]. Remarkably, an advanced age was obvious in the latter subjects (Table 3). It is supposed that individual factors contribute to the development of diving-induced pulmonary edema, because subjects affected once are at risk of further incidents. Thus, these subjects should be advised not to dive again. For those who refuse to accept this advice, the administration of nifedipine (5 mg) before the dive may prevent recurrence [167]. Pulmonary edema during scuba diving or swimming is more frequent than previously thought and must be considered in the differential diagnosis of diving-related injuries.

Fitness to dive with concomitant respiratory diseases

To meet the particular physiologic demands of the underwater environment adequately, a reasonable state of health is required for scuba diving. Certain medical conditions are incompatible with the safety of the individual and his or her diving partner (buddy) and may be made worse by the effects that diving has on health.

The respiratory system is of particular significance in the context of medical fitness to dive. First, exercise capacity at depth is primarily determined by ventilatory capacity because of the excessive work of breathing at higher gas densities [14]. Second, inert gas uptake and elimination are mainly driven by ventilation, gas exchange, and perfusion of the lungs. Any disturbances of these functions may increase the risk of DCI. Third, as the greatest gas-filled body cavity, the lungs are prone to rapid changes in pressure and thus may be subject to barotrauma. Any respiratory abnormalities that are associated with air trapping increase the risk for this potentially life-threatening injury.

When assessing the respiratory system for fitness to dive, a distinct point of view is necessary for recreational scuba diving versus commercial or military diving. In the latter occupations, diving medical examinations are performed to select diving candidates and to survey their health during the occupational exposure [168]. Thus, it is the privilege of the employer to prohibit from diving those individuals who have medical conditions that are associated with a significantly increased risk of diving-related medical complications. In contrast, the responsibility for the recreational dive is with the individual, and the environmental conditions of the dive are self-selected. Recreational divers should consult a physician to get medical advice on any significant

Table 3
Demographics and dive characteristics of cases of pulmonary edema during scuba diving

First author, year [reference]	n	Age (y)	Sex (M/F)	Temperature (°C)	Depth (msw)
Wilmshurst, 1989 [17]	11	45.6 ± 2.6	8/3	<12	N/A
Pons, 1995 [151]	3	30.7 ± 7.2	2/1	4.7–5.6	24–42
Hampson, 1997 [155]	5	43.3 ± 12.9	2/4	12–18	4.5–25
Gnadinger, 2001 [157]	1	52	1/0	25	3.3
Slade, 2001 [156]	8	52.4 ± 5.6	3/5	10–26	4.6–33.8
Hempe, 2003 [165]	1	49	0/1	Cold	8
Halpern, 2003 [166]	1	50	1/0	Mild	12

Figures presented as totals, means ± standard deviation, or ranges.
Abbreviations: F, female; M, male; N/A, not applicable.

associated risks in case there is a medical condition that may affect diving safety. Admittedly, some individuals only aim to get medical clearance. It is therefore important to ensure that the individual acknowledges and understands the associated risks of scuba diving.

In most recreational diving injuries, no preexisting medical problems are apparent [26], and the question has been raised of why people who want to dive should be restricted. Scuba diving has become a popular recreational activity throughout the world, and persons suffering from highly prevalent diseases, such as bronchial asthma, may want to start diving. Increasing data on subpopulations of divers diving safely with certain diseases have emerged, and evidence of significantly increased risks for diving-related injuries in these populations was lacking. This has led to a change in views on diving in persons with respiratory diseases over the past decade. A couple of thoracic societies have published recommendations on respiratory aspects of fitness to dive [169,170]. An increasing number of peer-reviewed articles have addressed the respiratory system and scuba diving in general [171–178] or asthma in particular [172,174, 179–182]. For example, a diagnosis of asthma has historically been considered an absolute contraindication to diving [28,61]. A differentiated approach with a trend toward being less restrictive is obvious from more recent recommendations [172,179–182]. The discussion on fitness to dive with respiratory diseases, however, remains controversial, mostly because of the issue that ethical considerations preclude randomized controlled trials in human beings. The analysis of risks therefore largely relies on empirically derived data and anecdotal reports.

Diving with respiratory diseases: epidemiology and clinical considerations

Among possible hazards to subjects diving with respiratory diseases, the risk for DCI is of major concern. Diving accident statistics may help to evaluate whether there is an increased risk. Unfortunately, there is no worldwide database on recreational diving accidents, and many reports rely on estimates or population surveys [73,119,120]. Divers Alert Network (DAN), located at Duke University in Durham, North Carolina, prospectively investigates dive profiles, medical history, and outcome in a growing number of recreational scuba divers in North America [26]. These data now comprise more than 36,000 dives by 3750 divers. The current incidence of DCI is 0.06% of dives, or 0.59% of divers, with

one fatality reported (0.03% of divers) [26]. These figures are slightly higher than previous ones that had been obtained from patient surveys and estimates but perfectly match figures reported from single operations in military and/or commercial scuba diving, such as the recovery of Trans World Airways Flight 800, which crashed off the coast of Long Island in 1996. An incidence of 0.05% had been reported for 3992 scuba dives to a mean depth of 35 msw performed by 350 divers [183]. Because most respiratory medical conditions have been considered absolute restrictions for military or commercial diving [168], however, epidemiologic data on subjects diving with respiratory diseases are available for recreational scuba diving only. Previous DAN accident statistics had revealed odds ratios of 1.98 for AGE and 1.16 for DCS in current asthmatics compared with case controls, but the data did not reach statistical significance [184]. Of the injury cases reported annually to the DAN by hyperbaric facilities, there are approximately 6% asthmatics, and asthma was present in less than 0.5% of diving fatalities [26]. Remarkably, there are no data available for other respiratory conditions of similar prevalence, such as chronic obstructive pulmonary disease (COPD), albeit up to 20% of divers do smoke actively [185,186].

Population surveys indicate that divers are diving with respiratory diseases. Whereas 9.7% of subjects diving in Western Australia are reported to have asthma currently, only 0.6% are reported to have COPD [187]. Surveys among sport scuba divers in the United States consistently found that approximately 4% of divers currently had asthma and another 4% had childhood asthma only [188,189]. A survey among British sport divers revealed that there are asthmatics who dive uneventfully, including those reporting daily asthma symptoms [190]. Surprisingly, more than half of the respondents did not know or even ignored the current recommendations for safe diving. In a recent survey among sports divers from continental Europe, 8.7% of the respondents indicated that they dive with current asthma and 42.4% of those with asthma were regularly using drugs to relieve or control their symptoms [186]. In that population, there were subjects who used drugs without bronchodilating activity as prophylaxis before diving and others who reported continued dyspnea but did not use bronchodilators, thus supporting the need for better education and disease management of asthmatic divers.

There are few data on subjects diving with less prevalent respiratory conditions. Population surveys among Australian and European sport divers indicate that there are few subjects diving with a history of spontaneous or traumatic pneumothorax or chronic bronchitis and that up to 5% of divers reported a history of pneumonia [186,191]. Beyond epidemiology, some curiosities may be found in the literature. There is one case report of a 28-year-old man who dived uneventfully for several months at depths between 3 and 50 msw with pneumothorax [192]. In accordance with what would be expected from the physiology, the diver was described as feeling best while diving, and he even felt better the deeper he went. A 58-year old man was reported to dive well except for the problem of "keeling," or swimming with a buoyancy-related tilt, after a right-sided pneumonectomy for squamous cell carcinoma of the lung [193]. He had been able to counteract the asymmetric buoyancy with weights attached to the left side. There are subjects diving with fibrosing pulmonary diseases, such as sarcoidosis, but no reports are available that provide systematic data on figures and outcomes. One case of a diver with stage III sarcoidosis, who suffered from symptomatology matching that of AGE during decompression from a 50-msw hyperbaric chamber exposure, has been reported [194]. Against medical advice, that diver continued to scuba dive and had a recurrent incident 2 years later after a dive to 30 msw in a lake. Regrettably, residual symptoms remained even after repeated hyperbaric oxygen treatments (Hanjo Roggenbach, MD, personal communication, 2004).

Respiratory assessment of fitness to dive

Because abnormalities of the respiratory system are obviously associated with an increased risk of suffering from underwater hazards, such as DCI or drowning, the investigation of the lung deserves particular attention. The routine assessment should comprise a medical history, physical examination, and spirometry. The need for routine medical examinations has been questioned recently, because conditions preventing subjects from diving were mostly detected by questionnaire [185], but physical examination is useful to document the physical state at the beginning of a diving career and to evaluate possible deviations during follow-up. This may, in fact, have legal implications in the case of residual damage from diving injuries. Spirometry should rule out any ventilatory abnormalities. There is no general consensus on particular limits; however, most reasonably, FEV_1 and FVC should exceed 80% of their respective predicted values [169,170,195]. The quotient of FEV_1/FVC should be greater than 70%, but it must be kept in mind that diving may increase the VC

because of respiratory muscle training, and lower than predicted FEV_1/FVC ratios have been found in experienced commercial divers [196,197].

Any history or detection of respiratory abnormalities should prompt further investigation. In fact, approximately 30% of diving candidates are reported to be referred for a specialist opinion because of respiratory conditions [185]. The British Thoracic Society has recently suggested an algorithm for further assessment [170], which recommends a chest radiograph in case of current respiratory symptoms or a history of lung disease or chest trauma. If radiography, in combination with the physical examination and spirometry, is normal, the candidate may be approved unless specific respiratory conditions apply. These conditions may comprise but are not restricted to obstructive airways diseases, such as asthma and COPD, pulmonary fibrosis, sarcoidosis, infectious diseases, and previous chest trauma. Asthma is the most prevalent of these conditions and thus the most important clinical pulmonary condition to be considered in an assessment of fitness to dive; therefore, a differentiated approach to diving eligibility is now recommended [170,180,181]. Table 4 provides recommendations on fitness to dive in asthmatics based on the current severity classification published by the National Institutes of Health [198,199]. Individual factors, such as self-management of the disease and compliance with treatment, must be taken into account when assessing fitness to dive, however, and these recommendations may only guide the physician's advice. The asthmatic diving candidate should be aware of the risks and dive accordingly (ie, avoid fast ascents and exertion). Airway hyperresponsiveness with a significant response to hyperpnea or hypertonic aerosols precludes diving because of the stimuli experienced by the diver, such as hyperpnea of dry gas during exercise and possible aspiration of seawater. Indirect bronchial challenges, such as eucapnic voluntary hyperpnea, are preferred over direct pharmacologic tests, because the latter are less specific for identifying asthma and exercise-induced bronchoconstriction [200]. A history of atopy alone (without respiratory symptoms and with normal lung function) has not been of concern for the evaluation of fitness to dive yet; in fact, there are many subjects diving uneventfully who have a sensitization to common aeroallergens [186,191,201]. One experimental study in human beings indicated postdive pulmonary function changes in asymptomatic subjects with hay fever and airway hyperreactivity to methacholine [202], however, and another study showed an increased postdive response to methacholine challenge in atopic subjects [203].

Table 4
Recommendations regarding fitness to dive for asthmatics

Step	Symptoms (day/night)[a]	PEF or FEV$_1$ (PEF variability %)[a]	Fitness to dive
Childhood only	None	≥80 <20	Yes
Mild intermittent	≤2 d/wk ≤2 nights/mo	≥80 <20	Yes, if >48 h since last reliever intake
Mild persistent	<Daily >2 nights/mo	≥80 20–30	Yes, if regular controller medication and >48 h since last reliever intake
Moderate persistent	Daily >1 night/wk	<80 >30	No
Severe persistent	Continual Frequent	≤60 >30	No

Abbreviation: PEF, peak expiratory flow.
[a] Clinical features before treatment.

Divers must have a certain aerobic capacity to be able to cope with the increased work of breathing at depth, which may be aggravated by exercise (eg, when swimming against a strong underwater current). Thus, further investigation of diving candidates with a history of respiratory disease or symptoms or abnormalities during routine assessment should include cardiopulmonary exercise testing. Any ventilatory abnormalities or impaired gas exchange during exercise should preclude diving, and a peak oxygen uptake of at least 25 and 27 mL/kg^{-1}/min^{-1} should be achieved in women and men, respectively.

Smoking is associated with the development of inflammatory airway changes even in the asymptomatic state, and a certain percentage of smokers get COPD [204]. Thus, it is worth questioning whether smokers are fit to dive. A recent analysis of DCI cases in the DAN database from 1989 through 1997 revealed that smokers with DCI tended to present with more severe symptoms than their nonsmoking counterparts [205]. Moreover, significant adjusted odds ratios for the comparison of heavy smokers, as defined by a history of more than 15 pack-years, with those who have never smoked showed some correlation with the severity of DCI in a dose-dependent fashion. It was therefore suggested that a history of smoking per se may justify further pneumatologic evaluation of the diving candidate [206].

Long-term effects of diving on the lung

Diving is associated with exposure to several factors that, independently of each other, have been shown to have effects on pulmonary function. Some of these, such as hyperoxia and VGM filtered in the pulmonary circulation, may induce inflammatory reactions in the lung, whereas others, such as increased breathing resistance and blood and/or fluid redistribution during immersion, may induce mechanical or physiologic stress only without tissue damage.

Studies of some experimental dives have provided insights into the mechanisms of changes in pulmonary function associated with diving and the time course of the changes attributable to different exposure factors. Such studies are not suitable for predicting long-term effects, however, because the effects of subsequent dives add to the effects of the experimental dives. It is easy to monitor the exposure in a well-controlled experimental dive, but one of the great challenges in epidemiologic studies is to define a measure of cumulative diving exposure over time to which any outcome measure can be related.

The basic physical parameters characterizing any dive are pressure, time, and gas mixture. These parameters are independent of the method of diving and form the basis for calculation of diving exposure, including oxygen exposure, decompression stress, and respiratory mechanical load. Differences between diving methods are quantitative rather than qualitative. In epidemiologic studies, there are difficulties in obtaining accurate estimates of cumulative exposure, even in prospective longitudinal studies. The number of dives encountered by different diving methods, number of days in saturation, or only the number of years as a diver is what has been achieved with some accuracy in the epidemiologic studies that have been reported to date. These simple measures of exposure are related to the basic physical parameters of the dives, however, and reflect the cumulative exposure to the more specific exposure factors in some way.

The first studies characterizing pulmonary function in divers showed that divers had larger than predicted VCs [196,197,207]. There was a significant correlation between FVC and the maximal depth ever dived to up to the age of 30 years [208], consistent with an effect of respiratory muscle training. After the age of 30 years, FVC declined despite continued diving. The FEV_1 was, however, not increased in proportion to the FVC, resulting in a lower than predicted FEV_1/FVC ratio. Initially this was not considered to be a result of airway obstruction, but the same studies did show lower than predicted maximal expiratory flow rates at low lung volumes. Later cross-sectional studies have shown lower FEV_1 and maximal expiratory flow rates at low lung volumes in divers compared with matched control groups and that the reductions in these variables are related to cumulative diving exposure in saturation divers as well as in air bounce divers [209–211].

The large VC in divers can be a result of the selection of subjects with large lungs [212] or that of adaptation to the hyperbaric environment with an increased load of breathing and respiratory muscle training. In a study on a group of apprentice divers, the FVC at the beginning of a diving education was larger than predicted [213] without a difference between subjects who had and subjects who did not have diving experience at the start of their education. There was a further small increase in FVC in the first year only of their professional career, with no further increase after 3 years.

The results of the 6-year longitudinal follow-up up of these apprentice divers confirm the results from the cross-sectional studies in that FEV_1 and maximal expiratory flow rates were reduced in the divers over the follow-up period when compared with a control group of policemen and that the reduction was related to diving exposure [214].

Other longitudinal studies included small groups of selected divers only but support the findings of the study in apprentice divers. After experimental saturation dives to 300 msw or more, 26 divers were followed for 4 years and compared with 28 saturation divers who had not taken part in deep dives to depths of 180 m or more. One year after the deep dive, there was a significant reduction in FEV_1 and maximal expiratory flow rates at low lung volumes, after which the rates of change were not different between the two groups [215]. The reduction in FEV_1 as a consequence of exposure to hyperoxia only, which was the same as in a deep saturation dive, has been shown to persist for 3 years in subjects who did not take part in any diving activity during the follow-up period [216]. That study indicated the exposure to hyperoxia contributes significantly to the short-term as well as long-term effects of diving on lung function.

There are few studies on lung function variables other than FVC, FEV_1, and the maximal expiratory flow rates, but there seems to be a reduction in transfer factor for carbon monoxide as well, which is related to cumulative diving exposure [209,214,217]. Exercise capacity and peak oxygen uptake do not seem to be reduced in divers, but when compared with control groups, divers have larger ventilatory equivalents for oxygen uptake and carbon dioxide output [207,218]. These changes and the reduction in Tl_{CO} may indicate small gas exchange abnormalities.

The long-term changes, although small and hardly influencing the quality of life of active professional divers who were subjected to the studies, may have some consequences, however. A reduced FEV_1 is associated with a reduced ventilatory capacity, even more so when gas density is increased under pressure, encroaching on the diver's underwater exercise capacity. A reduced FEV_1 may increase the risk of PBT as well, at least theoretically.

The epidemiologic studies have been conducted in professionally active divers. If the reduction in FEV_1 persists into retirement, the prevalence of respiratory symptoms is expected to increase by aging. In a group of retired Norwegian divers working in the North Sea before 1990 and experiencing saturation as well as mixed gas bounce diving, the prevalence of respiratory symptoms and spirometric airflow limitation, with a FEV_1/FVC ratio less than 70% and an FEV_1 less than 80% of predicted, was almost double that in the general population, and it was not related to smoking habits, atopy, or other occupational activities like welding [219]. The mean age of these retired divers was 52 years only, and mean time since retiring from diving was 12 years. Further follow-up of other groups of divers into retirement thus seems necessary.

References

[1] National Sporting Goods Assocation. Available at: http://www.nsga.org. Accessed June 22, 2005.
[2] Clarke JM. Pulmonary limits of oxygen tolerance in man. Exp Lung Res 1988;14:897–912.
[3] Harabin AL, Homer LD, Weathersby PK, et al. An analysis of decrements in vital capacity as an index of pulmonary oxygen toxicity. J Appl Physiol 1987;63:1130–5.

[4] Suzuki S. Probable lung injury by long term exposure to oxygen close to 50 kilopascals. Undersea Hyperb Med 1994;21:235–43.

[5] Thorsen E, Segadal K, Reed JW, et al. Contribution of hyperoxia to reduced pulmonary function after deep saturation dives. J Appl Physiol 1993;75:657–62.

[6] Clark JM, Jackson RM, Lambertsen CJ, et al. Pulmonary function in men after oxygen breathing at 3.0 ATA for 3.5 hours. J Appl Physiol 1991;71:878–85.

[7] Fracica PJ, Knapp MJ, Piantadosi CA, et al. Responses of baboons to prolonged hyperoxia: physiology and qualitative pathology. J Appl Physiol 1991;71:2352–62.

[8] Hlastala MP, Robertson HT, Ross BK. Gas exchange abnormalities produced by venous gas emboli. Respir Physiol 1979;36:1–17.

[9] Albertine JJ, Wiener-Kronish JP, Koike K, et al. Quantification of damage by air emboli to lung microvessels in anesthetized sheep. J Appl Physiol 1984;57:1360–8.

[10] Flick MR, Perel A, Staub NC. Leukocytes are required for increased lung microvascular permeability after microembolization in sheep. Circ Res 1981;48:344–51.

[11] Butler BD, Katz J. Vascular pressures and passage of gas emboli through the pulmonary circulation. Undersea Biomed Res 1988;15:203–9.

[12] Thorsen E, Risberg J, Segadal K, et al. Effects of venous gas microemboli on pulmonary gas transfer function. Undersea Hyperb Med 1995;22:347–53.

[13] Dujic Z, Eterovic D, Denoble A, et al. Effect of a single air dive on pulmonary diffusing capacity in professional divers. J Appl Physiol 1993;74:55–61.

[14] Maio DA, Farhi LE. Effect of gas density on mechanics of breathing. J Appl Physiol 1967;23:687–93.

[15] Van Liew H, Thalmann ED, Sponholtz DK. Hindrance to diffusive gas mixing in the lung in hyperbaric environments. J Appl Physiol 1981;51:243–7.

[16] Thorsen E, Skogstad M, Reed JW. Subacute effects of inspiratory resistive loading and head-out water immersion on pulmonary function. Undersea Hyperb Med 1999;26:137–41.

[17] Wilmshurst PT, Nuri M, Crother A, et al. Cold-induced pulmonary oedema in scuba-divers and swimmers and subsequent development of hypertension. Lancet 1989;1:62–5.

[18] O'Cain CF, Dowling NB, Slutsky AS, et al. Airway effects of respiratory heat loss in normal subjects. J Appl Physiol 1980;49:875–80.

[19] Burnet H, Lucciano M, Jammes Y. Respiratory effects of cold-gas breathing in humans under hyperbaric environment. Respir Physiol 1990;142:413–24.

[20] Rønnestad I, Thorsen E, Segadal K, et al. Bronchial response to breathing dry gas at 3.7 MPa ambient pressure. Eur J Appl Physiol 1994;69:32–5.

[21] Cotes JE, Davey IS, Reed JW, et al. Respiratory effects of a single saturation dive to 300 m. Br J Ind Med 1987;44:76–82.

[22] Suzuki S, Ikeda T, Hashimoto A. Decrease in the single breath diffusing capacity after saturation dives. Undersea Biomed Res 1991;18:103–9.

[23] Thorsen E, Segadal K, Påsche A, et al. Pulmonary mechanical function and diffusion capacity after deep saturation dives. Br J Ind Med 1990;47:242–7.

[24] Skogstad M, Thorsen E, Haldorsen T, et al. Divers' pulmonary function after open-sea bounce dives to 10 and 50 meters. Undersea Hyperb Med 1996;23:71–5.

[25] Tetzlaff K, Friege L, Koch A, et al. Effects of ambient cold and depth on lung function in humans after a single scuba dive. Eur J Appl Physiol 2001;85:125–9.

[26] Divers Alert Network. Report on decompression illness, diving fatalities and project dive exploration. The DAN annual review of recreational scuba diving injuries and fatalities based on 2001 data. Durham, NC: Divers Alert Network; 2003.

[27] Strauss MB, Wright PW. Thoracic squeeze diving casualty. Aerosp Med 1971;42:673–5.

[28] Strauss RH. Diving medicine. Am Rev Respir Dis 1979;119:1001–23.

[29] Schaefer KE, McNulty WP, Carey C, et al. Mechanisms in development of interstitial emphysema and air embolism on decompression from depth. J Appl Physiol 1958;13:15–29.

[30] Malhotra MS, Wright HC. The effects of a raised intrapulmonary pressure on the lungs of fresh unchilled cadavers. J Pathol Bacteriol 1961;82:198–202.

[31] Liebow AA, Stark JE, Vogel J, et al. Intrapulmonary air trapping in submarine escape training casualties. US Armed Forces Med J 1959;10:265–89.

[32] Schriger DL, Rosenberg G, Wilder RJ. Shoulder pain and pneumoperitoneum following a diving accident. Ann Emerg Med 1987;16:1281–4.

[33] Oh ST, Kim W, Jeon HM, et al. Massive pneumoperitoneum after scuba diving. J Korean Med Sci 2003;18:281–3.

[34] Muth CM, Shank ES. Gas embolism. N Engl J Med 2000;342:476–82.

[35] Dutka AJ. A review of the pathophysiology and potential application of experimental therapies for cerebral ischemia to the treatment of cerebral arterial gas embolism. Undersea Biomed Res 1985;12:403–21.

[36] Zwillich CW, Pierson DJ, Creagh CE, et al. Complications of assisted ventilation: a prospective study of 354 consecutive episodes. Am J Med 1974;57:161–70.

[37] Broome CR, Jarvis LJ, Clark RJ. Pulmonary barotrauma in submarine escape training. Thorax 1994;49:186–7.

[38] Friehs I, Friehs M, Friehs GB. Air embolism with bilateral pneumothorax after a five-meter dive. Undersea Hyperb Med 1993;20:155–7.

[39] Hamad A, Alghadban A, Ward L. Seizure in a scuba diver. Chest 2001;119:285–6.

[40] Neuman TS, Jacoby I, Bove AA. Fatal pulmonary barotrauma due to obstruction of the central circulation with air. J Emerg Med 1998;16:413–7.

[41] Roobottom CA, Hunter JD, Bryson PJ. The diagnosis of fatal gas embolism: detection by plain film radiography. Clin Radiol 1994;49:805–7.

[42] Carstairs S. Arterial gas embolism in a diver using a closed-circuit oxygen rebreathing apparatus. Undersea Hyperb Med 2001;28:229–31.

[43] Tetzlaff K, Neubauer B, Reuter M, et al. Pulmonary barotrauma of a diver using an oxygen rebreathing diving apparatus. Aviat Space Environ Med 1996;67:1198–200.

[44] Raymond LW. Pulmonary barotrauma and related events in divers. Chest 1995;107:1648–52.

[45] Benton PJ, Woodfine JD, Westwood PR. Arterial gas embolism following a 1-meter ascent during helicopter escape training: a case report. Aviat Space Environ Med 1996;67:63–4.

[46] Weiss LD, Van Meter KM. Cerebral air embolism in asthmatic scuba divers in a swimming pool. Chest 1995;107:1653–4.

[47] Zaugg M, Kaplan V, Widmer U, et al. Fatal air embolism in an airplane passenger with a giant intrapulmonary bronchogenic cyst. Am J Respir Crit Care Med 1998;157:1686–9.

[48] Rudge FW. Altitude-induced arterial gas embolism: a case report. Aviat Space Environ Med 1992;63:203–5.

[49] Cable GG, Keeble T, Wilson G. Pulmonary cyst and cerebral arterial gas embolism in a hypobaric chamber: a case report. Aviat Space Environ Med 2000;71:172–6.

[50] Rios-Tejada F, Azofra-Garcia J, Valle-Garrido J, et al. Neurological manifestation of arterial gas embolism following standard altitude chamber flight: a case report. Aviat Space Environ Med 1997;68:1025–8.

[51] Lee CT. Cerebral arterial gas embolism in air force ground maintenance crew—a report of two cases. Aviat Space Environ Med 1999;70:698–700.

[52] Hickey MJ, Zanetti CL. Delayed-onset cerebral arterial gas embolism in a commercial airline mechanic. Aviat Space Environ Med 2003;74:977–80.

[53] Unsworth IP. Pulmonary barotraumas in a hyperbaric chamber. Anaesthesia 1973;28:675–8.

[54] Wolf HK, Moon RE, Mitchell PR, et al. Barotrauma and air embolism in hyperbaric oxygen therapy. Am J Forensic Med Pathol 1990;11:149–53.

[55] Mueller PHJ, Tetzlaff K, Neubauer B, et al. Pulmonary barotrauma during hyperbaric oxygen therapy: a case report [abstract]. Undersea Hyperb Med 1998;25(Suppl):34.

[56] James RE. Extra-alveolar air resulting from submarine escape training: a post-training roentgenographic survey of 170 submariners. Report No. 550. Groton, CT: US Naval Submarine Medical Center; 1968.

[57] Yanir Y, Abramovich A, Beck-Razi N, et al. Telephone diagnosis of a strange voice. Chest 2003;123:2112–4.

[58] Kizer KW. Dysbaric cerebral air embolism in Hawaii. Ann Emerg Med 1987;16:535–41.

[59] Tetzlaff K, Reuter M, Leplow B, et al. Risk factors for pulmonary barotrauma in divers. Chest 1997;112:654–9.

[60] Leitch DR, Green RD. Pulmonary barotrauma in divers and the treatment of cerebral arterial gas embolism. Aviat Space Environ Med 1986;57:931–8.

[61] Melamed Y, Shupak A, Bitterman H. Medical problems associated with underwater diving. N Engl J Med 1992;326:30–5.

[62] Collins JJ. An unusual case of air embolism precipitated by decompression. N Engl J Med 1962;266:595–8.

[63] Tirpitz D, Schipke JD. Delayed recompression after scuba diving-induced pulmonary barotraumas: a case report. Aviat Space Environ Med 1996;67:266–8.

[64] Harker CP, Neuman TS, Olson LK, et al. The roentgenographic findings associated with air embolism in sport scuba divers. J Emerg Med 1993;11:443–9.

[65] Dick APK, Massey EW. Neurologic presentation of decompression sickness and air embolism in sport divers. Neurology 1985;35:667–71.

[66] Krzyzak J. A case of delayed-onset pulmonary barotrauma in a scuba diver. Undersea Biomed Res 1987;14:553–61.

[67] Moloff AL. Delayed onset arterial gas embolism. Aviat Space Environ Med 1993;64:1040–3.

[68] Clarke D, Gerard W, Norris T. Pulmonary barotrauma-induced cerebral arterial gas embolism with spontaneous recovery: commentary on the rationale for therapeutic recompression. Aviat Space Environ Med 2002;73:139–46.

[69] Neuman TS. Arterial gas embolism and decompression sickness. News Physiol Sci 2002;17:77–81.

[70] Williamson JA, King GK, Callanan VI, et al. Fatal arterial gas embolism. Detection by chest radiography and imaging before autopsy. Med J Aust 1990;153:97–100.

[71] Elliott DH, Harrison JAB, Barnard EEP. Clinical and radiological features of 88 cases of decompression barotrauma. In: Shilling CW, Beckett MW, editors. Proceedings of the VI Symposium on Underwater Physiology. Bethesda (MD): FASEB; 1978. p. 527–35.

[72] Lindemark C, Adolfson J. Lung rupture as a complication in free escape. In: Örnhagen H, Carlsson AL, editors. Proceedings of the XI Annual Meeting of the European Undersea Biomedical Society. Bromma (Sweden): Kugel Tryckeri AB; 1985. p. 81–4.

[73] Arness MK. Scuba decompression illness and diving fatalities in an overseas military community. Aviat Space Environ Med 1997;68:325–33.

[74] Calder IM. Autopsy and experimental observations on factors leading to barotrauma in man. Undersea Biomed Res 1985;12:165–82.

[75] Saywell WR. Submarine escape training, lung cysts

and tension pneumothorax. Br J Radiol 1989;62: 276–8.

[76] Mellem H, Emhjellen S, Horgen O. Pulmonary barotrauma and arterial gas embolism caused by an emphysematous bulla in a scuba diver. Aviat Space Environ Med 1990;61:559–62.

[77] Reuter M, Tetzlaff K, Warninghoff V, et al. Computed tomography of the chest in diving-related pulmonary barotrauma. Br J Radiol 1997;70:440–5.

[78] Le Vot J, Solacroup JC, Muyard B, et al. Le thorax de l'accidente de plongée. J Radiol 1989;70:357–63.

[79] Toklu AS, Kiyan E, Aktas S, et al. Should computed chest tomography be recommended in the medical certification of professional divers? A report of three cases with pulmonary air casts. Occup Environ Med 2003;60:606–8.

[80] Heritiér F, Schaller MD, Fitting JW, et al. Manifestations pulmonaires des accidents de plongée. Schweiz Z Sportmed 1993;41:115–20.

[81] Jego C, Berard H, Moulin P, et al. Des bulles qui ne doivent plus plonger. Rev Mal Respir 2003;20: 144–6.

[82] Leitch DR, Green RD. Recurrent pulmonary barotrauma. Aviat Space Environ Med 1986;57:1039–43.

[83] Carpenter CR. Recurrent pulmonary barotrauma in scuba diving and the risks of future hyperbaric exposures: a case report. Undersea Hyperb Med 1997; 24:209–13.

[84] Tetzlaff K, Reuter M, Warninghoff V, et al. Dive-related pulmonary barotrauma in the differential diagnosis of pneumologic outpatients. Pneumologie 1996;50:902–5.

[85] Colebatch HJ, Ng CK. Decreased pulmonary distensibility and pulmonary barotrauma in divers. Respir Physiol 1991;86:293–303.

[86] Benton PJ, Francis TJR, Pethybridge RJ. Spirometric indices and the risk of pulmonary barotraumas in submarine escape training. Undersea Hyperb Med 1999;26:213–7.

[87] Moon RE, Vann RD, Bennett PB. The physiology of decompression illness. Sci Am 1995;273:70–7.

[88] Doolette DJ, Mitchell SJ. The physiological kinetics of nitrogen and the prevention of decompression sickness. Clin Pharmacokinet 2001;40:1–14.

[89] Butler BD, Hills BA. The lung as a filter for microbubbles. J Appl Physiol 1979;47:537–43.

[90] Eckenhoff RG, Olstad CS, Carrod G. Human dose-response relationship for decompression and endogenous bubble formation. J Appl Physiol 1990;69: 914–8.

[91] Carturan D, Boussuges A, Vanuxem P, et al. Ascent rate, age, maximal oxygen uptake, adiposity, and circulating venous bubbles after diving. J Appl Physiol 2002;93:1349–56.

[92] Glen SK, Georgiadis D, Grosset DG, et al. Transcranial Doppler ultrasound in commercial air divers: a field study including cases with right-to-left shunting. Undersea Hyperb Med 1995;22:129–35.

[93] Gerriets T, Tetzlaff K, Liceni T, et al. Arteriove-

nous bubbles following cold water sport dives: relation to right-to-left shunting. Neurology 2000; 55:1741–3.

[94] Bove AA, Hallenbeck JM, Elliott DH. Circulatory responses to venous air embolism and decompression sickness in dogs. Undersea Biomed Res 1974;1: 207–20.

[95] Neuman TS, Spragg RG, Wagner PD, et al. Cardiopulmonary consequences of decompression stress. Respir Physiol 1980;41:143–53.

[96] Peterson BT, Grauer SE, Hyde RW, et al. Response of pulmonary veins to increased intracranial pressure and pulmonary air embolization. J Appl Physiol 1980;48:957–64.

[97] Levin LL, Stewart GJ, Lynch PR, et al. Blood and blood vessel wall changes induced by decompression sickness in dogs. J Appl Physiol 1981;50:944–9.

[98] Ward CA, McCullough D, Fraser WD. Relation between complement activation and susceptibility to decompression sickness. J Appl Physiol 1987;62: 1160–6.

[99] Ohkuda K, Nakahara K, Binder A, et al. Venous air emboli in sheep: reversible increase in lung microvascular permeability. J Appl Physiol 1981;51: 887–94.

[100] Buttolph TB, Dick EJ, Toner CB, et al. Cutaneous lesions in swine after decompression: histopathology and ultrastructure. Undersea Hyperb Med 1998;25: 115–21.

[101] Francis TJ, Pezeshkpour GH, Dutka AJ, et al. Is there a role for the autochthonous bubble in the pathogenesis of spinal cord decompression sickness? J Neuropathol Exp Neurol 1988;47:475–87.

[102] Francis TJ, Griffin JL, Homer LD, et al. Bubble-induced dysfunction in acute spinal cord decompression sickness. J Appl Physiol 1990;68:1368–75.

[103] Palmer AC. Nature and incidence of bubbles in the spinal cord of decompressed goats. Undersea Hyperb Med 1997;24:193–200.

[104] Broome JR, Dick EJ. Neurological decompression illness in swine. Aviat Space Environ Med 1996;67: 207–13.

[105] Dick EJ, Broome JR, Hayward IJ. Acute neurologic decompression illness in pigs: lesions of the spinal cord and brain. Lab Anim Sci 1997;47:50–7.

[106] Reuter M, Tetzlaff K, Brasch F, et al. Computed chest tomography in an animal model for decompression sickness: radiologic, physiologic, and pathologic findings. Eur Radiol 2000;10:534–41.

[107] Neuman TS, Bove AA. Combined arterial gas embolism and decompression sickness following no-stop dives. Undersea Biomed Res 1990;17:429–36.

[108] Broome JR. Reduction of decompression illness risk in pigs by use of non-linear ascent profiles. Undersea Hyperb Med 1996;23:19–26.

[109] Broome JR. Climatic and environmental factors in the aetiology of decompression sickness in divers. J R Nav Med Serv 1993;79:68–74.

[110] Jankowski LW, Nishi RY, Eaton DJ, et al. Exercise

during decompression reduces the amount of venous gas emboli. Undersea Hyperb Med 1997;24:59–65.

[111] Broome JR, Dutka AJ, McNamee GA. Exercise conditioning reduces the risk of neurologic decompression illness in swine. Undersea Hyperb Med 1995;22:73–85.

[112] Wisløff U, Brubakk AO. Aerobic endurance training reduces bubble formation and increases survival in rats exposed to hyperbaric pressure. J Physiol 2001; 537:607–11.

[113] Dujic Z, Duplancic D, Marinovic-Terzic I, et al. Aerobic exercise before diving reduce venous gas bubbles formation in humans. J Physiol 2004;555:637–42.

[114] Doolette DJ. Exercise fizzy-ology. J Physiol 2001; 537:330.

[115] Dembert ML, Jekel JF, Mooney LW. Health risk factors for the development of decompression sickness among US Navy divers. Undersea Biomed Res 1984;11:395–406.

[116] Carturan D, Boussuges A, Burnet H, et al. Circulating venous bubbles in recreational diving: relationships with age, weight, maximal oxygen uptake and body fat percentage. Int J Sports Med 1999;20:410–4.

[117] Vann RD. Mechanisms and risks of decompression. In: Bove AA, editor. Bove and Davis' diving medicine. 3rd edition. Philadelphia: WB Saunders; 1997. p. 146–58.

[118] Dunford RG, Vann RD, Gerth WA, et al. The incidence of venous gas emboli in recreational diving. Undersea Hyperb Med 2002;29:247–59.

[119] Hagberg M, Örnhagen H. Incidence and risk factors for symptoms of decompression sickness among male and female dive masters and instructors—a retrospective cohort study. Undersea Hyperb Med 2003;30:93–102.

[120] St Leger Dowse M, Bryson P, et al. Comparative data from 2250 male and female sports divers: diving patterns and decompression sickness. Aviat Space Environ Med 2002;73:743–9.

[121] Freiberger JJ, Denoble PJ, Pieper CF, et al. The relative risk of decompression sickness during and after air travel following diving. Aviat Space Environ Med 2002;73:980–4.

[122] Sheffield PJ. Flying after diving guidelines: a review. Aviat Space Environ Med 1990;61:1130–8.

[123] Catron PW, Flynn ET, Yaffe Y, et al. Morphological and physiological responses of the lungs of dogs to acute decompression. J Appl Physiol 1984;57: 467–74.

[124] Butler BD, Luehr S, Katz J. Venous gas embolism: time course of residual pulmonary intravascular bubbles. Undersea Biomed Res 1989;16:21–9.

[125] Atkins CE, Lehner CE, Beck KA, et al. Experimental respiratory decompression sickness in sheep. J Appl Physiol 1988;65:1163–71.

[126] Nossum V, Koteng S, Brubakk AO. Endothelial damage by bubbles in the pulmonary artery of the pig. Undersea Hyperb Med 1999;26:1–8.

[127] Nossum V, Hjelde A, Brubakk AO. Small amounts of venous gas embolism cause delayed impairment of endothelial function and increase polymorphonuclear neutrophil infiltration. Eur J Appl Physiol 2002; 86:209–14.

[128] Nossum V, Hjelde A, Bergh K, et al. Anti-C5a monoclonal antibodies and pulmonary polymorphonuclear leukocyte infiltration—endothelial dysfunction by venous gas embolism. Eur J Appl Physiol 2003;89:243–8.

[129] Zwirewich CV, Müller NL, Abboud RT, et al. Noncardiogenic pulmonary edema caused by decompression sickness: rapid resolution following hyperbaric therapy. Radiology 1987;163:81–2.

[130] Wirjosemito SA, Touhey JE, Worman WT. Type II altitude decompression sickness (DCS): US Air Force experience with 133 cases. Aviat Space Environ Med 1989;60:256–62.

[131] Butler BD, Hills BA. Transpulmonary passage of venous air emboli. J Appl Physiol 1985;59:543–7.

[132] Vik A, Brubakk AO, Hennessy TR, et al. Venous air embolism in swine: transport of gas bubbles through the pulmonary circulation. J Appl Physiol 1990;69: 237–44.

[133] Vik A, Jenssen BM, Eftedal O, et al. Relationship between venous bubbles and hemodynamic responses after decompression in pigs. Undersea Hyperb Med 1993;20:233–48.

[134] Vik A, Jenssen BM, Brubakk AO. Arterial gas bubbles after decompression in pigs with patent foramen ovale. Undersea Hyperb Med 1993;20:121–32.

[135] Moon RE, Camporesi EM, Kisslo JA. Patent foramen ovale and decompression sickness in divers. Lancet 1989;1:513–4.

[136] Wilmshurst PT, Byrne JC, Webb-Peploe MM. Relation between interatrial shunts and decompression sickness in divers. Lancet 1989;2:1302–6.

[137] Germonpré P, Dendale P, Unger P, et al. Patent foramen ovale and decompression sickness in sports divers. J Appl Physiol 1998;84:1622–6.

[138] Ries S, Knauth M, Kern R, et al. Arterial gas embolism after decompression: correlation with right-to-left shunting. Neurology 1999;52:401–4.

[139] Glen SK, Georgiadis D, Grosset DG, et al. Transcranial Doppler ultrasound in commercial air divers: a field study including cases with right-to-left shunting. Undersea Hyperb Med 1995;22:129–35.

[140] Bove AA. Risk of decompression sickness with patent foramen ovale. Undersea Hyperb Med 1998;25: 175–8.

[141] Wilmshurst P, Bryson P. Relationship between the clinical features of neurological decompression illness and its causes. Clin Sci 2000;99:65–75.

[142] Moon RE, Sheffield PJ. Guidelines for treatment of decompression illness. Aviat Space Environ Med 1997;68:234–43.

[143] Moon RE, Dear G de L, Stolp BW. Treatment of decompression illness and iatrogenic gas embolism. Respir Care Clin N Am 1999;5:93–135.

[144] Tetzlaff K, Shank ES, Muth CM. Evaluation and

management of decompression illness—an intensivists' perspective. Intensive Care Med 2003;29: 2128–36.

[145] Smith RM, Van Hoesen KB, Neuman TS. Arterial gas embolism and hemoconcentration. J Emerg Med 1994;12:147–53.

[146] Smith RM, Neuman TS. Elevation of serum creatine kinase in divers with arterial gas embolization. N Engl J Med 1994;330:19–24.

[147] Warren LP, Djang WT, Moon RE, et al. Neuroimaging of scuba diving injuries to the CNS. Am J Radiol 1988;151:1003–8.

[148] Reuter M, Tetzlaff K, Hutzelmann A, et al. MR imaging of the central nervous system in diving-related decompression illness. Acta Radiol 1997;38: 940–4.

[149] Tibbles PM, Edelsberg JS. Hyperbaric-oxygen therapy. N Engl J Med 1996;334:1642–8.

[150] Moon RE, Gorman DF. Treatment of the decompression disorders. In: Brubakk AO, Neuman TS, editors. Bennett and Elliott's physiology and medicine of diving. 5th edition. Philadelphia: WB Saunders; 2003. p. 600–50.

[151] Pons M, Blickenstorfer D, Oechslin E, et al. Pulmonary oedema in healthy persons during scuba-diving and swimming. Eur Respir J 1995;8:762–7.

[152] Balk M, Goldman JM. Alveolar hemorrhage as a manifestation of pulmonary barotrauma after scuba diving. Ann Emerg Med 1990;19:930–4.

[153] Harris JB, Stern EJ, Steinberg KP. Scuba diving accident with near drowning and decompression sickness. Am J Radiol 1995;164:592.

[154] Weiler-Ravell D, Shupak A, Goldenberg I, et al. Pulmonary oedema and haemoptysis induced by strenuous swimming. BMJ 1995;311:361–2.

[155] Hampson NB, Dunford RG. Pulmonary edema of scuba divers. Undersea Hyperb Med 1997;24:29–33.

[156] Slade JB, Hattori T, Ray CS, et al. Pulmonary edema associated with scuba diving. Chest 2001;120: 1686–94.

[157] Gnadinger CA, Colwell CB, Knaut AL. Scuba diving-induced pulmonary edema in a swimming pool. J Emerg Med 2001;21:419–21.

[158] Shupak A, Weiler-Ravell D, Adir Y, et al. Pulmonary oedema induced by strenuous swimming: a field study. Respir Physiol 2000;121:25–31.

[159] West JB. Invited review: pulmonary capillary stress failure. J Appl Physiol 2000;89:2483–9.

[160] Hopkins SR, Schoene RB, Martin TR, et al. Intense exercise impairs the integrity of the pulmonary blood-gas barrier in elite athletes. Am J Respir Crit Care Med 1997;155:1090–4.

[161] Hopkins SR, Schoene RB, Henderson WR, et al. Sustained submaximal exercise does not alter the integrity of the lung blood-gas barrier in elite athletes. J Appl Physiol 1998;84:1185–9.

[162] Mahon RT, Kerr S, Amundson D, et al. Immersion pulmonary edema in special forces combat swimmers. Chest 2002;122:383–4.

[163] Lund KL, Mahon RT, Tanen DA, et al. Swimming-induced pulmonary edema. Ann Emerg Med 2003; 41:251–6.

[164] Shupak A, Guralnik L, Keynan Y, et al. Pulmonary edema following closed-circuit oxygen diving and strenuous swimming. Aviat Space Environ Med 2003;74:1201–4.

[165] Hempe S, Lierz P. Akutes Lungenödem bei einer Taucherin. Anasthesiol Intensivmed Notfallmed Schmerzther 2003;38:648–50.

[166] Halpern P, Gefen A, Sorkine P, et al. Pulmonary oedema in scuba divers: pathophysiology and computed risk analysis. Eur J Emerg Med 2003;10:35–41.

[167] Wilmshurst P. Cardiovascular problems in divers. Heart 1998;80:537–8.

[168] Elliott DH. Medical evaluation for commercial diving. In: Bove AA, editor. Bove and Davis' diving medicine. 3rd edition. Philadelphia: WB Saunders; 1997. p. 361–71.

[169] Jenkins C, Anderson SD, Wong R, et al. Compressed air diving and respiratory disease. Med J Aust 1993; 158:275–9.

[170] British Thoracic Society Fitness to Dive Group. A subgroup of the British Thoracic Society Standards of Care Committee. British Thoracic Society guidelines on respiratory aspects of fitness for diving. Thorax 2003;58:3–13.

[171] Heritiér F, Russi E. Scuba diving: barotrauma, decompression sickness, pulmonary contraindications. Schweiz Med Wochenschr 1993;123:161–5.

[172] Neuman TS, Bove AA, O'Connor RD, et al. Asthma and diving. Ann Allergy 1994;73:344–50.

[173] Twarog F, Weiler JM, Wolf SI, et al. Discussion of risk of scuba diving in individuals with allergic and respiratory diseases. J Allergy Clin Immunol 1995; 96:871–3.

[174] Anderson AD, Brannan J, Trevillion L, et al. Lung function and bronchial provocation tests for intending divers with a history of asthma. SPUMS J 1995; 25:233–48.

[175] Heritiér F. Lungs and underwater diving. Rev Med Suisse Romande 1997;117:475–8.

[176] Russi EW. Diving and the risk of barotrauma. Thorax 1998;53(Suppl 2):S20–4.

[177] Tetzlaff K, Reuter M. Pneumologische Aspekte der Tauchmedizin. Pneumologie 1998;52:489–500.

[178] Dillard TA, Ewald FW. The use of pulmonary function testing in piloting, air travel, mountain climbing, and diving. Clin Chest Med 2001;22: 795–816.

[179] Krieger BP. Diving: what to tell the patient with asthma and why. Curr Opin Pulm Med 2001;7:32–8.

[180] Coëtmeur D, Briens E, Dassonville J, et al. Asthme et pratique de la plongée sous-marine. Contre-indication absolue pour quells asthmas? Rev Mal Respir 2001; 18:381–6.

[181] Tetzlaff K, Muth CM, Waldhauser LK. A review of asthma and scuba diving. J Asthma 2002;39: 557–66.

[182] Koehle M, Lloyd-Smith R, McKenzie D, et al. Asthma and recreational scuba diving. Sports Med 2003;33:109–16.

[183] Leffler CT, White JC. Recompression treatments during the recovery of TWA Flight 800. Undersea Hyperb Med 1997;24:301–8.

[184] Corson KS, Dovenbarger JA, Moon RE, et al. Risk assessment of asthma for decompression illness [abstract]. Undersea Biomed Res 1991;18(Suppl): 16–7.

[185] Glen S, White S, Douglas J. Medical supervision of sport diving in Scotland: reassessing the need for routine medical examinations. Br J Sports Med 2000; 34:375–8.

[186] Tetzlaff K, Muth CM. Demographics and illness prevalence of scuba diving asthmatics [abstract]. Eur Respir J 2003;22(Suppl 45):418s.

[187] Cresp R, Grove C, Lalor E, et al. Health status of recreational scuba divers in Western Australia. SPUMS J 2000;30:226–30.

[188] Bove AA, Neuman T, Kelsen S, et al. Observation on asthma in the recreational diving population [abstract]. Undersea Biomed Res 1992;19(Suppl):18.

[189] Hanson E, Fleisher J, Jackman R, et al. Demographics and illness prevalence in a recreational scuba diver population: fitness to dive [abstract]. Undersea Hyperb Med 1999;26(Suppl):48.

[190] Farrell PJS, Glanvill P. Diving practices of scuba divers with asthma. BMJ 1990;300:166.

[191] Taylor DM, O'Toole KS, Ryan CM. Experienced, recreational scuba divers in Australia continue to dive despite medical contraindications. Wilderness Environ Med 2002;13:187–93.

[192] Ziser A, Väänänen A, Melamed Y. Diving and chronic spontaneous pneumothorax. Chest 1985;87:264–5.

[193] Robinson LA, Rolfe MW. Keeling syndrome—a late complication of pneumonectomy. N Engl J Med 1996;335:1074.

[194] Tetzlaff K, Reuter M, Kampen J, et al. Hyperbaric chamber-related decompression illness in a patient with asymptomatic pulmonary sarcoidosis. Aviat Space Environ Med 1999;70:594–7.

[195] South Pacific Underwater Medicine Society. The SPUMS recreational diving medical. Reprinted December 1999. Available at: http://www.spums.org.au/SPUMS_Medical_1999_web.pdf. Accessed June 22, 2005.

[196] Crosbie WA, Clarke MB, Cox RAF, et al. Physical characteristics and ventilatory function of 404 commercial divers working in the North Sea. Br J Ind Med 1977;34:19–25.

[197] Crosbie WA, Reed JW, Clarke MC. Functional characteristics of the large lungs found in divers. J Appl Physiol 1979;46:639–45.

[198] National Asthma Education and Prevention Program. Expert panel report 2. Guidelines for the diagnosis and management of asthma. National Institutes of Health Publication No. 97–4051. Bethesda (MD): National Institutes of Health; 1997.

[199] National Asthma Education and Prevention Program. Expert panel report 2. Guidelines for the diagnosis and management of asthma. Update on selected topics 2002. National Institutes of Health Publication No. 02–5074. Bethesda (MD): National Institutes of Health; 2003.

[200] Holzer K, Anderson SD, Douglass J. Exercise in elite summer athletes: challenges for diagnosis. J Allergy Clin Immunol 2002;110:374–80.

[201] Tetzlaff K, Neubauer B, Reuter M, et al. Atopy, airway reactivity and compressed air diving in males. Respiration (Herrlisheim) 1998;65:270–4.

[202] Tetzlaff K, Staschen CM, Struck N, et al. Respiratory effects of a single dive to 50 meters in sport divers with asymptomatic respiratory atopy. Int J Sports Med 2001;22:85–9.

[203] Cirillo I, Vizzaccaro A, Crimi E. Airway reactivity and diving in healthy and atopic subjects. Med Sci Sports Exerc 2003;35:1493–8.

[204] Bohadana A, Teculescu D, Martinet Y. Mechanisms of chronic airway obstruction in smokers. Respir Med 2004;98:139–51.

[205] Buch DA, El Moalem H, Dovenbarger JA, et al. Cigarette smoking and decompression illness severity: a retrospective study in recreational divers. Aviat Space Environ Med 2003;74:1271–4.

[206] Dillard TA, Ewald FW. Should divers smoke and vice versa? Aviat Space Environ Med 2003;74:1275–6.

[207] Davey IS, Cotes JE, Reed JW. Relationship of ventilatory capacity to hyperbaric exposure in divers. J Appl Physiol 1984;56:1655–8.

[208] Watt S. Effect of commercial diving on ventilatory function. Br J Ind Med 1985;42:59–62.

[209] Thorsen E, Segadal K, Kambestad B, et al. Divers' lung function: small airways disease? Br J Ind Med 1990;47:519–23.

[210] Tetzlaff K, Friege L, Reuter M, et al. Expiratory flow limitation in compressed air divers and oxygen divers. Eur Respir J 1998;12:895–9.

[211] Dmitrouk AI, Gulyar SA, Ilyin VN, et al. Physiological mechanisms of adaptation of divers to the condition of deepwater in the Antarctic. In: Sterk W, Geeraedts L, editors. Proceedings of 16th Annual Meeting of the European Biomedical Society. Amsterdam; 1990. p. 311–9.

[212] Bouhuys A, Beck GJ. Large lungs in divers? J Appl Physiol 1979;47:1136–7.

[213] Skogstad M, Thorsen E, Haldorsen T. Lung function over the first 3 years of a professional diving career. Occup Environ Med 2000;57:390–5.

[214] Skogstad M, Thorsen E, Haldorsen T, et al. Lung function over six years among professional divers. Occup Environ Med 2002;59:629–33.

[215] Thorsen E, Segadal K, Kambestad BK, et al. Pulmonary function one and four years after a deep saturation dive. Scand J Work Environ Health 1993; 19:115–20.

[216] Thorsen E, Kambestad BK. Persistent small air-

ways dysfunction after exposure to hyperoxia. J Appl Physiol 1995;78:1421–4.

[217] Bermon S, Lapoussiere JM, Dolisi C, et al. Pulmonary function of a firemen-diver population: a longitudinal study. Eur J Appl Physiol 1994;69:32–5.

[218] Thorsen E, Segadal K, Kambestad B. Characteristics of the response to exercise in professional saturation divers. Undersea Biomed Res 1991;18:93–101.

[219] Thorsen E, Irgens Å, Grønning M, et al. Prevalence of obstructive lung disease among retired North Sea divers [abstract]. Undersea Hyperb Med 2003; 30(Suppl):223.

ELSEVIER
SAUNDERS

Clin Chest Med 26 (2005) 381–394

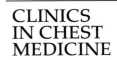

CLINICS
IN CHEST
MEDICINE

Physiological and Clinical Aspects of Apnea Diving

Claus-Martin Muth, MD*, Ulrich Ehrmann, MD, Peter Radermacher, MD

Sektion Anaesthesiologische Pathophysiologie und Verfahrensentwicklung, Universitaetsklinikum, Parkstrasse 11, D-89073 Ulm (Donau), Germany

Apnea diving, also known as breath-hold diving, is the oldest known form of diving. Early records of the ancient Greek historian, Herodotus, tell about warriors of the Persian king Xerxes who recovered sunken treasures in the fifth century BC [1]. Furthermore, for the past 2000 years along the coasts of Japan (Ama) and Korea, mainly female apnea divers (Hae Nyo) earn their living by harvesting seafood and collecting pearls from shellfish [2]. Professional apnea divers also are found in Greece (sponge divers) and on the Tuamotu Archipelago (pearl divers). Today, these professional divers do their work with repeated breath-hold dives daily, over several hours, regardless of the weather or the water temperature. During their daily working practice, they dive between 150 and 250 times to depths of 5 to 20 meters of seawater (msw) (66 ft) and stay there for in average 1 to 2 minutes. These dives are interspersed by surface intervals of 2 to 3 minutes' duration to recover [3]. In addition, the past few decades have seen the growing popularity of apnea diving for sport spear fishing in many areas, including along the Mediterranean coast. These activities are performed by breath-hold diving and have a long tradition of regular competition games. Over time, the subsistence food hunting aspects of apnea diving have been replaced by the sport aspects, and the search for maximum diving depth and longest diving duration has become an important feature.

Apnea diving has become popular in the past decade [4]. When the Italian Enzo Maiorca and French Jacques Mayol reached a depth of 50 msw (165 ft) in 1960, and then 100 msw (333 ft) in 1983, only a few enthusiasts were active in this sport. This has changed dramatically over the past decade, and today it is a sport with a growing community, official championships, and an active list of impressive records [5]. There are five main disciplines of competitive freediving [5]. The first is constant weight diving, where competitors have to swim down underwater and back upwards with one breath of air and the help of masks, fins, wetsuit, and weights but without any help from external devices. In free immersion, competitors have to pull along a measuring rope to their depth and back again. In variable weight diving, divers descend by a sleigh loaded up to a maximum of 30 kg (approximately 66 lb) along a rope. Athletes have to swim upwards on their own but are allowed to use the rope for assistance. Static apnea deals with breath-holding in a pool. Athletes lay in the pool with their face immersed in the water and hold their breath for as long as possible. Wetsuits, masks, and weights are allowed. Dynamic apnea is performed with or without fins. After one deep breath, athletes swim as far as possible horizontally under water. Finally, there is no limit freediving, probably the most dangerous of all the freediving disciplines. Deep divers descend along a guide rope with the aid of a 60-kg loaded sleigh. On the ascent, divers are drawn toward the surface with an air balloon. This type of freediving requires little to no physical activity and is focused on the ability of the divers to cope with the extreme water pressure at depth and with descending and ascending

---

* Corresponding author.
E-mail address: claus-martin.muth@medizin.uni-ulm.de (C.-M. Muth).

as quickly as possible while holding their breath. No limit freediving is not approved as a competitive discipline because of its inherent danger [5] and, therefore, is more of an exhibition sport for free-diving extremists.

The current records in the various diving disciplines include no limit diving: 171 msw (561 ft), with an unofficial record at a remarkable 200 msw (656 ft); static diving: 8:58 minutes duration; and dynamic apnea diving: 212 m (695 ft). It is doubtful that the absolute limits have yet been reached [5].

Unlike self-contained underwater breathing apparatus (scuba) divers, breath-hold divers usually cannot stay underwater for more than 3 to 5 minutes. Even during this short diving period, however, profound changes in the physiologic functions of the cardiovascular and the respiratory systems take place. This article describes these pathophysiologic effects and outlines the potential hazards associated with apnea diving.

Theoretic limits of diving depth

Until recently, it was believed that the maximum diving depth in apnea diving should be approximately 30 to 50 msw (according to 100–165 ft or 4–6 ata [atmospheres absolute]) [6]. This assumption was based Boyle's law, which states that if the temperature of a fixed mass of gas is kept constant, the relationship between the volume and pressure varies in such a way that the product of the pressure and volume remains constant [7]. Thus, at a constant temperature and mass, the volume of a gas is inversely proportional to the pressure exerted on the gas. For example, when the pressure is doubled, the volume is reduced to one half of the original volume. With regard to the air-filled lungs, and based on the theoretic calculations described previously, the lung volume should decrease continuously during decent. Furthermore, it has been assumed that a reduction in lung volume below residual volume (RV) would result in a lung squeeze and, therefore, potentially be harmful [6,8]. Thus, the ratio of total lung capacity (TLC) to RV for a longer period of time was believed to determine the depth limit (TLC:RV = maximum diving depth, in atmospheres of pressure). If, for instance, average parameters for lung volumes are taken, with a TLC of 6 L and a RV of 1.5 L, the maximum diving depth is 30 msw (100 ft), as 6 L/1.5 L = 4 (ie, 4 ata or 30 msw). Until the 1970s, most diving records were compatible with this concept, and in those athletes who exceeded this depth mark-

edly, exceptionally high vital capacities were found, such as in Bob Croft, a former United States Navy diver, who reached a depth of 73 meters [1,4].

As described previously, today's records are far beyond Bob Croft's record from the late 1960s, and depths of approximately 170 msw now are reached (Fig. 1). The prior, rather simple physiologic considerations are inadequate, and other factors have to be considered.

One of these factors is the redistribution of blood from the periphery to the intrapulmonary vessels, which allows the RV to decrease. Immersion in water already leads to such an increase in intrathoracic blood volume [9,10], and this effect is pronounced further by the depth-dependent compression of the alveoli (described previously) [11].

In air, the pressure surrounding the body equals the pressure within the lungs (Fig. 2). With immersion in water to the neck, the immersed part of the body is under the influence of an elevated pressure (atmospheric pressure plus the hydrostatic pressure of the water, which is directly proportional to the distance from the water surface) (see Fig. 2), whereas the intrapulmonary pressure still is near 1 ata, creating a pressure gradient between the intra- and extrathoracic regions, thereby increasing venous return [9,10]. This immersion into water suffices to explain a redistribution of approximately 700 mL of blood into the thorax. In addition, Ferretti shows radiologic findings in apnea divers under water, including a substantial reduction in lung volume, an elevation of the diaphragm, and an engorgement of the lung blood vessels (see Fig. 2) [4]. Currently,

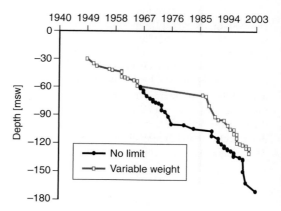

Fig. 1. Evolution of the diving depth in apnea. The figure shows the enormous increase in diving depth from 1949 until today in the specialties of no limit and variable weight (see text). The most profound increase has taken place in the past 10 years.

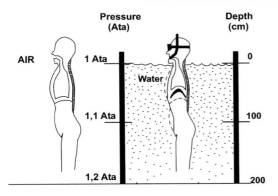

Fig. 2. Immersion effects. Immersion in water to the neck already leads to a reduction in lung volume, an elevation of the diaphragm (*right*) and a redistribution of blood into the thorax. With increasing depth, these effects are more pronounced. (*Modified from* Hong SK. Breath-hold diving. In: Bove AA, Davis JC, editors. Diving medicine. Philadelphia: W.B. Saunders; 1997. p. 66.)

the redistribution of blood during deep apnea dives is assumed to reach approximately 1 to 1.5 L, whereas the maximum for possible blood redistribution into the thorax still is unknown.

According to the previously described calculation of the TLC:RV, this increase in thoracic blood volume provides a physiologic explanation for diving depths below 100 msw. Pipin Ferreiras, a Cuban apnea diver and world-famous record holder, has a documented TLC of 9.6 L and a RV of 2.2 L. Without taking into account the blood redistribution, his predicted maximal diving depth is $9.6/2.2 = 4.4$ (ie, 4.4 ata = 34 msw). Including a redistribution of 1.5 L of blood, the RV can decrease to 0.7 L (2.2 L − 1.5 L), and the "new" depth is approximately 127 msw ($9.6/0.7 = 13.7$, 13.7 ata = 127 msw) (Fig. 3).

There seems to be no upper limit of this redistribution affect except for the resistance of the lung capillaries to mechanical stress. This resistance is described as high and, therefore, is likely to prevent lung disruption and alveolar hemorrhage in most cases [12]. Nevertheless, alveolar hemorrhage and hemoptysis are described in extreme apnea divers during training and competition [13,14]. This is not necessarily related to overdistension of pulmonary vessels but can be explained by an elevation of the pulmonary capillary pressure resulting from the previously described immersion- and submersion-induced increasing blood shift in apnea divers. This may lead to a fluid shift from the capillary lumen into the alveolar interstitium and, subsequently, the alveolar space (see Fig. 3) [13]. Another possible

explanation for this phenomenon refers to the intense involuntary diaphragmatic contractions in breath-hold divers during the so-called "struggle phase" at the end of dives [14]. In the first phase of a dive, apnea divers are completely relaxed and do not feel any urge to breathe. This phase of dives is called the "easy-going phase," with the glottis closed at a stable intrathoracic pressure [1,15]. The end of this phase, called the physiologic "breaking point," depends on physiologic factors, such as $PaCO_2$, which triggers the respiratory center [1,15,16]. Beyond this physiologic breaking point, the glottis remains closed, but involuntary rhythmic contractions of the inspiratory muscles and the diaphragm evolve and progress [15]. During this struggle phase, which is determined primarily by divers' psychologic tolerance to such unpleasant sensations [17], these contractions progressively increase in frequency and intensity, creating a negative intrathoracic pressure as a result of the forced attempts to breathe. Therefore, these maneuvers might contribute to alveolar hemorrhage because of damage to pulmonary capillaries [14]. Finally, hemorrhage need not necessarily originate from the lung but can come from the tracheobronchial tree or even the sinuses. During descent, the trachea collapses almost totally wheras the mucosal vessels become engorged, which in some cases can lead to an overdistension and bleeding [18]. There-

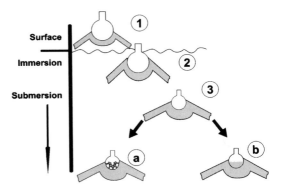

Fig. 3. Blood shift. At surface (1), the alveoli of the lung and the pulmonary blood vessels have their normal diameters. Immersion (2) to the neck creates a negative intrathoracic pressure and, thus, an increased venous return into the pulmonal vessels. Submersion while breath-holding (3) leads to a compression of alveoli (Boyle's law) and a further redistribution of blood into the thoracic vessels, leading to engorgement of these vessels. In greater depth, this mechanism may lead either to a rupture of vessels from overdistension (a) or to an intraalveolar edema (b) from the very high hydrostatic pressure.

fore, especially if symptoms are mild, barotrauma of the sinuses may be the source of the blood [19].

In an effort to increase maximum diving depths further, a technique known as lung packing or buccal pumping has become popular within the apnea diving community [1,4]. This technique enables divers to increase their lung volume above total TLC. After a complete maximum inspiration, athletes take a mouthful of air with the glottis closed. The air in the mouth is compressed using the oral and pharyngeal muscles, then the glottis is opened and the air forced into the lungs (Fig. 4A, B) [20]. This pumping

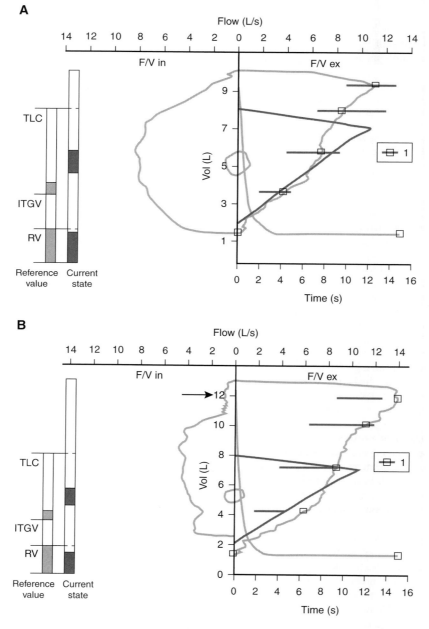

Fig. 4. Buccal pumping maneuver. The bodyplethysmographic findings in an elite apnea diver without (*A*) and with (*B*) buccal pumping maneuver (*arrow*), which enables hyperinflation of the lungs and increased TLC.

movement is repeated several times. Buccal pumping has been developed by spearfishing breath-hold divers in the Mediterranean and was introduced to sport diving by Bob Croft. Informal personal measurements and data from the literature demonstrate that buccal pumping can increase TLC by 30% to 50% (on average, by 1.5 to 3 L) [20,21]. When applied to the calculation (described previously), this technique allows deeper diving. If the TLC in the prior example of Pipin is increased by 2 L from 9.6 to 11.6 L, then, based on the blood shift–corrected RV of 0.7 L, the new maximal diving depth is approximately 156 msw (11.6/0.7 = 16.6; 16.6 ata = 156 msw). Neither for the redistribution of blood into the thorax nor for the hyperinflation of the lungs is the absolute upper limit known, however.

Increasing the volume of air in the lungs above TLC, however, carries a theoretic risk of inducing pulmonary barotrauma. Although there are reports of the cardiovascular effects, there is limited information on the pulmonary effects of buccal pumping [22]. Because of the elastic recoil of the chest wall, the intrathoracic pressure is increased during breath-holding at TLC with relaxed respiratory muscles, which in turn reduces venous return and thus cardiac output. Andersson and colleagues report that these effects are accentuated by the buccal pumping maneuver, possibly resulting in fainting among breath-hold divers [22]. Indeed, a substantial reduction of blood pressure was shown in the early phase of breath-holding, especially when buccal pumping was maximal [22].

Furthermore, it is shown that relaxed airway pressure, reflecting intrathoracic pressure, is increased considerably by buccal pumping [20]. According to the mechanisms of pulmonary barotrauma during ascent in scuba divers, in whom an ascent of only 1 meter with full lungs can cause a rupture of the lungs from overinflation (explained by Boyle's law) [23,24], this buccal pumping–induced increase in intrathoracic pressure is interpreted as a possibly substantial risk of lung rupture in apnea divers. Little data is available on the effects of buccal pumping on transpulmonary pressure. Simpson and coworkers [25] report no increase in transpulmonary pressure after buccal pumping, assessed by direct measurements in an individual subject, and suggest a considerable increase in intrapleural pressure during buccal pumping. This seems analogous to the protective effects afforded by thoracoabdominal binding in fresh, unchilled human cadavers, where it is shown that the intratracheal pressure at which pulmonary rupture occurs is higher in cadavers whose chests and abdomen are bound tightly than in unbound cadavers [23].

Therefore, buccal pumping, in general, does not seem major risk for pulmonary barotrauma per se, although compliance heterogeneities within the lung [26,27] and the high pressures generated in the oropharynx and used to force air through the glottis into the lung may result in lung damage [28]. Nevertheless, although many freedivers in the world are performing this maneuver, to date there are no reports of pulmonary barotrauma associated with buccal pumping. In fact, the intrathoracic hypertension syndrome reported in a single case appeared during ascent and, therefore, more likely was related to a redistribution of the expanding gases together with an air-trapping mechanism [27].

Finally, competitive apnea divers train the elasticity of their chest wall and their diaphragm with special exercises to achieve the best ratio of TLC to RV, as this ratio to a significant extent still defines the ability to dive to greater depth. Therefore, optimal chest wall elasticity and a special ability to reduce the RV further at deep expiration are major factors contributing to the impressive, and progressive, deep diving records.

Changes in the partial pressures of the breathing gases during descent and ascent

The effects of apnea diving on PO_2 and PCO_2 are substantially different from mere breath-holding at the surface, because, in addition to the usual physiologic gas effects (ie, oxygen uptake from the lung into the blood and carbon dioxide elimination from blood to alveoli), the lungs of apnea divers are compressed during descent, as a result of the increasing ambient pressure, and are decompressed during ascent. In the early 1960s, alveolar gas exchange during breath-hold diving was a focus of physiologic research [29–39], but scientific findings were limited until recently. Particularly in the field of extreme apnea diving, relevant physiologic investigations have been undertaken only recently [4,21,40,41].

Typically, the arterial gas partial pressures in well-trained, nonhyperventilating apnea divers immediately before dives do not differ from the normal values in a nondiving population, with a PCO_2 of approximately 35 mm Hg and a PO_2 of 100 mm Hg. Because of the increase in ambient pressure while descending, divers' lung volume is reduced, according to Boyle's law. During dives, the alveolar partial pressures of nitrogen, oxygen, and carbon dioxide increase, according to Dalton's law: the total pressure of a gas mixture is the sum of the partial pressures of each individual gas [7]. Together with Boyle's law, it follows that the partial pressures of the single gases in a gas mixture double if the total pressure is doubled, so that an increased amount of all three gases dissolves in the blood [10]. Therefore, the PO_2 at a depth of 5 and 20 msw theoretically are approximately 130 and 250 mm Hg, respectively (Fig. 5) [21,37], ensuring an adequate delivery of oxygen to the blood so that hypoxia is unlikely at depth. During the descent, the direction of carbon dioxide diffusion theoretically is reversed at a depth of approximately

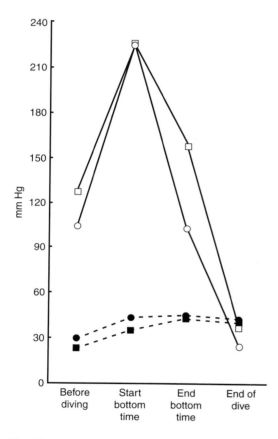

Fig. 5. PaO_2 and $PaCO_2$ values in apnea divers in a simulated dive to 20 msw. The PaO2 (*solid lines*) increases while descending (gas laws of Dalton and Boyle), although theoretically predicted values were not reached. This most likely is the result of immersion and blood-shift induced changes in ventilation-perfusion relations with increased shunting of venous blood. In contrast, the $PaCO_2$ (*dotted lines*) increased by only less than 20 mm Hg even after 4 minutes at 3 ata, most likely because of high carbon dioxide storage capacities in blood and rapid tissues. Furthermore, the Haldane effect attenuates the $PaCO_2$ at surfacing. (*Modified from* Muth CM, Radermacher P, Pittner A, et al. Arterial blood gases during diving in elite apnea divers. Int J Sports Med 2003;24:106.)

8 msw. Because of the compression-induced rise of the $PACO_2$, it was theorized that carbon dioxide would follow its new pressure gradient from alveoli to the blood rather than be eliminated from the blood to the alveoli [10]. Recent study findings and the authors' results suggest that a theoretic estimation solely based on Boyle's law, which predicts linear increase or decrease of alveolar partial pressures for the respiratory gases as a result of compression and decompression, respectively, does not sufficiently explain the time course and movement of arterial blood gases during apnea dives. It seems that the gas partial pressure predictions are erroneous, particularly in the case of carbon dioxide (see Fig. 5). To explain these data satisfactorily, the blood solubilities of the respiratory gases have to be considered. A substantial rise in $PaCO_2$ is prevented by the large amount of this relatively high soluble gas taken up by the blood with increasing ambient pressure, which thereby blunts the compression effect on the blood-gas tension [21]. In addition, the significant immersion-induced blood shift into the thorax contributes further to this effect, as the compression-induced increase of the intrapulmonary blood volume enhances the blood pool available for gas uptake from the alveolar space [42,43]. Finally, during ascent, an increase in $PaCO_2$ is blunted by the Haldane effect: as a result of decompression, the marked fall in PaO_2 is associated with a substantial reduction of the hemoglobin-oxygen saturation, which, in turn, increases blood carbon dioxide solubility [44]. Indeed, during 75 seconds of simulated apnea dives to ambient pressures equivalent to a depth of 20 msw, Linér and colleagues predict PCO_2 values of approximately 50 mm Hg [34], although the theoretic level, as derived from Boyle's law, is beyond 100 mm Hg. Measurements of arterial blood-gas tensions during short-term dives to shallow depths in the professional Korean apnea divers and in aquatic mammals (freediving Wedell seals) correspond with these observations [37,45,46]. $PaCO_2$ values did not increase to the levels predicted from the depth-induced increase in alveolar pressure in these studies. The authors' findings in professional apnea divers during simulated wet dives to the same depth with a duration of 4 to 5 minutes confirms these findings, revealing a $PaCO_2$ of only 40 to 45 mm Hg (see Fig. 5) [21]. In the latter study, the athletes hyperventilated to a certain extent and started dives from $PaCO_2$ levels of approximately 30 mm Hg [21].

When divers start to ascend at the end of the bottom phase, the lung volume increases as a result of decompression. Simultaneously, PAO_2 and $PACO_2$ decrease continuously, and the normal flow direction for carbon dioxide is restored [31]. PAO_2 decreases until it equals the mixed venous PO_2 and, consequently, oxygen diffusion from the alveoli to the blood ceases. The direction of oxygen transfer may be reversed so that oxygen moves from the pulmonary capillary into the alveolar gas. Critical hypoxia may occur, especially after extended diving duration at significant depth [47]. Protocols of apnea diving accidents show that loss of motor control and consciousness in most cases appears immediately before or shortly after surfacing.

Finally, according to Ferretti, there is some evidence that elite apnea divers are able to tolerate a lower PaO_2 and oxygen saturation than controls [4] and, furthermore, are more tolerant to carbon dioxide, as documented by the reduced carbon dioxide reactivity in Korean diving women, Japanese Ama, underwater hockey players, and elite apnea divers [48–53]. The question, however, remains whether or not this finding is an example of adaptation or if people who have low sensitivity to carbon dioxide self-select for breath-hold diving activities.

Excessive hyperventilation

It is well known by active divers that hyperventilation immediately before apnea dives prolongs the breath-hold duration substantially. Because the $PACO_2$ and consequently the $PaCO_2$ are inversely proportional to the alveolar ventilation, increasing the minute ventilation increases the carbon dioxide elimination rate. Therefore, after hyperventilation, the $PaCO_2$ is decreased, thus it takes a longer time for the $PaCO_2$ to reach the breaking point of approximately 55 to 60 mm Hg that triggers the brainstem respiratory center [16]. Alternatively, any extension of the apnea time decreases the PaO_2 further. At surface, the urge to breathe is triggered not only by the $PaCO_2$ but also by a reduced PO_2 to approximately 50 to 60 mm Hg. Therefore, pure oxygen also prolongs the apnea time substantially. Klocke and Rahn report that after normobaric oxygen breathing, even untrained subjects reached breath-hold times of up to 8.5 minutes, and after oxygen breathing, together with hyperventilating, up to 14 minutes [54]. Deep diving in apnea is somewhat similar to breath-holding with oxygen prebreathing. As discussed previously, PAO_2 and PaO_2 increase as a result of compression of the lung and reach hyperoxic values, although the blood oxygen content increases only marginally because of the sigmoid shape of the hemoglobin-oxygen dissociation curve. Under this condition, an increased $PaCO_2$ is the only remaining

trigger mechanism to stimulate breathing. Hyperventilation before diving, therefore, enables divers to stay longer under water until such a $PaCO_2$ level is reached. The prolonged oxygen uptake during apnea, however, results in a decreased PaO_2. While ascending, the rapid decompression of the lungs causes a marked fall of PAO_2 and PaO_2, often with significant hypoxia. Arterial blood samples taken from apnea divers just before resuming respiration after apnea dives of 4 to 5 minutes show PO_2 values of 25 to 30 mm Hg [21]. Hyperventilating before apnea dives is dangerous particularly if divers are engaged in strenuous activity, because oxygen consumption is increased. In this case, even when still at depth, the PaO_2 may become critically low, and the ascent-related decompression (and hypoxia) makes a loss of consciousness likely [47]. This phenomenon, known as shallow-water blackout, also known in the apnea diving community as samba (a hypoxia-induced type of seizure) frequently is implicated in apnea diving accidents. The majority of fatal accidents in apnea diving are recorded in competition or record attempts. Therefore, excellent and close supervision of the athletes in those situations is crucial. Unfortunately, a well-defined threshold PO_2 that is considered safe does not exist.

Nitrogen narcosis and decompression sickness

As with oxygen, the nitrogen partial pressure (PN_2) of the breathing gas is increased by compression. Therefore, during descent, not only PaO_2 but also PN_2 rises. Consequently, according to Henry's law [7], which states that at a given temperature, the amount of gas dissolved in a solute is directly proportional to the pressure of the gas above the solution, tissue nitrogen uptake occurs [10,55,56]. Facing depths far below 50 msw, elite apnea divers become susceptible to nitrogen narcosis ("rapture of the depth"), although the time for PN_2 equilibration in blood and brain is short. Up until now, few data exist on this issue, but the anecdotal behavioral and sensory experiences described by elite apnea divers can be interpreted as symptoms of a nitrogen narcosis. In contrast, the possibility of decompression sickness in apnea divers after repeated dives is well documented. A single apnea dive does not lead to a significant nitrogen uptake into the tissues, so even after a deep dive, symptoms of decompression sickness are unlikely to occur. According to the Haldane principles of inert gas kinetics during compression and decompression, the nitrogen elimination always is slower than the uptake (Fig. 6) [57]. Therefore,

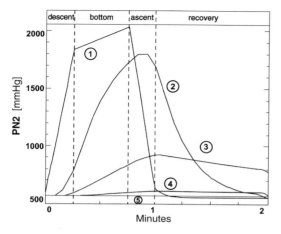

Fig. 6. Theoretic PN_2 in different tissues during and after a simulated apnea dive to a depth of 20 msw over 1 minute. The tissues are marked with numbers: lung (1); kidney (2); brain, heart, and viscera (3); muscle (4); and fat (5). Even after the dive, increased tissue PN_2 is present indiciating that nitrogen accumulates after repetitive dives. The increase in Pn_2 in the lung during the bottom time is the result of oxygen consumption and the concentration of nitrogen of resulting from the respiratory quotient of 0.8. (*Modified from* Olzowski AJ, Rahn H. Gas stores during repetitive breath-hold diving. In: Shiraki K, Yousef MK, editors. Man in stressful environment—diving, hyper- and hypobaric environment. Springfield (IL): Thomas; 1987. p. 52.)

with repetitive dives, especially with short surface intervals and diving depths beyond 15 to 20 msw (50–66 ft), nitrogen accumulates progressively in the tissues (Fig. 7) [10,55,58,59]. The level of nitrogen tissue loading not only depends on the diving depth but also is determined by the ratio of dive duration to recovery period at the surface. Using this ratio, an effective diving depth can be calculated, which reflects the tissue inert gas loading that occurs in scuba divers breathing compressed air at this depth [55]. Decompression sickness, therefore, is possible in apnea divers when repetitive dives are performed [56,58,60–63]. Although in apnea diving training and competition such incidents are reported only anecdotally, one case is reported of neurologic decompression sickness in an apnea diver after repeated apnea dives to a depth of approximately 20 msw (66 ft); complete recovery was seen after hyperbaric treatment [61]. This dramatic response to a recompression treatment was considered indirect evidence that bubble formation was the cause of this incident. Furthermore, neurologic symptoms of decompression sickness among Polynesian apnea pearl divers are known as taravana, which means "to fall crazy" [63,64]. This expression refers to a symptom complex, which occurs after repeated apnea dives to depths from 20 to 30 msw (66 to 100 ft), and includes vertigo, nausea, and mental anguish. Some divers become paralyzed, partially or completely, and fatalities are described [63,64]. Nevertheless, although there is some evidence that, dependent on dive depth, venous nitrogen partial pressures may reach values

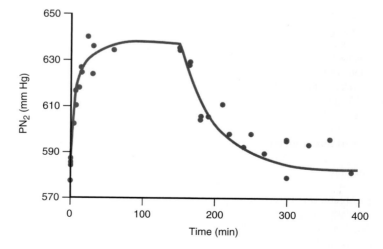

Fig. 7. Time course of venous N_2 during and after work shift in Korean Amas. Data are pooled measurements from nine volunteer subjects (*Modified from* Radermacher P, Falke KJ, Park YS, et al. Nitrogen tensions in brachial vein blood of Korean Ama divers. J Appl Physiol 1992;73:2593.)

that may lead to bubble formation in blood during decompression, the only available study of apnea divers immediately after ascent fails to detect circulating bubbles using the Doppler ultrasound method. Boussuges and coworkers used continuous Doppler sonography and transthoracic 2-D echocardiography to detect circulating bubbles after breath-hold diving in 10 underwater fishing divers who performed repeated breath-hold dives for periods ranging from 2 to 6 hours, with a mean maximum depth of 35 msw [65]. In this study, no circulating bubbles were detected in the right heart cavities with the 2-D echocardiography or in the pulmonary artery with continuous Doppler sonography. The investigators acknowledged, however, that the study had some limits, as only a few subjects were studied and the earliest detection was 3 minutes after immersion. Further studies on bubble formation in apnea divers are required.

In contrast to diving humans, diving mammals do not experience decompression sickness, although the diving depths are greater. Weddell seals reach approximately 500 msw (1650 ft) and stay up to 30 minutes under water; sperm whales can dive to 3000 msw (9900 ft) or more, with maximum dive times of approximately 120 minutes [66]. Several physiologic adaptations contribute to this phenomenon. First, as whales and seals do not have a sternum, the rib cage prevents the lung from squeezing. Furthermore, the lungs of these animals can collapse completely, so that the PN_2 ceases to increase at a certain depth (approximately 150 msw in Weddell seals) and, consequently, blood and tissue nitrogen uptake ceases [66–68]. Vasoconstriction in all organ systems (except for the brain and the adrenals) further limits the nitrogen uptake in peripheral tissues [46,69,70]. Finally, the contraction of the spleen, associated with a marked release of red blood cells into the systemic circulation, results in increased blood nitrogen solubility, thereby reducing blood PN_2 and markedly limiting bubble formation [45,46,70].

Cardiovascular effects of apnea diving

More than a century ago, the French physiologist Paul Bert described a fall in heart rate in diving ducks. This diving-related bradycardia, present to a variable degree in all homoeothermic animals [71–73], is called the diving reflex and usually is associated with peripheral vasoconstriction.

Many mechanisms may trigger this reflex [74,75], but breath-holding at elevated lung volume and stimulation of facial trunks of the trigeminal nerve by

water are considered the most important [15,74,76]. In this context, the dependence of the diving bradycardia on the water temperature is of special interest. Whether or not real breath-hold dives or simple face immersions in water are performed, the lower the water temperature, the more pronounced the bradycardia [74,77]. This aspect is underscored by the observation that the diving reflex is less marked in swimmers with immersion only to the neck and in divers wearing a face mask covering most parts of the facial skin [78]. Other mechanisms, such as the compression-induced increase of PaO_2 and immersion-induced redistribution of blood into the thoracic vessels that leads to enhanced cardiac preload, also contribute to the diving reflex [79].

Normally, the initial fall in heart rate during a breath-hold dive is to approximately 60% to 70% of the predive level. Heart rates as low as 10 to 15 beats per minute, however, are reported in elite apnea divers diving to depths of 65 msw (214.5 ft) [41,80,81].

In contrast to diving animals, in humans, the diving reflex usually is not associated with a fall in cardiac output [69], which in turn may cause arterial hypertension as a result of the intense diving-induced vasoconstriction [15,74,79,82]. The hormonal and metabolic regulatory adaptations related to the cardiovascular responses during apnea diving are studied in freediving Wedell seals [83]. Epinephrine and norepinephrine levels increase markedly during dives and fall to baseline levels during recovery. In contrast, cyclic guanine monophosphate concentrations—which can be considered a marker of nitric oxide release—increased during recovery. These changes in catecholamine concentrations are considered part of the diving-induced peripheral vasoconstriction leading to anaerobic metabolism and tissue lactate accumulation [83]. In the early recovery phase, plasma lactate concentrations rise when peripheral perfusion resumes and are associated with a vasodilatation-induced lactate washout into the systemic circulation [83]. The catecholamine release is considered responsible for the splenic contraction observed in these animals [84]. To assess similar effects in human divers, plasma lactate levels are measured in apnea divers. Although a comparable increase in blood lactate concentrations are found in Australian pearl divers [85], researchers could not confirm this result in short repetitive dives of 1 to 2 minutes of duration to a depth of 1.4 meters (4.6 ft) [36]. The authors' investigations in breath-hold dives to 20 meters (66 ft) of durations of 4 and 5 minutes also do not show any increase in lactate concentrations [86]. Lactate values in this study remained within the normal range during the whole investigation period. In particular, no increase was seen at the end of dives or during recovery, which makes a significant degree of anaerobic metabolism unlikely. This was confirmed further by measurement of the arterial lactate-to-pyruvate ratios, a parameter of the cytosolic redox potential, which also remained unchanged. In the subjects in this study, blood catecholamine levels were high from the beginning (ie, in the predive phase) and remained unchanged in all subsequent measurements. Thus, an increase and decline similar to that in seals was not detectable. The emotional state of the subjects of this study [86], a certain excitement resulting from the special situation and high personal motivation, may have assumed importance in this context.

As discussed previously, the diving reflex is strongly related to water temperature [77,87] and may lead to cardiac dysrhythmias with increasing incidence of supraventricular extrasystoles, particularly at the end of the dives (Fig. 8) [41,88,89]. This phenomenon is believed caused by the cardiac dilatation resulting from the dive-related increase in intrathoracic blood volume [4,41,90]. Furthermore, the incidence of such arrhythmias markedly increases at low water temperatures [74]. In summary, the diving response (ie, bradycardia and peripheral vasoconstriction in response to apneic submersion) is acknowledged as an oxygen-conserving reflex in diving species that maintains perfusion to the brain, reduces cardiac work and blood flow to viscera and muscle and, thus, limits overall oxygen consumption [91,92].

Humans clearly are not able to sustain apnea dives even remotely as long as diving mammals. This may be the result of a less developed diving response in humans. The more modest bradycardia and less

effective reduction of cardiac output in humans in the face of peripheral vasoconstriction results in an increase in blood pressure during apnea, rather than an unchanged blood pressure, as observed in diving animals [10]. These effects likely result in a greater metabolic rate in humans than in diving mammals during dives and reduce the possible duration of apnea dives in humans. There is at present no clear evidence to indicate that there is a significant oxygen-conserving mechanism operating in humans during apnea diving. Nevertheless, some recent studies of humans support the possible existence of such a functional oxygen-conserving effect of the diving response. Andersson and colleagues demonstrate a significant benefit of apnea-induced cardiovascular responses with a much slower decline of SaO_2 [93]. In their study, after 30 seconds of apnea during medium-intensity dynamic leg exercise, subjects who had the most marked cardiovascular responses (ie, the most pronounced responses to the diving reflex) had a 4- to 5-times slower decline in SaO_2 than subjects who had the least marked cardiovascular response.

As additional possible support for an adaptive energy-conservation effect of diving in humans, there is evidence that the diving response can be trained. Several investigators show that there is a negative correlation between the number of dives and the heart rate during dives, or a more pronounced decrease in heart rate and vasoconstriction in well-trained divers compared with those who have lesser training [49,89, 94,95]. These observations also may contribute to the presence of an oxygen-conserving effect.

In Weddell seals, spleen contraction with subsequent injection of red blood cells into the peripheral circulation is well documented and results in increases of hemoglobin concentration from approximately 17.5 g/dl to approximately 22 g/dl (equiva-

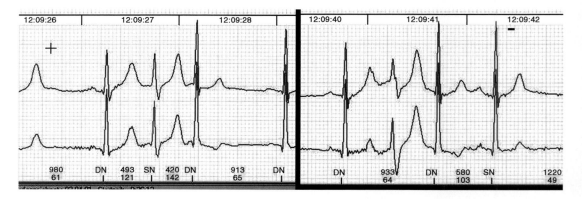

Fig. 8. ECG recordings in an elite apnea diver in a simulated dive to 20 msw and with 5-minute duration. At the end of the dive, an increasing incidence of supraventricular extrasystoles is seen in the diver.

lent to an increase in hematocrit from 44% to 55%) when measured directly after surfacing [84]. Thus, this spleen contraction seems an integral part of the diving response in these animals. The question has been raised as to whether or not spleen contraction exists and plays any significant role in adaptation to diving in humans. Spleen contraction and increased hematocrit during breath-hold diving are shown in Japanese Ama divers [96]. In healthy volunteers and splenectomized subjects, the interaction between short-term adaptation to apnea with face immersion and erythrocyte release from the spleen was investigated [97]. In the intact subjects, hematocrit and hemoglobin concentrations increased by 6.4% and 3.3%, respectively, over the serial apneas and returned to baseline 10 minutes after the series. Furthermore, the interval until reaching the physiologic breaking point of apnea was prolonged by 30.5% after these adaptive serial dives. In contrast, no change was observed in a splenectomized study subject group. Furthermore, Bakovic and coworkers recently showed that the reduced spleen size during breath-hold apnea was the result of an active contraction rather than a passive collapse secondary to reduced arterial blood flow [98]. Spleen contraction, hence, also occurs in humans as a part of the diving response [99] and may help prolong apnea times.

Summary

Apnea diving has been a subject of active interest to physiologists for more than 50 years and remains an area of physiologic inquiry because of the unique and at times extreme aspects of the diving environment and the associated physiology. Today, apnea divers have exceeded almost all previously predicted limits. Physiologists and clinicians have been successful in establishing explanations for the apparent conflict between the theoretic limits of diving physiology and the remarkable performance of human divers beyond those theoretic limits. Even in the short time of a human apnea dive, profound cardiovascular, respiratory, and gas exchange effects are observed in divers. The marked alterations of alveolar and arterial blood gas tensions are the result of the interaction of metabolism and the rapid sequence of compression and decompression, thereby helping to explain most of the apnea-related accidents. Decompression sickness is possible with repetitive apnea dives to greater depths. Apnea divers can reach depths beyond the theoretic physiologic limits because of the immersion-related blood shift into the thorax together with the increased TLC resulting from deliberate pulmonary overinflation using the lung-packing maneuver, which, however, increases the risk of pulmonary barotrauma. Similar to diving mammals and birds, human apnea divers exhibit a fall in heart rate, particularly and more pronounced at low water temperature. This phenomenon is called the diving reflex, can be trained to a degree, and serves as an oxygen-conserving effect, but increases the incidence of ventricular arrhythmia.

Despite advances in the understanding of diving physiology and clinical problems, important questions remain unanswered. Many of the subjects discussed in this article would benefit from the illumination of further investigation. In addition, virtually nothing is known about the long-term effects of extreme apnea diving, especially regarding adverse health effects. Finally, although the absolute limits of apnea diving are not yet known, it is increasingly clear that the quest by extreme apnea divers to find those limits could come at a potentially high physiologic and medical price if those limits are exceeded.

References

[1] Ferrigno M, Lundgren CEG. Human breath-hold diving. In: Lundgren CEG, Miller JN, editors. The lung at depth. Lung biology in health and disease, volume 132. New York: Marcel Dekker; 1999. p. 529–85.

[2] Hong SK, Rahn H. The diving women of Korea and Japan. Sci Am 1967;216:34–43.

[3] Hong SK, Henderson J, Olszowka A, et al. Daily diving patterns of Korean and Japanese breath-hold divers (Ama). Undersea Biomed Res 1991;18:433–43.

[4] Ferretti G. Extreme human breath-hold diving. Eur J Appl Physiol 2001;84:254–71.

[5] AIDA (Association Internationale pour le Développement de l'Apnée). Available at: http://www.aida-international.org/. Accessed 2003.

[6] Craig AB. Depth limits of breath hold diving (an example of Fennology). Respir Physiol 1968;5:14–22.

[7] Flook V. Physics and physiology in the hyperbaric environment. Clin Phys Physiol Meas 1987;8:197–230.

[8] Carey CR, Schaefer KE, Alvis H. Effect of skin diving on human lung volumes. J Appl Physiol 1956;8:519–23.

[9] Arborelius M, Ballidin UI, Lilja B, et al. Hemodynamic changes in man during immersion with the head above water. Aerosp Med 1972;43:592–8.

[10] Hong SK. Breath-hold diving. In: Bove AA, Davis JC, editors. Diving medicine. Philadelphia: W.B. Saunders; 1997. p. 65–74.

[11] Schaefer KE, Allison RD, Dougherty JH, et al. Pulmonary and circulatory adjustments determining

the limits of depths in breath hold diving. Science 1968;162:1020–3.

[12] West JB, Mathieu-Costello O. Strength of the pulmonary blood-gas barrier. Respir Physiol 1992;88: 141–8.

[13] Boussuges A, Pinet C, Thomas P, et al. Haemoptysis after breath-hold diving. Eur Respir J 1999;13: 697–9.

[14] Kiyan E, Aktas S, Toklu AS. Hemoptysis provoked by voluntary diaphragmatic contractions in breath-hold divers. Chest 2001;120:2098–100.

[15] Andersson J, Schagatay E. Effects of lung volume and involuntary breathing movements on the human diving response. Eur J Appl Physiol 1998;77:19–24.

[16] Lin YC, Lally DA, Moore TO, et al. Physiological and conventional breath-hold breaking points. J Appl Physiol 1974;37:291–6.

[17] Rigg JR, Rebuck AS, Campbell EJ. A study of factors influencing relief of discomfort in breath-holding in normal subjects. Clin Sci Mol Med 1974;47:193–9.

[18] Lindholm P, Nyrén S. MRI studies of the glossopharyngeal breathing used by breath-hold divers. In: Jansen EC, Mortensen CR, Hyldegaard O, editors. Abstracts and Proceedings of the 29th Annual Scientific Meeting of the European Underwater and Baromedical Society. Copenhagen (Denmark): European Underwater and Baromedical Society; 2003. p. 40.

[19] Fagan P, McKenzie B, Edmonds C. Sinus barotrauma in divers. Ann Otol Rhinol Laryngol 1976;85(1 Pt 1): 61–4.

[20] Örnhagen H, Schagatay E, Andersson J, et al. Mechanisms of "buccal pumping" ("lung packing") and its pulmonary effects. In: Gennser M, editor. Manuscripts for XXIVth Annual Scientific Meeting of the European Underwater and Baromedical Society. Stockholm (Sweden): European Underwater and Baromedical Society; 1998. p. 80–3.

[21] Muth CM, Radermacher P, Pittner A, et al. Arterial blood gases during diving in elite apnea divers. Int J Sports Med 2003;24:104–7.

[22] Andersson J, Schagatay E, Gustafsson P, et al. Cardiovascular effects of "buccal pumping" in breath-hold divers. In: Gennser M, editor. Manuscripts for XXIVth Annual Scientific Meeting of the European Underwater and Baromedical Society. Stockholm (Sweden): European Underwater and Baromedical Society; 1998. p. 103–6.

[23] Malhotra MS, Wright HC. The effects of a raised intrapulmonary pressure on the lungs of fresh unchilled cadavers. J Pathol Bacteriol 1961;82:198–202.

[24] Tetzlaff K, Reuter M, Leplow B, et al. Risk factors for pulmonary barotrauma in divers. Chest 1997;112: 654–9.

[25] Simpson G, Ferns J, Murat S. Pulmonary effects of "lung packing" by buccal pumping in an elite breath-hold diver. SPUMS J 2003;33:122–6.

[26] Dahlbäck GO, Lundgren CEG. Pulmonary air-trapping induced by water immersion. Aerosp Med 1972;43: 768–74.

[27] Sala-Sanjaume J, Desola Ala J, Geronimo Blasco C. The intrathoracic hypertension syndrome in a breath-hold diver. Med Clin (Barc) 1998;111:798.

[28] Bayne CG, Wurzbacher T. Can pulmonary barotrauma cause cerebral air embolism in a non-diver? Chest 1982;81:648–50.

[29] Craig AB, Harley AD. Alveolar gas exchanges during breath-hold dives. J Appl Physiol 1968;24:182–9.

[30] Craig AB, Medd WL. Oxygen consumption and carbon dioxide production during breath-hold diving. J Appl Physiol 1968;124:190–202.

[31] Hong SK, Rahn H, Kang DH, et al. Diving pattern, lung volumes, and alveolar gas of the Korean diving women (Ama). J Appl Physiol 1963;18:457–65.

[32] Landsberg PG. Alveolar and peripheral venous gas changes during breath-hold diving. S Afr Med J 1982;62:902–4.

[33] Lanphier EH, Rahn H. Alveolar gas exchange during breath-hold diving. J Appl Physiol 1963;18:471–7.

[34] Linér MH, Ferrigno M, Lundgren CEG. Alveolar gas exchange during simulated breath-hold diving to 20 m. Undersea Hyperb Med 1993;20:27–38.

[35] Linér MH. Cardiovascular and pulmonary responses to breath-hold diving in humans. Acta Physiol Scand Suppl 1994;620:1–32.

[36] Olsen CR, Fanestil DD, Scholander PF. Some effects of apneic underwater diving on blood gases, lactate, and pressure in man. J Appl Physiol 1962;17:938–42.

[37] Qvist J, Hurford WE, Park YS, et al. Arterial blood gas tensions during breathhold diving in the Korean ama. J Appl Physiol 1993;75:285–93.

[38] Schaefer KE, Carey CR. Alveolar pathways during 90-foot breath-hold dives. Science 1962;137:1051–2.

[39] Tibes U, Stegemann J. Behaviour of the end tidal respiratory gas pressure, O_2 uptake and CO_2 output following simple apnea in water, on land and apneic diving. Pflugers Arch 1969;311:300–11.

[40] Ferretti G, Costa M, Ferrigno M, et al. Alveolar gas composition and exchange during deep breath-hold diving and dry breath-holds in elite divers. J Appl Physiol 1991;70:794–802.

[41] Ferrigno M, Grassi B, Feretti G, et al. Electrocardiogram during deep breath-hold dives by elite divers. Undersea Biomed Res 1991;18:81–91.

[42] Chang LP, Lundgren CEG. Maximal breath-holding time and immediate tissue CO_2 storage capacity during head-out immersion in humans. Eur J Appl Physiol 1996;73:210–8.

[43] Linér MH, Linnarsson D. Tissue oxygen and carbon dioxide stores and breath-hold diving in humans. J Appl Physiol 1994;77:542–7.

[44] Christiansen J, Douglas CG, Haldane JS. The absorption and dissociation of carbon dioxide by human blood. J Physiol Lond 1914;48:244–77.

[45] Qvist J, Hill RD, Schneider RC, et al. Hemoglobin concentrations and blood gas tensions of free-diving Weddell seals. J Appl Physiol 1986;61:1560–9.

[46] Zapol WM, Hill RD, Qvist J, et al. Arterial gas tensions and hemoglobin concentrations of the freely

diving Weddell seal. Undersea Biomed Res 1989;16: 363–73.

[47] Craig AB. Underwater swimming and loss of consciousness. JAMA 1961;176:255–8.

[48] Tatai K. Comparisons of ventilatory capacities among fishing divers, nurses, and telephone operators in Japanese females. Jpn J Physiol 1957;7:37–41.

[49] Davis FM, Graves MP, Guy HJ, et al. Carbon dioxide response and breath-hold times in underwater hockey players. Undersea Biomed Res 1987;14:527–34.

[50] Masuda Y, Yoshida A, Hayashi F, et al. Attenuated ventilatory responses to hypercapnia and hypoxia in assisted breath-hold drivers (Funado). Jpn J Physiol 1982;32:327–36.

[51] Masuda Y, Yoshida A, Hayashi F, et al. The ventilatory responses to hypoxia and hypercapnia in the Ama. Jpn J Physiol 1981;31:187–97.

[52] Grassi B, Ferretti G, Costa M, et al. Ventilatory responses to hypercapnia and hypoxia in elite breath-hold divers. Respir Physiol 1994;97:323–32.

[53] Delapille P, Verin E, Tourny-Chollet C, et al. Ventilatory responses to hypercapnia in divers and non-divers: effects of posture and immersion. Eur J Appl Physiol 2001;86:97–103.

[54] Klocke FJ, Rahn H. Breath holding after breathing of oxygen. J Appl Physiol 1959;14:689–93.

[55] Lanphier EH. Application of decompression tables to repeated breath-hold dives. In: Rahn H, Yokoyama T, editors. Physiology of breath-hold diving and the Ama of Japan. Washington (DC): National Academy of Sciences; 1965. p. 225–34.

[56] Paulev PE. Nitrogen tissue tensions following repeated breath-hold dives. J Appl Physiol 1967;22:714–8.

[57] Hempleman HV. History of decompression procedures. In: Bennett P, Elliott D, editors. The physiology and medicine of diving. London: W.B. Saunders; 1993. p. 342–75.

[58] Radermacher P, Falke KJ, Park YS, et al. Nitrogen tensions in brachial vein blood of Korean Ama divers. J Appl Physiol 1992;73:2592–5.

[59] Olzowski AJ, Rahn H. Gas stores during repetitive breath-hold diving. In: Shiraki K, Yousef MK, editors. Man in stressful environment—diving, hyper- and hypobaric environment. Springfield (IL): Thomas; 1987. p. 41–56.

[60] Fanton Y, Grandjean B, Sobrepère G. Accident de décompression en apnée [Decompression accident under apnea]. Presse Med 1994;23:1094 [in French].

[61] Paulev P. Decompression sickness following repeated breath-hold dives. J Appl Physiol 1965;20:1028–31.

[62] Spencer MP, Okino H. Venous gas emboli following repeated breath-hold dives [abstract]. Fed Proc 1972; 31:355.

[63] Wong R. Breath-hold diving can cause decompression illness. SPUMS J 2000;30:2–6.

[64] Cross ER. Taravana diving syndrome in the Tuamoto diver. In: Rahn H, Yokoyama T, editors. Physiology of breath-hold diving and the ama of Japan. Washington (DC): National Academy of Sciences; 1965. p. 205–17.

[65] Boussuges A, Abdellaoui S, Gardette B, et al. Circulating bubbles and breath-hold underwater fishing divers: a two-dimensional echocardiography and continuous wave Doppler study. Undersea Hyperb Med 1997;24:309–14.

[66] Kooyman GL, Ponganis PJ. The challenges of diving to depth. Am Scientist 1997;85:530–9.

[67] Chouteau J, Corriol JH. Physiological aspects of deep sea diving. Endeavour 1971;30:70–6.

[68] Falke KJ, Hill RD, Qvist J, et al. Seal lungs collapse during free diving: evidence from arterial nitrogen tensions. Science 1985;229:556–8.

[69] Zapol WM, Liggins GC, Schneider RC, et al. Regional blood flow during simulated diving in the conscious Weddell seal. J Appl Physiol 1979;47: 968–73.

[70] Zapol WM. Diving adaptations of the Weddell Seal. Sci Am 1987;285:100–5.

[71] Butler PJ, Jones DR. Physiology of diving of birds and mammals. Physiol Rev 1997;77:837–99.

[72] Lin YC. Breath-hold diving in terrestrial mammals. Exerc Sport Sci Rev 1982:270–307.

[73] Strauss MB. Physiological aspects of mammalian breath-hold diving: a review. Aerosp Med 1970;41: 1362–81.

[74] Gooden BA. Mechanism of the human diving response. Integr Physiol Behav Sci 1994;29:6–16.

[75] Manley L. Apnoeic heart rate response in humans. A review. Sports Med 1990;9:286–310.

[76] Lindholm P, Sundbald P, Linnarsson D. Oxygen-conserving effects of apnea in exercising men. J Appl Physiol 1999;87:2122–7.

[77] Folinsbee L. Cardiovascular response to apneic immersion in cool and warm water. J Appl Physiol 1974;36:226–32.

[78] Schagatay E, Andersson J, Holm B. The triggering of the human diving response. In: Gennser M, editor. Manuscripts for XXIVth Annual Scientific Meeting of the European Underwater and Baromedical Society. Stockholm (Sweden): European Underwater and Baromedical Society; 1998. p. 80–3.

[79] Ferrigno M, Hickey DD, Linér M, et al. Simulated breath-hold diving to 20 meters: cardiac performance in humans. J Appl Physiol 1987;62:2160–7.

[80] Arnold RW. Extremes in human breath hold, facial immersion bradycardia. Undersea Biomed Res 1985; 12:183–90.

[81] Strømme SB, Ingier F. Comparison of diving bradycardia and maximal aerobic power. Aviat Space Environ Med 1978;49:1267–70.

[82] Andersson J, Schagatay E, Gislén A, et al. Cardiovascular responses to cold-water immersions of the forearm and face, and their relationship to apnoea. Eur J Appl Physiol 2000;83:566–72.

[83] Hochachka PW, Liggins GC, Guyton GP, et al. Hormonal regulatory adjustments during voluntary diving in Weddell seals. Comp Biochem Physiol [B] 1995; 112:361–75.

[84] Hurford WE, Hochachka PW, Schneider RC, et al.

Splenic contraction, catecholamine release, and blood volume redistribution during diving in the Weddell seal. J Appl Physiol 1996;8:298–306.

[85] Scholander PF, Hammel HT, LeMessurier H, et al. Circulatory adjustment in pearl diver. J Appl Physiol 1962;17:184–90.

[86] Ehrmann U, Pittner A, Paulat K, et al. Herzfrequenz und metabolische Parameter beim Apnoetauchen [Heart rate and metabolic effects during apnea diving]. Dtsch Z Sportmed 2004;55:295–8 [in German].

[87] Gooden BA. Why some people do not drown. Hypothermia versus the diving response. Med J Aust 1992; 157:629–32.

[88] Olsen CR, Fanestil DD, Scholander PF. Some effects of breath holding and apneic underwater diving on cardiac rhythm in man. J Appl Physiol 1962;17:461–6.

[89] Bonneau A, Friemel F. Arrythmia and vago-sympathetic equilibrium in athletic divers. [Troubles du rhythme et équilibre vago-symapthique chez le plongeur sportif]. Arch Mal Cœur Vaiss 1989;82:99–105 [in French].

[90] Ferrigno M, Ferretti G, Ellis A, et al. Cardiovascular changes during deep breath-hold dives in a pressure chamber. J Appl Physiol 1997;83:1282–90.

[91] Sterba JA, Lundgren CEG. Diving bradycardia and breath-holding time in man. Undersea Biomed Res 1985;12:139–50.

[92] Sterba JA, Lundgren CEG. Breath-hold duration in man and the diving response induced by face immersion. Undersea Biomed Res 1988;15:361–75.

[93] Andersson JP, Liner MH, Runow E, et al. Diving response and arterial oxygen saturation during apnea and exercise in breath-hold divers. J Appl Physiol 2002;93:882–6.

[94] Schagatay E, Andersson J. Diving response and apneic time in humans. Undersea Hyperb Med 1998;25: 13–9.

[95] Schagatay E, van Kampen M, Emanuelsson S, et al. Effects of physical and apnea training on apneic time and the diving response in humans. Eur J Appl Physiol 2000;82:161–9.

[96] Hurford WE, Hong SK, Park YS, et al. Splenic contraction during breath-hold diving in the Korean ama. J Appl Physiol 1990;69:932–6.

[97] Schagatay E, Andersson JPA, Hallén M, et al. Selected contribution: role of spleen emptying in prolonging apneas in humans. J Appl Physiol 2001;90:1623–9.

[98] Bakovic D, Valic Z, Eterovic D, et al. Spleen volume and blood flow response to repeated breath-hold apneas. J Appl Physiol 2003;95:1460–6.

[99] Espersen K, Frandsen H, Lorentzen T, et al. The human spleen as an erythrocyte reservoir in diving-related interventions. J Appl Physiol 2002;92:2071–9.

ELSEVIER
SAUNDERS

Clin Chest Med 26 (2005) 395 – 404

CLINICS
IN CHEST
MEDICINE

Epidemiology, Risk Factors, and Genetics of High-Altitude–Related Pulmonary Disease

James P. Maloney, MD[a,*], Ulrich Broeckel, MD[b]

[a]*Division of Pulmonary and Critical Medicine, University of Colorado Health Sciences Center, 4220 East 9th Avenue, C-272, Denver, CO 80262, USA*
[b]*Division of Cardiovascular Medicine, Human and Molecular Genetics Center, Medical College of Wisconsin, Milwaukee, WI, USA*

Human illness at high altitudes has been an area of fascination for centuries. Marco Polo recognized the problems of "the headache mountains" in 1272 when crossing the Pamir mountains of Asia with his party, giving an early description of acute mountain sickness (AMS) [1]. AMS, high-altitude–related pulmonary edema (HAPE), and attributable deaths were major problems for Indian and Pakistani troops engaged in their 1965 war over Kashmir, when troops and artillery crews lived for prolonged periods at 5800 m [2]. In this conflict it was recognized that some individuals were more susceptible to illness at high altitude, whereas others were resistant. Although military campaigns and mountaineering at extreme altitudes strikingly demonstrate the limitations humans face in such environments, most high-altitude–related pulmonary illness occurs in subjects engaged in recreation at moderate alpine altitudes (2200–4400 m).

The spectrum of high-altitude pulmonary illness is comprised of AMS, HAPE, pulmonary hypertension resulting from chronic hypoxia, and chronic mountain sickness (CMS) [3]. High-altitude cerebral edema (HACE) is considered the end stage of severe AMS [4]. This review discusses predominantly AMS and HAPE as high-altitude–related pulmonary diseases, with some discussion of high-altitude pulmonary hypertension and CMS. Although uncertainty persists and opinions vary as to whether or not AMS has a major pulmonary component, many patients who have HAPE also have AMS and it often is difficult to study subjects who have purely one or the other because of this overlap [5]. Furthermore, evidence suggests that AMS and HAPE risk are tied to the hypoxic ventilatory response (HVR), and HVR reflects pulmonary and neural components [6,7]. The study of AMS also provides many of the foundations of high-altitude science useful for the understanding of the pulmonary response to high altitude.

The risk for high-altitude pulmonary illness likely is determined by environmental and genetic factors. Recent studies have helped improve understanding of the epidemiology and susceptibility factors (including genetic factors) that underlie high-altitude–related pulmonary diseases. The pathophysiology, prevention, and treatment of AMS and HAPE are reviewed in this issue and elsewhere and discussed only as needed [3,8]. The study of high-altitude illness provides insight into the human response to global tissue hypoxia. The study of high-altitude illness also should be translatable to the understanding of common causes of death that are the result of regional hypoxia and ischemia [9].

Supported by National Institutes of Health grants RO1HL071618-01 (to J.P. Maloney), R01HL74321 (to U. Broeckel), and General Clinical Research Center grant M01-RR00058 (Medical College of Wisconsin).

* Corresponding author.
E-mail address: james.maloney@uchsc.edu
(J.P. Maloney).

Epidemiology

Demographics of high-altitude–related pulmonary disease

High-altitude pulmonary illness resulting from chronic hypoxia

Although in developed countries the focus of high-altitude research is on the acute illnesses of sojourners, it is important to remember that an estimated 140 million people live at high altitude in less developed countries (Tibet, Peru, and others) [10]. These high-altitude dwellers sustain distinct illnesses related to chronic hypoxia, such as having low birthweight children [11] or developing chronic right heart failure from hypoxic pulmonary hypertension [12]. Most of these chronic illnesses fall under the umbrella of CMS. CMS has a more important human impact worldwide than AMS and HAPE. Differences in the prevalence of CMS between inbred populations suggest that inherited factors may confer physiologic protection in some populations [10,13,14]. As the cause of chronic illness in residents of these regions often is multifactorial, it is difficult to attribute all their problems to the effects of chronic hypoxia. In comparison, few residents of developed countries make their homes at high altitude. Some exceptions occur, such as in Leadville, Colorado, a town of 3000 residents, at 10,430 ft (3180 m). Study of residents of these areas provides valuable insight into the physiology and consequences of chronic high-altitude exposure [15].

Pulmonary hypertension in high-altitude residents

The typical physiologic consequences of chronic hypobaric hypoxia in humans residing at high altitude are asymptomatic chronic pulmonary arterial hypertension (PAH) and a variable degree of polycythemia. Autopsy studies and cardiac catheterizations document that pulmonary vascular remodeling and PAH can occur after prolonged residence at altitudes, such as in Leadville, Colorado (3180 m) [16]. Elevated mean pulmonary arterial pressures (mPAP) of 24 ± 7 mm Hg are typical in high-altitude residents (normal mPAP, 13–15 mm Hg). Such residence usually is well tolerated, acclimatization occurs in the majority, and there is no evidence that the physiologic changes at these moderate altitudes are permanent for the majority of residents if and when they return to living at low altitude [17]. Because of increased pulmonary vascular muscularization and chronic PAH, however, some high-altitude residents develop symptoms. After a period at low altitude, some high-altitude residents also experience more severe pulmo-

nary hypertension, even the development of HAPE, on returning to their usual high-altitude residence [15]. Such events show that acclimatization is not a permanent phenomenon. Sarybaev and colleagues investigated Kyrgyzstan miners whose schedules alternated a 1-month residence at low-altitude homes with 1 month working at mines at 3700–4200 m. These miners developed levels of PAH at the end of their work month similar to those seen in Leadville residents, but during their 1-month hiatus at low altitude, their pulmonary pressures returned to normal. No evidence of permanent PAH was seen even after 3 years of this intermittent hypoxic exposure in these miners [17].

Adult subacute mountain sickness

This illness is uncommon and seen in subjects who typically are from altitude nonadapted populations and who migrate to high altitudes for months, such as Indian soldiers camped at 5800 m during the 1965 India-Pakistan War [2]. Manifestations resemble those of CMS but with an accelerated presentation. A similar illness, subacute infantile mountain sickness, occurs in children born to mothers from nonadapted populations who move to high altitude, such as Han Chinese lowland residents who migrate to highlands in Tibet [18].

Chronic mountain sickness

CMS occurs in individuals from populations that typically are adapted to high altitude but who develop eventual sequelae of polycythemia, fatigue, and right heart failure from pulmonary hypertension in adulthood after decades of life in a hypoxic environment [12]. This seems more common in South American highland dwellers than in Tibetan highland dwellers [19].

Acute high-altitude pulmonary illness in sojourners

The epidemiology of illness in transient visitors (sojourners) to high altitude is well described. This subset of high-altitude illness reflects an acute physiologic response.

Acute mountain sickness

AMS is a response to a single environment stimulus, namely hypobaric hypoxia. AMS occurs in up to 25% of sojourners who travel for short duration to a typical 8000-ft (2440-m) base ski resort, sleep there, and recreate at higher altitudes of up to 3964 m (eg, Colorado) during the day [20,21]. At typical resort base altitudes of 2400–3100 m, the inspired fraction of oxygen remains stable at 21%, but the lower barometric pressure produces an average partial pressure of oxygen in the alveoli (PAO_2) in the range of 70 mm Hg and hemoglobin arterial oxygen saturations (SaO_2) of 92%–93% when awake. At 3660 m, an altitude common in higher regions of many ski resorts, typical SaO_2 percentages are in the low 80s. Those who sleep at high altitudes are exposed to more severe hypoxia during sleep because of nocturnal periodic breathing, when saturations decline another 5%–8% below awake values [22]. This is the basis for the adage, "climb high, sleep low," known to mountaineers; this avoids the greater initial hypoxemia and arterial desaturation encountered in nonacclimatized individuals during sleep. At typical Himalayan trekking altitudes (3000–4500 m), the incidence of AMS approaches 50%· [23]. Sojourners typically arrive from sea level altitudes and travel directly to their high-altitude destination in a short period of time, which is a modifiable behavior.

Features of acute mountain sickness

Onset of AMS occurs within 24 hours of hypoxic exposure, often within the first few hours. The hallmark symptoms of AMS are neurologic, including headache and malaise. The standardized diagnostic clinical criteria are embodied in the Lake Louise scoring system, which uses a symptom set as primary clinical criteria. This self-reported score consists of questions that rank symptom severity on a 0- to 3-point scale for headache, gastrointestinal complaints (appetite, nausea, fatigue, and vomiting), lightheadedness, insomnia, and malaise. A Lake Louise score greater than 4 has a sensitivity of 78% and a specificity of 93% for the diagnosis of AMS [24]. An additional clinical assessment score is a part of the Lake Louise questionnaire and registers change in mental status, ataxia, and peripheral edema on a similar severity scale.

Most of those who develop AMS have mild to moderate symptoms that abate in 2–3 days without specific treatment. The prominence of neurologic symptoms in AMS led to the theory that cerebral edema is a cardinal event in AMS pathogenesis [4], which is reasonably supported by animal and human studies [25–27]. Such a mechanism of pathogenesis explains the most severe form of AMS: HACE. The acuity of onset of AMS suggests that AMS may be the result of hypoxia-induced changes in the expression of multiple genes, particularly those capable of causing brain edema, such as vascular endothelial growth factor. Furthermore, the phenomena of re-ascent HAPE and re-ascent AMS (discussed previously) [28] show that acclimatization in residents of high-altitude communities is not permanent and can change over time, likely reflecting altered gene expression resulting from differences in ambient oxygen in the environment.

Most sojourners who have mild to moderate AMS do not seek or receive specific treatment, although several therapies are efficacious in hastening recovery (acetazolamide, dexamethasone, oxygen, and descent) [3]. A minority develops more severe or persistent manifestations of AMS (eg, HACE) and needs to be transported to lower altitudes or receive medical treatment. Vacationers who have had AMS and choose to take prophylactic medications (such as dexamethasone or acetazolamide) on return ascents are in the minority, as AMS usually is mild. Most learn to ascend more slowly to allow acclimatization [29]. Residents of moderate altitudes (eg, Denver, Colorado or Salt Lake City, Utah) are acclimatized partially and have a lower risk for AMS [21]. Sojourners who develop AMS (or other high-altitude illness) are considered susceptible and usually have a recurrence with future ascents unless they take preventative measures. AMS rarely results in death, unless evacuation of rare patients who have HACE to lower altitude is not possible.

Features of high-altitude–related pulmonary edema

HAPE is defined (in the setting of acute altitude-related hypoxic exposure) based on symptoms and signs. Symptom requirements are at least two of these four: dyspnea at rest, cough, weakness or decreased exercise performance, and chest congestion or tightness. A diagnosis of HAPE requires the presence of at least two of the following four criteria: (1) crackles or wheezing, (2) central cyanosis, (3) tachypnea, and (4) tachycardia [30]. The incidence of HAPE is lower than that of AMS and is identified in 0.1%–1% of sojourner ascents at typical mountain resorts, although incidence increases with rapid and higher ascents [3]. Unlike AMS, HAPE onset often is not manifest in the first day at high altitude, although HAPE usually occurs within the first 5 days. The most compelling theory of the pathogenesis of HAPE is that of PAH with uneven hypoxic vasoconstriction in susceptible subjects leading to focal areas of pressure and flow-related vascular shear and overperfusion, resulting in endothelial failure, capillary leak, and eventual noncardiogenic pulmonary edema [3,31]. Acute PAH is a central feature of HAPE and resolves with oxygen and descent. HAPE-prone subjects also are shown to develop higher PAP during an acute hypoxic challenge than HAPE-resistant subjects [32,33]. HAPE easily can result in death if descent and adequate oxygen cannot be provided. Underlying chronic PAH may be a risk factor for

HAPE [34], as is a congenital single pulmonary artery [35]. These findings highlight the role of stress-induced capillary failure in HAPE pathogenesis. In susceptible subjects, effective preventative treatments are available, including oral vasodilators (nifedipine) and inhaled salmeterol [3]. These agents act by mechanisms of lowering pulmonary pressures or increasing alveolar fluid clearance, respectively. Failure to use these agents as prophylaxis by HAPE-susceptible individuals is a modifiable risk factor.

Risk factors for high-altitude–related pulmonary disease

Risk factors for high-altitude–related pulmonary disease are listed in Box 1 and include demographic, modifiable, and nonmodifiable (including genetic) risk factors.

Demographic factors

There is no clear effect of sex, race, or age on the incidence of these illnesses (at least in sojourner populations living at low altitudes). Limited evidence suggests that advanced age may lower AMS susceptibility, possibly because older patients tolerate cerebral edema better because of age-related encephalomalacia [20,36]. Nonadapted (historically lowland dwelling) populations with a recent mass migration to high-altitude residence seem to have a higher incidence of CMS and related illnesses [18]. High-altitude residents may develop accommodation to altitude exposure with lessened altitude-related illness prevalences. Adaptation can occur in a population, is not modifiable, and reflects inheritance through long periods of natural selection for beneficial traits in a particular environment (such as over centuries in the Nepalese highlands). In contrast, acclimatization occurs in individuals, is modifiable, and reflects the short-term physiologic effects of residence at higher altitude [37].

Modifiable risk factors

Sojourners can modify their risk of high-altitude illness easily by slowing their rate of ascent, choosing a lower destination altitude, and sleeping at the lowest practical altitude during the period of acclimatization [38]. All of these measures improve acclimatization success. This is evident particularly in subjects who had AMS or HAPE: a lower altitude ski resort is tolerated better than a higher altitude resort. In addition, medications are available for the prevention of AMS and HAPE in susceptible subjects. Failure to use these medications is a modifiable risk factor. Oxygen enrichment in sleeping rooms is an effective preventative measure, although it is not practical for the majority of sojourners [39]. The roles of dehydration [29,40], increased fluid balance [41], fitness [42], and athletic activity [43] in AMS pathogenesis are controversial and studies are contradictory. In high-altitude Peruvian residents who have environmental cobalt exposure from nearby mine drainage, half of a group of 27 polycythemic men were found to have elevated serum cobalt concentrations. None of the 53 low-altitude or nonpolycythemic high-altitude control residents had detectable serum cobalt. As cobalt stabilizes hypoxia-inducible factor (HIF) 1α (the central transcription factor of the hypoxia cascade) and slows its degradation, such

---

Box 1. Risk factors for high-altitude pulmonary illness

Modifiable factors

Rapid rate of ascent
Failure to acclimatize at lower altitude
Failure to use preventative medication
Increased sleeping altitude

Unmodifiable factors

Increased elevation of destination
History of AMS and HAPE
Unadapted ancestry or genetics
Lower HVR (reported for AMS only)
Residence near sea level
Single pulmonary artery (reported for HAPE only)
Pulmonary hypertension (reported for HAPE only)

Controversial factors

Dehydration (reported for AMS only)
Decreased fitness
Younger age (reported for AMS only)
Strenuous exercise first day
Cobalt exposure (miners) (reported for CMS only)
Sex
Respiratory infection
Decreased exhaled nitric oxide (NO) during hypoxia (reported for HAPE only)

environmental cobalt exposure could be a risk for CMS [44].

Unmodifiable factors

Unmodifiable factors, likely genetic (discussed later), include an inherent susceptibility to AMS or HAPE in some individuals. A history of altitude-related disease frequently is associated with a persistent increased risk of recurrent disease with hypoxic exposure (although medications or slower ascent are helpful). Also, the altitude of a destination cannot be modified if the unwavering goal (as in mountaineers) is to ascend to that level. Risk factors based on innate physiologic responses, such as HVR, also seem to be important unmodifiable factors (unless a preventative medication, such as acetazolamide, is used).

Circulating mediators and physiologic risk factors

Several circulating mediators have been studied as potential biomarkers for gaining insight into the physiology, prevention, and treatment of high-altitude illness. Most of these are evaluated in small studies of limited power, and none are validated clinically or available commonly as predictive or diagnostic blood tests for risk of high-altitude illness [45–47]. Because subjects exposed to hypoxic environments hyperventilate as a compensatory response to raise their PAO_2, a lower HVR or a lower SaO_2 percentage (by pulse oximetry) between individuals exposed to hypoxic environments is investigated as a risk factor for AMS. Studies evaluating HVR as a risk factor for AMS are not definitive [48], although a recent study of 150 mountaineers (known to be either AMS susceptible or resistant) finds that the decline in SaO_2% during 20–30 minutes of hypoxia was 4.9% more in AMS-susceptible subjects [6]. Some of the influences on HVR seem to be genetic (discussed later). HAPE-susceptible subjects are shown to have lower pulmonary production of NO in response to acute hypoxia [32], enhanced pulmonary pressures with exercise or hypoxic challenge [33,49], some evidence of worse nocturnal desaturation [22], and augmented sympathetic activity during acute hypoxia [50].

Genetic risk factors

The risk for high-altitude pulmonary illness, like any complex illness, is determined by environmental and genetic factors. Despite decades of research of high-altitude illness, it is not yet clearly known if susceptibility to AMS and HAPE in sojourners is, to an important degree, a heritable genetic trait. The limited knowledge of the genetics of high-altitude illness comes mostly from studies of relevant traits in inbred (genetically homogenous) populations, candidate gene association studies in noninbred populations (such as Europeans and Japanese), and studies of hypoxic phenotypes using inbred and genetically engineered animal strains (Box 2). Evolving knowledge of the hypoxia response cascade and of human genetic variation through the Human Genome Project is facilitating investigations of genetic risk for high-altitude pulmonary illness in high-altitude residents

Box 2. Genetic variation factors implicated in high-altitude pulmonary illness

Human studies

Inbred populations
HVR in identical twins
HVR[a]
Polycythemia[a]
ACE[a]
GST[a]

Noninbred populations
HIF1α[a]
eNOS (NOS3)[b]
HLA DR6, DQ4[b]
ACE[b]

Animal studies

Strain risk for hypoxic pulmonary hypertension
Cattle
Rodents
Chickens

Genetically-engineered mice:
eNOS
HIF1
HIF2
HO-1
HO-2
Serotonin transporter

[a] Implicated for CMS, hypoxic pulmonary hypertension, or adaptation.
[b] Implicated for HAPE.

and sojourners. Significant inroads into the genetics of high-altitude illness can be expected over the next decade.

Insights from studies of inbred populations

Inbred populations always are of particular interest for genetic study, as members have a homogeneous genetic background. Such groups are less likely to inject troublesome confounding factors from genetic heterogeneity that complicate data analysis (such as racial admixture) [51]. Sojourners, in contrast, usually are genetically heterogeneous (eg, Europeans and North Americans).

High-altitude traits in inbred populations

Clear differences in the prevalence of polycythemia, low infant birthweight, SaO2%, HVR, and pulmonary hypertension between genetically, relatively constrained highland populations, such as Tibetans in Lhasa (less susceptible) and Bolivian Aymara (more susceptible), suggest that inherited (genetic) factors in these populations confer physiologic protection (adaptation) [37]. Adapted Tibetans may show no evidence of pulmonary hypertension or altered pulmonary vascular responses to acute hypoxia, however, despite life at an altitude higher than residents of Leadville, Colorado (most of whom have PAH) [52]. The HVR may be an important determinant of risk, and there is evidence that this has an important genetic-based variability. Collins and colleagues studied 12 pairs of identical twins and 12 pairs of fraternal twins and found that HVR was correlated within identical twin pairs but not within fraternal twin pairs [53].

Genetic association studies of candidate genes for high-altitude tolerance in genetically restricted populations

Variants of the angiotensin-converting enzyme (ACE) gene have been investigated widely as candidates for genetic risk of high-altitude illness. The results are contradictory, however, and highlight the greatest problem that plagues genetic association studies: small group sizes that lead to insufficient power and flawed conclusions. The severity of chronic PAH at high altitude is associated with specific ACE alleles in highland residents of the Pamir Mountains of Asia (where Marco Polo had AMS) [54]. In this study, residents who had PAH were threefold more likely to carry the ACE intron 16 insertion-insertion genotype (II), although the number of subjects studied was small for a genetic association

study (48 had PH; 30 were normal). This insertion (I) allele is shown to have functional consequences on ACE activity [55]. A study of highland Andeans does not detect any difference in allele frequency at this locus compared with lowland natives [56], whereas another study of well-adapted highland Asians finds an increase in the I allele versus lowland dwellers (suggesting it was associated with increased fitness at altitude) [57]. Similar studies have been done in heterogeneous populations (discussed later). Evaluating a different candidate gene, Suzuki and colleagues find a higher frequency of the $(GT)_{14}$ dinucleotide repeat allele in intron 13 of the HIF1α gene in Nepalese Sherpas compared with Japanese and suggest this is an adaptation allele [58]. No functional effects of this allele are known and, combined with the small group sizes, it seems unlikely that this is a true adaptation allele. In a fascinating study, Gelfi and colleagues studied extracts of muscle biopsy proteins from well-adapted high-altitude–dwelling Tibetans and compared them to muscle biopsy extracts of low-altitude dwelling Tibetans and Nepali controls. Using a proteomic approach, they found seven differentially regulated proteins, most impressive of which was a 380% upregulation of glutathione-S-transferase (GST), a key enzyme for managing oxidant stress [59]. This study does not evaluate if well-described GST gene polymorphisms explain these results [60], and these findings may or not be relevant to high-altitude pulmonary disease.

Insights from genetic studies in heterogenous populations

A candidate gene approach mainly is used to identify DNA variants influencing the risk of AMS. Although the association study method is a powerful approach to investigate the influence of genetic markers on a particular disease or phenotype, the results of studies have to be interpreted with caution, largely because of limited sample size, population heterogeneity, and the difference in disease definition and phenotyping [51]. Nevertheless, these studies may provide initial leads for replication in other populations and more comprehensive evaluations.

Genetic association studies of candidate genes for acute mountain sickness susceptibility

The ACE intron 16 insertion (I) allele displays no association with AMS incidence or severity in a study of 159 European mountaineers ascending to 4559 m [61]. Other studies of candidate gene variants with possible disease relevance for AMS are published only in abstract or letter form.

Genetic association studies of candidate genes for high-altitude–related pulmonary edema susceptibility

NO is a potent pulmonary vasodilator that seems important for HAPE pathogenesis. NO production seems to be diminished in HAPE-susceptible individuals compared with those who are HAPE resistant [32,49], and inhaled NO is an effective (although impractical) HAPE treatment [62]. Thus, genetic variation in the endothelial NO synthase (eNOS or NOS3) pathway is an area of intense interest for HAPE. NOS3 polymorphisms are associated with HAPE susceptibility but only in a Japanese population. Droma and colleagues report a higher prevalence of two NOS3 variant polymorphisms in 41 HAPE-susceptible Japanese climbers compared with 51 healthy climbers [63]. This is not replicated in a European study of mountaineers that evaluated 51 HAPE-susceptible and 52 HAPE-resistant controls for three NOS3 polymorphisms [64]. The ACE intron 16 insertion (I) allele displays no association with HAPE incidence or severity in a study of 159 mountaineers ascending to 4559 m [61] or in a study of 49 HAPE-susceptible Japanese climbers [65]. Tyrosine hydroxylase is highly expressed in the carotid body, where it seems responsive to hypoxia. In a study of 43 HAPE-susceptible Japanese climbers and 51 HAPE-resistant controls, two tyrosine hydroxylase polymorphisms also show no association with HAPE susceptibility or HVR [66]. The HLA DR6 and DQ4 antigens are reported as associated with HAPE susceptibility in a Japanese study of 30 HAPE-susceptible subjects compared with 100 healthy controls [67].

Insights from animal studies into genetic risk of high-altitude pulmonary illness

Because the diagnosis of AMS and HAPE involve an assessment of symptoms, relevant animal models are difficult to develop [68]. The disparate responses of animal models to hypobaric hypoxia, however, are relevant, yield interesting insights, and are a starting point for generating hypotheses on appropriate candidate genes whose common variants can be evaluated in genetic association studies as risk factors for these illnesses in humans.

Animal models of hypoxic pulmonary hypertension

Most of these models evaluate the effects of chronic hypoxia on PAP and right heart hypertrophy or failure. Rodent strains used in research are inbred specifically to minimize the effects of a heterogeneous genetic background on experimental results.

Such commonly used rat strains have widely different responses to chronic hypoxia. Hilltop strains develop severe PAH, right heart failure, polycythemia, and death during chronic hypoxia [69]. Madison strain rats do well during chronic hypoxia, with only mild to moderate sequelae. The genes that underlie these susceptibilities are unknown. The NOS pathway is an area of intense manipulation in genetically engineered mice. Given NO's apparent role in HAPE pathogenesis and that some NOS enzymes are upregulated by hypoxia [70], genetic variants of NOS are of substantial interest in the study of high-altitude illness. Mice that are null or heterozygous ($+/-$) for NOS3 develop more severe pulmonary hypertension during chronic hypoxia and display more prominent pulmonary hypertension and right ventricular hypertrophy with acute hypoxia than wild-type mice [71,72]. Another hypoxia-regulated gene, hemoxygenase 1 (HO-1), seems to be protective in a chronic hypoxic environment, as HO-1 null mice develop severe PAH and RV dilation [73], whereas overexpression of HO-1 in transgenic mice protects against hypoxic PAH [74]. Mice null for hemoxygenase 2 (HO-2) display a diminished HVR, suggesting that HO-2 functions in control of ventilation during hypoxia [75]. Mice that are heterozygous for defects in the hypoxia sensing transcription factors HIF1α or HIF2α are protected against chronic hypoxia-induced PAH and polycythemia [76], suggesting that a blunted HIF1-mediated hypoxic response may be beneficial at high altitude. Overexpression in transgenic mice of the serotonin transporter gene also increases chronic hypoxia PAH and RV hypertrophy [77], whereas serotonin transporter null mice conversely are protected against these changes [78].

Animal models of altered hypoxic ventilatory response

Like mice null for HO-2, mice partially deficient (heterozygous) for HIF1α also have defects in hypoxia sensing. These defects, however, are localized at the level of the carotid bodies in the HIF1α mice that result in a diminished HVR [79]. Defects in HVR are implicated in AMS pathogenesis.

Summary

The epidemiology for high-altitude–related pulmonary disease is well described, and effective preventative measures are available for AMS and HAPE. Although risk factors for high-altitude illness are known, overall little is understood of the genetic factors that seem to determine the wide disparities in the human ability to adapt or acclimatize to high altitude. Delineation of these genetic factors in the current "Genome Era" is a priority for gaining insight into the human response to hypoxia. Knowledge of the response to global hypoxia hopefully can be translated beyond prevention and treatment of high-altitude diseases toward a greater understanding of important diseases of regional hypoxia and ischemia, such as stroke, coronary artery disease, and peripheral vascular disease.

References

[1] Komroff M. The travels of Marco Polo. New York: Heritage Press; 1934.

[2] Singh I, Khanna PK, Srivastava MC, et al. Acute mountain sickness. N Engl J Med 1969;280:175–84.

[3] West JB. The physiologic basis of high-altitude diseases. Ann Intern Med 2004;141:789–800.

[4] Hackett PH, Roach RC. High altitude cerebral edema. High Alt Med Biol 2004;5:136–46.

[5] Bartsch P, Maggiorini M, Ritter M, et al. Prevention of high-altitude pulmonary edema by nifedipine. N Engl J Med 1991;325:1284–9.

[6] Burtscher M, Flatz M, Faulhaber M. Prediction of susceptibility to acute mountain sickness by SaO2 values during short-term exposure to hypoxia. High Alt Med Biol 2004;5:335–40.

[7] Hohenhaus E, Paul A, McCullough RE, et al. Ventilatory and pulmonary vascular response to hypoxia and susceptibility to high altitude pulmonary oedema. Eur Respir J 1995;8:1825–33.

[8] Hackett PH, Roach RC. High-altitude illness. N Engl J Med 2001;345:107–14.

[9] Semenza GL, Agani F, Feldser D, et al. Hypoxia, HIF-1, and the pathophysiology of common human diseases. Adv Exp Med Biol 2000;475:123–30.

[10] Moore LG. Human genetic adaptation to high altitude. High Alt Med Biol 2001;2:257–79.

[11] Niermeyer S, Yang P, Shanmina, et al. Arterial oxygen saturation in Tibetan and Han infants born in Lhasa, Tibet. N Engl J Med 1995;333:1248–52.

[12] Penaloza D, Sime F. Chronic cor pulmonale due to loss of altitude acclimatization (chronic mountain sickness). Am J Med 1971;50:728–43.

[13] Beall CM, Strohl KP, Blangero J, et al. Ventilation and hypoxic ventilatory response of Tibetan and Aymara high altitude natives. Am J Phys Anthropol 1997;104:427–47.

[14] Beall CM, Blangero J, Williams-Blangero S, et al. Major gene for percent of oxygen saturation of arterial hemoglobin in Tibetan highlanders. Am J Phys Anthropol 1994;95:271–6.

[15] Scoggin CH, Hyers TM, Reeves JT, et al. High-altitude pulmonary edema in the children and young adults of Leadville, Colorado. N Engl J Med 1977;297:1269–72.

[16] Grover RF, Vogel JH, Voigt GC, et al. Reversal of high altitude pulmonary hypertension. Am J Cardiol 1966;18:928–32.

[17] Sarybaev AS, Palasiewicz G, Usupbaeva DA, et al. Effects of intermittent exposure to high altitude on pulmonary hemodynamics: a prospective study. High Alt Med Biol 2003;4(4):4455–63.

[18] Anand IS, Wu T. Syndromes of subacute mountain sickness. High Alt Med Biol 2004;5:156–70.

[19] Beall CM, Brittenham GM, Strohl KP, et al. Hemoglobin concentration of high-altitude Tibetans and Bolivian Aymara. Am J Phys Anthropol 1998;106:385–400.

[20] Honigman B, Theis MK, Koziol-McLain J, et al. Acute mountain sickness in a general tourist population at moderate altitudes. Ann Intern Med 1993;118:587–92.

[21] Montgomery AB, Mills J, Luce JM. Incidence of acute mountain sickness at intermediate altitude. JAMA 1989;261:732–4.

[22] Eichenberger U, Weiss E, Riemann D, et al. Nocturnal periodic breathing and the development of acute high altitude illness. Am J Respir Crit Care Med 1996;154(6 Pt 1):1748–54.

[23] Hackett PH, Rennie D. Rales, peripheral edema, retinal hemorrhage and acute mountain sickness. Am J Med 1979;67:214–8.

[24] Maggiorini M, Muller A, Hofstetter D, et al. Assessment of acute mountain sickness by different score protocols in the Swiss Alps. Aviat Space Environ Med 1998;69:1186–92.

[25] Hackett PH, Yarnell PR, Hill R, et al. High-altitude cerebral edema evaluated with magnetic resonance imaging: clinical correlation and pathophysiology. JAMA 1998;280:1920–5.

[26] Morocz IA, Zientara GP, Gudbjartsson H, et al. Volumetric quantification of brain swelling after hypobaric hypoxia exposure. Exp Neurol 2001;168:96–104.

[27] Schoch HJ, Fischer S, Marti HH. Hypoxia-induced vascular endothelial growth factor expression causes vascular leakage in the brain. Brain 2002;125(Pt 11):2549–57.

[28] Scoggin CH, Hyers TM, Reeves JT, et al. High-altitude pulmonary edema in the children and young adults of Leadville, Colorado. N Engl J Med 1977;297:1269–72.

[29] Basnyat B, Lemaster J, Litch JA. Everest or bust: a cross sectional, epidemiological study of acute mountain sickness at 4243 meters in the Himalayas. Aviat Space Environ Med 1999;70:867–73.

[30] Lake Louise consensus definition and quantification of altitude illness. In: Sutton J, Coates G, Houson CS, editors. Hypoxia: mountain medicine. Burlington (VT): Quenn City Press; 1992. p. 327–30.

[31] Hopkins SR, Garg J, Bolar DS, et al. Pulmonary blood flow heterogeneity during hypoxia and high-altitude pulmonary edema. Am J Respir Crit Care Med 2005;171:83–7.

[32] Duplain H, Sartori C, Lepori M, et al. Exhaled nitric oxide in high-altitude pulmonary edema: role in the

regulation of pulmonary vascular tone and evidence for a role against inflammation. Am J Respir Crit Care Med 2000;162:221–4.

[33] Eldridge MW, Podolsky A, Richardson RS, et al. Pulmonary hemodynamic response to exercise in subjects with prior high-altitude pulmonary edema. J Appl Physiol 1996;81:911–21.

[34] Das BB, Wolfe RR, Chan KC, et al. High-altitude pulmonary edema in children with underlying cardio-pulmonary disorders and pulmonary hypertension living at altitude. Arch Pediatr Adolesc Med 2004; 158:1170–6.

[35] Hackett PH, Creagh CE, Grover RF, et al. High-altitude pulmonary edema in persons without the right pulmonary artery. N Engl J Med 1980;302:1070–3.

[36] Roach RC, Houston CS, Honigman B, et al. How well do older persons tolerate moderate altitude? West J Med 1995;162:32–6.

[37] Beall CM. Tibetan and Andean patterns of adaptation to high-altitude hypoxia. Hum Biol 2000;72:201–28.

[38] Murdoch DR, Curry C. Acute mountain sickness in the Southern Alps of New Zealand. N Z Med J 1998;111: 168–9.

[39] West JB. Oxygen enrichment of room air to relieve the hypoxia of high altitude. Respir Physiol 1995;99: 225–32.

[40] Basnyat B, Subedi D, Sleggs J, et al. Disoriented and ataxic pilgrims: an epidemiological study of acute mountain sickness and high-altitude cerebral edema at a sacred lake at 4300 m in the Nepal Himalayas. Wilderness Environ Med 2000;11:89–93.

[41] Westerterp KR, Robach P, Wouters L, et al. Water balance and acute mountain sickness before and after arrival at high altitude of 4,350 m. J Appl Physiol 1996;80:1968–72.

[42] Milledge JS, Beeley JM, Broome J, et al. Acute mountain sickness susceptibility, fitness and hypoxic ventilatory response. Eur Respir J 1991;4:1000–3.

[43] Roach RC, Maes D, Sandoval D, et al. Exercise exacerbates acute mountain sickness at simulated high altitude. J Appl Physiol 2000;88:581–5.

[44] Jefferson JA, Escudero E, Hurtado ME, et al. Excessive erythrocytosis, chronic mountain sickness, and serum cobalt levels. Lancet 2002;359:407–8.

[45] Tissot van Patot MC, Leadbetter G, Keyes LE, et al. Greater free plasma VEGF and lower soluble VEGF receptor-1 in Acute Mountain Sickness. J Appl Physiol 2005;98(5):1626–9.

[46] Maloney J, Wang D, Duncan T, et al. Plasma vascular endothelial growth factor in acute mountain sickness. Chest 2000;118:47–52.

[47] Goerre S, Wenk M, Bartsch P, et al. Endothelin-1 in pulmonary hypertension associated with high-altitude exposure. Circulation 1995;91:359–64.

[48] O'Connor T, Dubowitz G, Bickler PE. Pulse oximetry in the diagnosis of acute mountain sickness. High Alt Med Biol 2004;5:341–8.

[49] Busch T, Bartsch P, Pappert D, et al. Hypoxia decreases exhaled nitric oxide in mountaineers suscep-

tible to high-altitude pulmonary edema. Am J Respir Crit Care Med 2001;163:368–73.

[50] Duplain H, Vollenweider L, Delabays A, et al. Augmented sympathetic activation during short-term hypoxia and high-altitude exposure in subjects susceptible to high-altitude pulmonary edema. Circulation 1999;99:1713–8.

[51] Ioannidis JP, Ntzani EE, Trikalinos TA, et al. Replication validity of genetic association studies. Nat Genet 2001;29:306–9.

[52] Groves BM, Droma T, Sutton JR, et al. Minimal hypoxic pulmonary hypertension in normal Tibetans at 3,658 m. J Appl Physiol 1993;74:312–8.

[53] Collins DD, Scoggin CH, Zwillich CW, et al. Hereditary aspects of decreased hypoxic response. J Clin Invest 1978;62:105–10.

[54] Aldashev AA, Sarybaev AS, Sydykov AS, et al. Characterization of high-altitude pulmonary hypertension in the Kyrgyz: association with angiotensin-converting enzyme genotype. Am J Respir Crit Care Med 2002;166:1396–402.

[55] Rigat B, Hubert C, Alhenc-Gelas F, et al. An insertion/deletion polymorphism in the angiotensin I-converting enzyme gene accounting for half the variance of serum enzyme levels. J Clin Invest 1990;86:1343–6.

[56] Rupert JL, Kidd KK, Norman LE, et al. Genetic polymorphisms in the Renin-Angiotensin system in high-altitude and low-altitude Native American populations. Ann Hum Genet 2003;67(Pt 1):17–25.

[57] Qadar Pasha MA, Khan AP, Kumar R, et al. Angiotensin converting enzyme insertion allele in relation to high altitude adaptation. Ann Hum Genet 2001; 65(Pt 6):531–6.

[58] Suzuki K, Kizaki T, Hitomi Y, et al. Genetic variation in hypoxia-inducible factor 1alpha and its possible association with high altitude adaptation in Sherpas. Med Hypotheses 2003;61:385–9.

[59] Gelfi C, De Palma S, Ripamonti M, et al. New aspects of altitude adaptation in Tibetans: a proteomic approach. FASEB J 2004;18:612–4.

[60] Fryer AA, Bianco A, Hepple M, et al. Polymorphism at the glutathione S-transferase GSTP1 locus. A new marker for bronchial hyperresponsiveness and asthma. Am J Respir Crit Care Med 2000;161:1437–42.

[61] Dehnert C, Weymann J, Montgomery HE, et al. No association between high-altitude tolerance and the ACE I/D gene polymorphism. Med Sci Sports Exerc 2002;34:1928–33.

[62] Scherrer U, Vollenweider L, Delabays A, et al. Inhaled nitric oxide for high-altitude pulmonary edema. N Engl J Med 1996;334:624–9.

[63] Droma Y, Hanaoka M, Ota M, et al. Positive association of the endothelial nitric oxide synthase gene polymorphisms with high-altitude pulmonary edema. Circulation 2002;106:826–30.

[64] Weiss J, Haefeli WE, Gasse C, et al. Lack of evidence for association of high altitude pulmonary edema and polymorphisms of the NO pathway. High Alt Med Biol 2003;4:355–66.

[65] Hotta J, Hanaoka M, Droma Y, et al. Polymorphisms of renin-angiotensin system genes with high-altitude pulmonary edema in Japanese subjects. Chest 2004; 126:825–30.

[66] Hanaoka M, Droma Y, Hotta J, et al. Polymorphisms of the tyrosine hydroxylase gene in subjects susceptible to high-altitude pulmonary edema. Chest 2003; 123:54–8.

[67] Hanaoka M, Kubo K, Yamazaki Y, et al. Association of high-altitude pulmonary edema with the major histocompatibility complex. Circulation 1998;97:1124–8.

[68] Kleinsasser A, Levin DL, Loeckinger A, et al. A pig model of high altitude pulmonary edema. High Alt Med Biol 2003;4:465–74.

[69] Ou LC, Smith RP. Strain and sex differences in the cardiopulmonary adaptation of rats to high altitude. Proc Soc Exp Biol Med 1984;177:308–11.

[70] Jung F, Palmer LA, Zhou N, et al. Hypoxic regulation of inducible nitric oxide synthase via hypoxia inducible factor-1 in cardiac myocytes. Circ Res 2000;86: 319–25.

[71] Fagan KA, Fouty BW, Tyler RC, et al. The pulmonary circulation of homozygous or heterozygous eNOS-null mice is hyperresponsive to mild hypoxia. J Clin Invest 1999;103:291–9.

[72] Steudel W, Scherrer-Crosbie M, Bloch KD, et al. Sustained pulmonary hypertension and right ventricular hypertrophy after chronic hypoxia in mice with congenital deficiency of nitric oxide synthase 3. J Clin Invest 1998;101:2468–77.

[73] Yet SF, Perrella MA, Layne MD, et al. Hypoxia induces severe right ventricular dilatation and infarction in heme oxygenase-1 null mice. J Clin Invest 1999;103:R23–9.

[74] Christou H, Morita T, Hsieh CM, et al. Prevention of hypoxia-induced pulmonary hypertension by enhancement of endogenous heme oxygenase-1 in the rat. Circ Res 2000;86:1224–9.

[75] Adachi T, Ishikawa K, Hida W, et al. Hypoxemia and blunted hypoxic ventilatory responses in mice lacking heme oxygenase-2. Biochem Biophys Res Commun 2004;320:514–22.

[76] Brusselmans K, Compernolle V, Tjwa M, et al. Heterozygous deficiency of hypoxia-inducible factor-2alpha protects mice against pulmonary hypertension and right ventricular dysfunction during prolonged hypoxia. J Clin Invest 2003;111:1519–27.

[77] MacLean MR, Deuchar GA, Hicks MN, et al. Overexpression of the 5-hydroxytryptamine transporter gene: effect on pulmonary hemodynamics and hypoxia-induced pulmonary hypertension. Circulation 2004; 109:2150–5.

[78] Eddahibi S, Hanoun N, Lanfumey L, et al. Attenuated hypoxic pulmonary hypertension in mice lacking the 5-hydroxytryptamine transporter gene. J Clin Invest 2000;105:1555–62.

[79] Yu AY, Shimoda LA, Iyer NV, et al. Impaired physiological responses to chronic hypoxia in mice partially deficient for hypoxia-inducible factor 1alpha. J Clin Invest 1999;103:691–6.

ELSEVIER
SAUNDERS

Clin Chest Med 26 (2005) 405 – 414

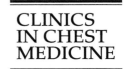

CLINICS
IN CHEST
MEDICINE

Limits of Respiration at High Altitude

Robert B. Schoene, MD

*Division of Pulmonary and Critical Care Medicine, University of California—San Diego, School of Medicine,
200 West Arbor Drive, San Diego, CA 92103, USA*

In healthy individuals who are at low altitude, the lung has enough redundancy in its structure and function that the obtaining of oxygen from the air into the blood is an easy task. The lungs' structure ensures a margin of safety during times of stress, either from disease or environment, such that individuals survive. During forays to or habitation at high altitude, however, the stress is pervasive and constant. Because humans have evolved primarily at low altitudes, the stress of living, working, or recreating at high altitudes is an unnatural state.

In this setting, the lungs are the first interface between the air in the environment and the tissues of the body, which require oxygen for existence. The steps required to ensure the transport of oxygen from the air to the mitochondria include convection of air in the conductive airways, mechanics of ventilation, diffusion of oxygen from the alveolar air to the blood by gas exchange at the alveolar-capillary barrier, convection of oxygen in the blood to the tissues, and diffusion of oxygen from the capillary across the cell membrane through the cytosol into the mitochondria. This article reviews the mechanisms that ensure the success of this process in an environment where the availability of oxygen is diminished compared to that at low altitude.

First, the chemo- and mechanoreceptors and the subsequent neurologic drive to breathe are reviewed. Second, the mechanics of respiration and the energy cost of that process to the body at high altitude are described. Third, the impairment of transfer from oxygen to air to the blood and the elimination of

carbon dioxide (ie, gas exchange) add understanding to the difficulty humans have resting and exercising in an environment of thin air. The fourth and final step of oxygen delivery to the tissues is outlined briefly. The article's structure is designed to provide insight into resourcefulness and adaptation during times of stress at high altitude, which will provide a better understanding of humans who have heart and lung disease at low altitude.

High-altitude environment

Anyone who has gone to altitudes above 7500 feet has incurred an inordinate sense of dyspnea. This breathlessness is a result of the higher demand on ventilation required to move enough air to supply oxygen to the body in an environment where the air density becomes lower with higher altitude. As altitude increases and barometric pressure decreases, more and more air movement is required to supply oxygen for gas exchange. This phenomenon imposes more demands on the mechanics of ventilation which may be limited. The remainder of the journey (ie, the transport of oxygen from the air to the mitochondria) is a complicated but integrated process that is essential for the survival of creatures on earth. The adaptations that occur at high altitudes optimize the transport of oxygen so that cellular respiration can proceed. All of these adaptations begin immediately but some may take months, years, or generations to come to full fruition; even then, the processes may never be complete. High altitudes, where the availability of oxygen is low and where humans sojourn for brief periods or for a lifetime, provide an excellent

E-mail address: rschoene@ucsd.edu

0272-5231/05/$ – see front matter © 2005 Elsevier Inc. All rights reserved.
doi:10.1016/j.ccm.2005.06.015

classroom for physiologists to understand this elegant process.

The drive to breathe

Ventilation increases immediately upon assent to high altitude and continues to increase over time [1–3]. This process is called ventilatory adaptation. The increase in ventilation is related directly to the oxygen and carbon dioxide concentrations in alveolar air, the barometric pressure, and alveolar ventilation. Ventilatory acclimatization is a complicated interaction of metabolic and mechanical signals that stimulate the central nervous system, which subsequently initiates the neuromuscular events resulting in the mechanics of ventilation.

The PO_2 in the arterial blood perfuses the carotid body, which is the sensor of hypoxemia. The carotid body then sends a signal by the carotid sinus nerve to the brainstem, where neural signals are sent to the muscles of respiration [4–7]. Although the acute response in ventilation to hypoxia is blunted in part by the resultant repository alkalosis, the carotid body continues to undergo adaptation, so that over time, the increase in ventilation is greater at any given PO_2. In a sojourner who is at high altitude for a period of weeks, ventilation continues to increase, presumably because of the increase sensitivity in the carotid body. This increase in ventilation results in a lower PCO_2, higher alveolar partial pressure of oxygen (PAO_2), and subsequent increase in the oxygen content of the arterial blood.

The measured response is called the hypoxic ventilatory response (HVR). HVR is an inherent characteristic and can be measured in a laboratory setting where subjects are exposed to gradually decreasing levels of oxygen; minute ventilation is plotted against the PO_2 or arterial oxygen saturation [8]. HVR is malleable in its adaptation but does increase during a stay at high altitude [7,9,10]. There is an association between HVR and subsequent exercise ventilation upon ascent: individuals who have high HVR values have higher resting and exercise ventilation and arterial oxygen saturation than those who with more blunted HVRs [11–13]. This inherent characteristic is related to climbers' success at climbing to extreme altitudes (26,000 feet or greater), because greater ventilation during rest and exercise results in a higher arterial oxygen saturation and higher oxygen delivery to the exercising muscles (Fig. 1).

This characteristic may be important particularly in extreme altitude climbing; for instance, on the summit of Mt. Everest, the barometric pressure is

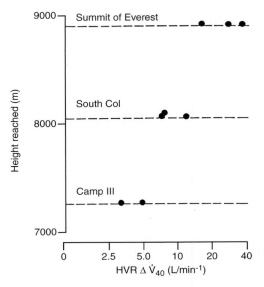

Fig. 1. Data from the 1981 AMREE showing that individuals who had higher HVRs performed better at higher altitudes than those who had lower HVRs. (*Data from* Schoene RB, Lahiri S, Hackett PH, et al. Relationship of hypoxic ventilatory response to exercise performance on Mt. Everest. J Appl Physiol 1984;56:1478–83.)

approximately 250 mm Hg, giving individuals an inspired PO_2 of approximately 42 mm Hg. Extraordinary ventilation is necessary to ensure a viable level of oxygen in the alveolus (measured at 32 mm Hg), which is accompanied by an alveolar partial pressure of carbon dioxide ($PACO_2$) of approximately 7.5 to 8.5 mm Hg, consistent with extreme hyperventilation. (Measurements were made by Pizzo on the summit of Mt. Everest in October, 1981 [14].) Several years after these measurements were made, a simulated ascent of Mt. Everest was made in a hypobaric chamber using subjects whose alveolar carbon dioxide levels ranged from 8 to 12 mm Hg and were related to individual resting HVR values [10,15]. This ventilatory response is vital for function and survival at moderate and extreme altitude, yet it extracts a metabolic price on exercising individuals. The work of breathing for any given level of work is proportionally greater the higher the ascent.

The ventilatory demand at high altitude

For any given energy expenditure, ventilation (VE_{BTPS}, liters/minute) increases proportionately with each elevation in altitude. Because barometric pressure decreases with increasing altitude, the volume of

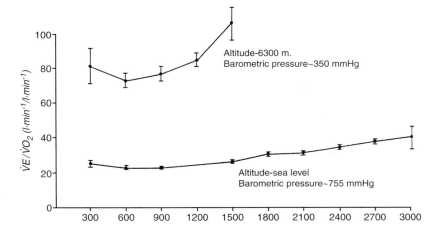

Fig. 2. Ventilatory equivalents for oxygen consumption (VE/VO2) during exercise in subjects at sea level and 21,000 feet demonstrating that at comparable workloads, exercise ventilation is almost four times greater at that altitude than at sea level. (*From* Schoene RB. Hypoxic ventilatory response in exercise ventilation at sea level and high altitude. In: West JB, Lahiri S, editors. High altitude and man. Bethesda (MD): American Physiologic Society; 1984. p. 25; with permission.)

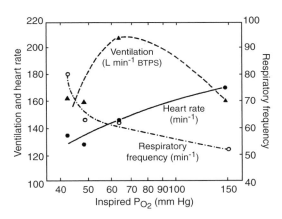

Fig. 3. Data from the 1981 AMREE showing that maximal exercise ventilation in liters per minute (BTPS) (*dashed line*) increased as the inspired PO_2 decreased from sea level values (150 mm Hg) to approximately 60 mm Hg at 21,000 feet but decreased as climbers approached the summit of Mt. Everest, where the inspired PO_2 was 42 mm Hg. The increase in ventilation is secondary to the hypoxic stimulation of exercise hyperpnea and the level of exercise, which was 200 W of work at 21,000 feet, whereas the hypoxia stimulus was greater at 29,000 feet, but the work capacity was reduced greatly. (*From* West JB, Hackett PH, Maret KH, et al. Pulmonary gas exchange on the summit of Mt. Everest. J Appl Physiol 1983;55:695; with permission.)

gas contains less oxygen than at sea level. Thus, supplying the same amount of oxygen for any given workload requires a greater total volume of ventilation. Studies of high-altitude environment and of hypobaric chambers document this ventilatory response. In 1981, on the American Medical Research Expedition to Everest (AMREE), and in a 1985 study in a hypobaric chamber, Operation Everest II (OE II), healthy subjects exercising at real or simulated altitudes of 21,000 feet (barometric pressure approximately 350 mm Hg) breathed approximately four times greater for any given workload at that altitude than at sea level (Figs. 2 and 3). On AMREE at 200 watts of work, the mean ventilation for all subjects was 207 liters per minute (BTPS [body temperature and pressure saturated]) compared with sea level values at that workload of approximately 65 liters per minute [14]. On OE II, at comparable simulated altitudes of 21,000 feet and sea level, minutes ventilation were approximately 160 liters per minute and 89 liters per minute, respectively [15]. The lower minute ventilation in the hypobaric chamber study may reflect less ventilatory acclimatization because of the shorter times spent at that altitude in the chamber study.

Energentics and work of breathing at high altitude

Even though overall minute ventilation is much higher at high altitude, there is a slightly decreased work of breathing at any given minute ventilation secondary to the decreased gas density at high altitude. It is conceivable that the decreased gas density could substantially decrease the resistive load of the convection of gas at high levels of exercise. This decrease in work of breathing is, however, modest and must be balanced against the increase in ventilatory demands from the hypoxic stimulation of exercise ventilation. Cibella and colleagues [16] studied a small number of subjects and showed that, in spite of the lower gas density, the net result was still a greater energy output while breathing at high altitude for any given workload than at low altitude (Figs. 4 and 5). It is no surprise then that it still requires more energy to breathe at high altitude.

When climbing at high altitude, there is only a finite amount of energy that can be expended. It takes muscles to perpetrate this work—the mechanical work of locomotion and the work of breathing—and all muscles require a certain amount of perfusion of blood to deliver oxygen for work. In a disproportionate manner, the muscles of respirations extract a higher percentage of the total oxygen consumption when at high altitude than at low altitude.

In an earlier study at low altitude, Hansen and coworkers [17] exercised 15 highly trained runners to maximum and measured the energy expenditure for the work of breathing. It was their conclusion that in spite of this high level of work, the net affects of the greater ventilatory response was an advantage and the improved gas exchange and respiratory alkalosis were worth the price of an increased work of breathing.

Johnson and coworkers [18] studied athletes at an exhaustive level of exercise and found that there was some flow limitation in the airways. In a subsequent study, using esophageal and gastric balloons and manometers, they then evaluated the function of the diaphragm of normal individuals at high levels of work. They measured transdiaphragmatic pressures at 85% of maximum oxygen consumption (VO_{2max}) and higher and found that the strength of the diaphragm, as measured with that technique, decreased by approximately 25% [19]. It seemed, therefore, that exercise at these high levels of work was not sustainable. Evidence of diaphragmatic fatigue was not apparent at exercise levels of 70% of VO_{2max} or less [20]. The high-altitude climber who needs extraordinary levels of ventilation to function may be limited regarding the intensity of exercise and sustainable exercise.

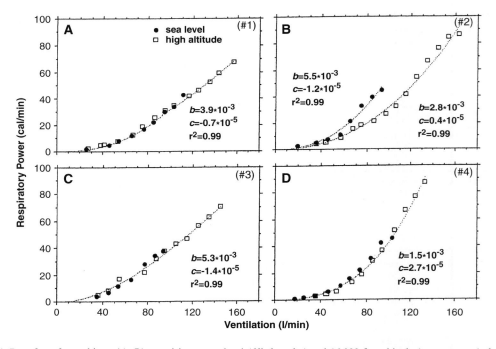

Fig. 4. Data from four subjects (*A−D*) exercising at sea level (*filled circles*) and 16,000-feet altitude (*open squares*) showing that the work of breathing, expressed as respiratory power (cal/min), was substantially greater at high altitude. (*From* Cibella F, Cuttitta G, Romano S, et al. Respiratory energetics during exercise at high altitude. J Appl Physiol 1999;86:1787; with permission.)

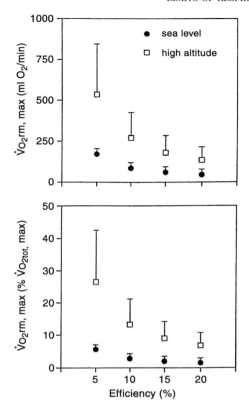

Fig. 5. (*Top*) Data from subjects exercising at sea level (*filled circles*) and 16,000 feet (*open squares*) demonstrating the maximal oxygen cost of breathing ($VO_{2rm, max}$) during maximal ventilation at physiologic levels of mechanical efficiency (range 5%–20%). (*Bottom*) Similar data except that $VO_{2rm, max}$ is expressed as a percentage of the total maximal rate of oxygen uptake ($VO_{2tot, max}$). These data show that the work of breathing is substantially higher at this altitude than at sea level. Values are means ± SEM. (*From* Cibella F, Cuttitta G, Romano S, et al. Respiratory energetics during exercise at high altitude. J Appl Physiol 1999;86:1788; with permission.)

Investigators turned to distribution of muscle perfusion during exercise. Because cardiac output is finite and all the muscles that are exercising require blood flow, the body needs to decide how to proportion that flow between the working muscles of locomotion and the muscles of respiration. The concept was that with high levels of ventilation during exercise, the respiratory muscles would "steal" a higher percentage of the cardiac output, thus depriving the muscles of locomotion of perfusion and, subsequently, oxygen. Babcock and colleagues [21] stimulated the diaphragm with supra-

maximal phrenic nerve stimulation at a frequency in humans comparable to 86% to 92% of VO_{2max} for approximately 13 minutes. After that period, there was a consistent fall of approximately 26% in the forced generated by the diaphragm at all levels of work. The investigators believe that competition for blood flow between the local motor muscles and the diaphragm eventually deprived the diaphragm of blood flow, which resulted in subsequent diaphragmatic muscle fatigue. Cibella and colleagues [16] estimate the mechanical efficiency of breathing at low and high (over 16,000 feet) altitudes and calculate that the oxygen cost of breathing amounts to 26% and 5.5% of VO_{2max}, respectively. These remarkable findings suggest that the work of breathing alone at high altitude may limit functional work; other than the slight decrease of gas density at that altitude, there is no reason to believe that mechanical efficiency is substantially different between the two altitudes.

Another complicating factor investigated in several studies shows that peripheral vascular resistance in the exercising muscle is increased as maximal exercise is approached. Blood flow may, therefore, be decreased to the muscles, which are generating the work and may be distributed further to the respiratory muscles (Fig. 6) [22–24].

A hypothetic situation taken from the data from AMREE suggests that at least 40% of energy expenditure when climbing above 26,000 feet is dedicated to the work of breathing. For instance, if the VO_{2max} of many of the subjects on an expedition is approximately 5 liters per minute at sea level, if the approximate work of breathing at maximum of exercise at low altitude is 8% to 10% of the total oxygen consumption, and if the VO_{2max} at that altitude is approximately 1 liter per minute with comparable maximum minute ventilations, then a phenomenal percentage of approximately 40% of total energy expenditure is dedicated merely to breathing. It is, thus, easy to conceptualize at least one of the major limitations to work at these altitudes.

The importance of a high ventilatory response to maintain adequate oxygenation during exercise at high altitude is, in part, offset by the disproportionate amount of energy needed to breathe compared with sea level. It, therefore, seems that one of the paramount reasons for the limitations to exercise at moderate to extreme altitudes is a matter of the finite amount of cardiac output and the body's decision of how to distribute that blood flow to balance adequate oxygenation and functional work. It is not difficult to imagine a similar analogy in patients who have moderate to severe restrictive and obstructive pulmo-

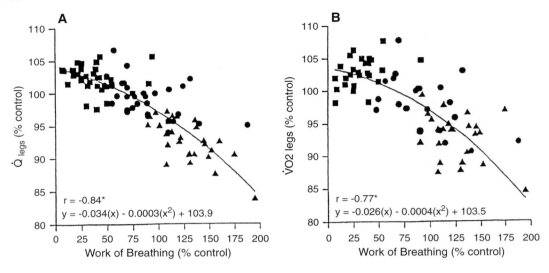

Fig. 6. Data from highly trained cyclists showing that, at maximal exercise, as the work of breathing increases, the blood flow to the legs ($\dot{Q}_{legs}$) (*A*) and the rate of oxygen consumption ($\dot{V}O_2$ legs) (*B*) of the legs decrease. These studies were performed at resting ventilation and maximal ventilation in a control state and with inspiratory loading. •, control; ■, inspiratory unload; ▲, inspiratory load. (*From* Harms C, Babcock M, McClaran S, et al. Respiratory muscle work compromises leg blood flow during maximal exercise. J Appl Physiol 1997;82:1577; with permission.)

nary disease whose work of breathing extracts a great deal of energy from the rest of their muscles.

Limitations of gas exchange in the lung

The low PO_2 in the air at high altitudes imposes a global limitation of transfer of oxygen from the alveolus to the blood. For this transfer to be successful, four conditions are necessary:

1. An adequate driving pressure for oxygen from the air to the blood
2. A sufficiently high surface area and low diffusion distance for gas exchange
3. An affinity of hemoglobin for oxygen
4. An adequate time for equilibration of oxygen from air to blood as the red blood cells traverse the pulmonary capillary

Although there is a surfeit of oxygen at low altitude, which essentially eliminates diffusion limitations as a reason for hypoxemia, at high altitude this driving pressure is, by definition, lower.

As discussed previously, the body's first response to ambient hypoxia is an increase in alveolar ventilation. With an increase in alveolar ventilation, there is a decrease in $PACO_2$ and an increase in the PAO_2, which increases the alveolar-capillary gradient

for oxygen. Although this increase in PAO_2 may not be a large amount (as discussed previously), at extreme altitude this increase is essential to ensure some diffusion from the pulmonary capillary to the hemoglobin in the red blood cells. With ongoing ventilatory adaptation to high altitude, there is further augmentation of ventilation and subsequently of PAO_2, thus increasing the driving pressure at the air-blood interface [14]. As discussed previously, individual HVR plays an important role in increasing the driving pressure for oxygen from air to the blood without which, at extreme altitudes, life is even more tenuous.

Another important factor that facilitates the loading of oxygen into the blood at the lung is the affinity of hemoglobin for oxygen, which is defined by the oxygen-hemoglobin dissociation curve (OHC). Because the driving pressure for oxygen at the lung at moderate or extreme altitude is low, the greater affinity that hemoglobin has for oxygen, the more oxygen is loaded onto hemoglobin at the pulmonary-capillary interface. In humans, the marked respiratory alkalosis, which occurs especially at very high altitudes, shifts the OHC to the left, increasing the affinity of hemoglobin for oxygen and improving loading of oxygen. A marked alkalemia is documented in climbers at extreme altitude [14]. Some animals who live at high altitude or birds who migrate at extreme altitude (the Bar-headed Goose of the Tibetan Plateau) have left-shifted OHCs that facilitate loading of oxygen from the air to hemoglobin, without which it is nearly impossible for these birds to fly at altitudes above 26,000 feet [14,25].

A further problem exists for the diffusion of oxygen from the air to the blood when there is a wide range of need for oxygen from rest to high levels of exercise. Large volumes of ambient air must come in contact with the alveolar-capillary surface area, where diffusion of oxygen of the air to the blood takes place. The lung is well designed for this purpose in that the alveolar-capillary interface provides a large surface area for gas exchange that responds rapidly to high levels of metabolic demand, such as intense exercise.

The blood flow across the pulmonary capillary with increases in cardiac output during exercise is, however, a limiting factor for oxygen flux as the body's demand for oxygen consumption increases. Success of the loading of oxygen depends on the proportion of diffusion capacity to perfusion of blood at the capillary level. Difficulties for gas exchange, therefore, are encountered at high altitude, where there is a decreased driving pressure for oxygen. Not only is the driving pressure for oxygen for air to the blood less, but also the transit time across the pulmonary capillary with exercise is shorter, and in spite of a left-shifted OHC, the loading process for oxygen takes places at a steep portion of that curve [14,15,26]. The marginal advantage to gas exchange at high altitude that is conveyed by an increase in

ventilation and a higher P_{AO_2} is, thus, mitigated in part by the decreased transit time of red blood cells across the pulmonary capillary when cardiac output increases when during exercise (Fig. 7) [27].

The degree to which cardiac output increases dictates the transit time across the pulmonary capillary, and limits to overall exercise at high altitudes cause lower cardiac output than would be achieved at low altitude; the decrease of transit time at the highest sustainable workloads is not as great as at low altitude. Other mechanisms play a role in the impairment of gas exchange at high altitude. One is the low mixed venous P_{O_2}, especially during exercise, which further decreases the rate of equilibration of oxygen of air to the blood.

In the 1980s, there was interest in defining the factors that affect the drop in arterial oxygen saturation during exercise at high altitude (Fig. 8) (at low altitude, arterial oxygen saturation does not decrease with exercise). The diffusion limitation and impairment of gas exchange and, thus, lower arterial oxygen saturation, drop to a greater degree with increasing altitude [14,15,28–31].

To quantitate gas exchange in the lung at low and high altitude, Wagner and colleagues undertook several studies using the multiple inert gas elimination technique (MIGET) [29–31]. This elegant method uses the infusion of six inert gases into the pulmonary artery, each with different blood solubil-

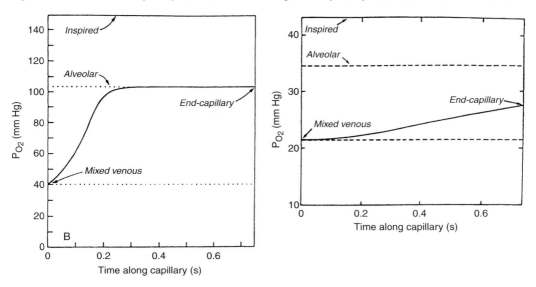

Fig. 7. Plots of the P_{O_2} (mm Hg) at sea level (*left*) and the summit of Mt. Everest (*right*) versus the transit time of blood across the pulmonary capillary. These schematic representations demonstrate that, with ascent, the driving pressure for oxygen from the air to the blood is lower; thus, there is not enough time for equilibration for oxygen across the pulmonary capillary. This phenomenon results in arterial oxygen desaturation, which is accentuated with higher levels of exercise. (*From* West JB, Wagner PD. Predicted gas exchange on the summit of Mt. Everest. Respir Physiol 1980;42:10; with permission.)

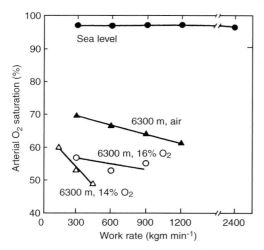

Fig. 8. Arterial oxygen saturation, as measured by ear oximetry, plotted against work rate at sea level and 21,000-feet altitude in humans exercising to maximal effort. The lower two lines were obtained with subjects breathing 16% and 14% oxygen at 21,000 feet. (*From* West JB, Hackett PH, Maret KH, et al. Pulmonary gas exchange on the summit of Mt. Everest. J Appl Physiol 1983;55:693; with permission.)

ity, such that the concentration of these gases can be measured on their arterial side after the blood has traversed the lung and in exhaled gas. For instance, if the lung is normal, the least soluble gases are exhaled in the lung and, thus, can be measured in exhaled air, whereas the soluble gases stay in the blood and can be measured in the arterial blood. Where there are areas of low ventilation and perfusion ratios or right-to-left intrapulmonary shunt, the quantification of these six gases can apportion the overall gas exchange into various high-to-low ventilation-perfusion units. For instance, lungs with an intrapulmonary shunt do not permit even insoluble gases to come in contact with air spaces. Thus, a high proportion of the insoluble gas can be measured in the arterial blood. Any degree of hypoxemia that cannot be quantitated by MIGET (and MIGET's ability to quantify ventilation and perfusion), therefore, is considered secondary to a diffusion limitation. With this elegant investigative tool in hand, studies were undertaken in hypobaric chambers. The first three studies [29–31] used acute exposure to 10,000- and 15,000-feet altitudes in healthy subjects who had high levels of exercise. The decrease in oxygen saturation during exercise that occurred in this experiment was found secondary to areas of low ventilation-perfusion units and diffusion limitations.

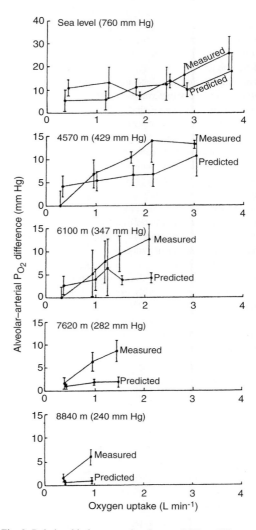

Fig. 9. Relationship between alveolar-arterial PO_2 difference and the rate of oxygen uptake in OE II, a high-altitude chamber study designed to simulate an ascent by humans of more than 40 days to the summit of Mt. Everest (29,028 feet). These data were obtained from the MIGET, which measures ventilation-perfusion relationships and shows that the predicted alveolar-arterial PO_2 difference (mm Hg) could be accounted for only in part by ventilation-perfusion inequality. The remaining difference was attributed to a diffusion limitation of oxygen from the air to the blood. Values are mean ± SEM. (*From* Wagner PD, Sutton JR, Reeves JT, et al. Operation Everest II: pulmonary gas exchange during a simulated ascent of Mt. Everest. J Appl Physiol 1987;63:2354; with permission.)

Some members of this investigative team were involved in OE II, a project that took healthy young individuals from sea level to a simulated ascent of Mt. Everest during 40 days [26]. Many studies were done, including using the MIGET technique to look at gas exchange during this simulated ascent. Measurements were made on the simulated summit where the barometric pressure was 250 mm Hg. There was some persistence of ventilation and perfusion inequality, but the higher the subjects went, the greater the contribution of diffusion limitations to hypoxemia. The increasing diffusion limitation was believed secondary to the marked decrease in driving pressure for oxygen from the air to the blood (Fig. 9).

At simulated altitudes early in the experiment, there was more ventilation and perfusion heterogeneity believed possibly to be secondary to interstitial edema, which can occur at high altitude and presumably clears with further acclimatization. The ventilation and perfusion mismatch correlated with the subject's pulmonary artery pressures and slight increases in the pulmonary capillary wedge pressures with exercise. Another explanation, other then left ventricular dysfunction, for the increase in wedge pressures is impairment of left ventricular function secondary to deviation of the ventricular septum into the left ventricle from the high right-sided pressures secondary to pulmonary hypertension. The explanation has yet to be determined. The phenomenon of extravascular lung water, which may evolve into the overt syndrome of high-altitude pulmonary edema, is associated with accentuated pulmonary artery pressures [32–37]. These increases in pulmonary vascular pressures impose an inordinate stress on the fragile pulmonary capillaries and may lead to capillary rupture and, thus, interstitial and alveolar hemorrhage [38–44]. Any degree of interstitial or alveolar edema that worsens gas exchange further is tolerated poorly at very high altitudes and, at times, is a lethal condition.

Summary

The lung is an extremely capable organ that under most conditions is capable of compensating for the stresses of illnesses to ensure adequate acquisition of oxygen from the atmosphere, ensuring delivery of oxygen to the mitochondria. Even with acute and chronic exposure to high altitude, the lungs' resourceful adaptations ensure that this process can take place. This process is challenged, however, by global hypoxia, especially if there is impairment in the three major processes needed for adequate tissue oxygenation:

1. An intact ventilatory drive to breathe
2. A sufficient increase in alveolar ventilation, which is stimulated by that drive
3. Intact gas exchange at the alveolar-capillary interface

This article reviewed some of the classic and recent physiologic mechanisms that make the study of high altitude fascinating and relevant to patients at low altitude who have heart or lung disease.

References

[1] Boycott AE, Haldane JS. The effects of low atmospheric pressure on respiration. J Physiol 1908;37: 355–77.

[2] Houston CS, Riley RL. Respiratory and circulatory changes during acclimatization to high altitude. Am J Physiol 1947;149:565–88.

[3] Rahn H, Otis AB. Man's respiratory response during and after acclimatization to high altitude. Am J Physiol 1946;157:445–59.

[4] Bisgard GE, Busch MA, Forster HV. Ventilatory acclimatization to hypoxia is not dependent of cerebral hypocapnic alkalosis. J Appl Physiol 1986;60: 1011–5.

[5] Vizek M, Pickett CK, Weil JV. Increased carotid body hypoxic sensitivity during acclimatization to hypobaric hypoxia. J Appl Physiol 1987;63:2403–10.

[6] Smith CA, Bisgard GE, Neilsen AM, et al. Carotid bodies are required for ventilatory acclimatization to chronic hypoxia. J Appl Physiol 1986;60:1011–5.

[7] Nielson AM, Bisgard GE, Vidruk EH. Carotid chemoreceptor activity during acute and sustained hypoxia in goats. J Appl Physiol 1998;65:1976–82.

[8] Weil JV, Byrne-Quinn E, Sodal IE, et al. Hypoxic ventilatory response in normal man. J Clin Invest 1970;49:1061–72.

[9] Forster HF, Dempsey JA, Birnbaum ML, et al. The effect of chronic exposure to hypoxia on ventilatory response to CO2 and hypoxia. J Appl Physiol 1971;31: 586–92.

[10] Schoene R, Roach RC, Hackett P, et al. Operation Everest II: ventilatory adaptation during gradual decompression to extreme altitude. Med Sci Sports Exerc 1990;22:804–10.

[11] Schoene RB, Lahiri S, Hackett PH, et al. Relationship of hypoxic ventilatory response to exercise performance on Mt. Everest. J Appl Physiol 1984;56: 1478–83.

[12] Schoene RB. Control of ventilation in climbers to extreme altitude. J Appl Physiol 1982;43:886–90.

[13] Matsuyama S, Kimura H, Sugita T, et al. Control of ventilation in extreme altitude climbers. J Appl Physiol 1986;61:400–6.

[14] West JB, Hackett PH, Maret KH, et al. Pulmonary gas exchange on the summit of Mt. Everest. J Appl Physiol 1983;55:678–87.

[15] Sutton JR, Reeves JT, Wagner PD, et al. Operation Everest II: oxygen transport during exercise at extreme simulated altitude. J Appl Physiol 1988;64:1309–21.

[16] Cibella F, Cuttitta G, Romano S, et al. Respiratory energetics during exercise at high altitude. J Appl Physiol 1999;86:1785–92.

[17] Hanson P, Claremont A, Dempsey J, et al. Determinants and consequences of ventilatory responses to competitive endurance running. J Appl Physiol 1982; 52:615–23.

[18] Johnson B, Snupe K, Dempsey J. Mechanical constraints on exercise hyperpnea in endurance athletes. J Appl Physiol 1992;73:874–86.

[19] Johnson B, Babcock M, Saman O, et al. Exercise-induced diaphragmatic fatigue in healthy humans. J Physiol 1993;460:385–405.

[20] Marciniuk D, Sanii M, Younes M. Role of central respiratory muscle fatigue in endurance exercise in normal subjects. J Appl Physiol 1994;76:236–41.

[21] Babcock M, Pegelow D, McClaran S, et al. Contribution of diaphragmatic power output to exercise-induced diaphragm fatigue. J Appl Physiol 1995;78:1710–9.

[22] Barclay J. A delivery-independent blood flow effect on skeletal muscle fatigue. J Appl Physiol 1986;61: 1084–90.

[23] Harms C, Babcock M, McClaran S, et al. Respiratory muscle work compromises leg blood flow during maximal exercise. J Appl Physiol 1997;82:1573–83.

[24] Wetter T, Harms C, Nelson W, et al. Influence of respiratory muscle work on VO2 and leg blood flow during submaximal exercise. J Physiol 1999;82:643–51.

[25] Black CP, Tenney SM. Oxygen transport during progressive hypoxia in high-altitude and sea-level water foul. Respir Physiol 1980;39:217–39.

[26] Wagner PD, Sutton JR, Reeves JT, et al. Operation Everest II: pulmonary gas exchange during a simulated ascent of Mt. Everest. J Appl Physiol 1987;63: 2348–59.

[27] West JB, Wagner PD. Predicted gas exchange on the summit of Mt. Everest. Respir Physiol 1980;42: 1–16.

[28] West JB, Boyer SJ, Graber DJ, et al. Maximal exercise at extreme altitudes on Mt. Everest. J Appl Physiol 1983;55:688–98.

[29] Gale GE, Torre-Bueno J, Moon RE, et al. Ventilation-prefusion inequality in normal humans during exercise at sea level and simulated altitutde. J Appl Physiol 1985;58:978–88.

[30] Torre-Bueno J, Wagner PD, Saltzman HA, et al. Prefusion limitation in normal humans during exercise at sea level in simulated altitude. J Appl Physiol 1985; 58:989–95.

[31] Wagner PD, Gale GE, Moon RE, et al. Pulmonary gas exchange in humans exercising at sea level in simulated high altitude. J Appl Physiol 1986;61:260–73.

[32] Fred HL, Schmidt AM, Bates T, et al. Acute pulmonary edema of altitude clinical and physiologic observations. Circulation 1962;25:929–37.

[33] Hutgren H, Grover R, Hartley L. Abnormal circulatory responses to high altitude in subjects with a previous history of high altitude pulmonary edema. Circulation 1971;44:759–70.

[34] Eldridge MW, Podolosi A, Richardson RS, et al. Pulmonary hemodynamic response to exercise in subjects with prior high altitude pulmonary edema. J Appl Physiol 1996;81:911–21.

[35] Mckechnie JK, Leary WP, Noakes TD, et al. Acute pulmonary edema in two athletes during a 90-km running race. S Afr Med J 1979;56:261–5.

[36] Pascoe JR, Ferraro GL, Cannon JH, et al. Exercise-induced pulmonary hemorrhage in racing horses: preliminary study. Am J Vet Res 1981;42:703–7.

[37] Whitwell KE, Greet TR. Collection and evaluation of tracheobronchial washes in the horse. Equine Vet J 1984;16:499–508.

[38] West JB, Tsukimoto K, Mathieu-Costello O, et al. Stress failure in pulmonary capillaries. J Appl Physiol 1991;70:1731–42.

[39] West JB, Mathieu-Costello O. Structure, strength, failure, and remodeling of the pulmonary blood-gas barrier. Annu Rev Physiol 1999;61:543–7.

[40] West JB, Matheiu-Costello O. Strength of pulmonary blood-gas barrier. Respir Physiol 1992;88:141–8.

[41] Hopkins SR, Schoene RB, Henderson WR, et al. Intense exercise impairs the integrity of the pulmonary blood-gas in elite athletes. Am Rev Respir Crit Care Med 1997;155:1090–4.

[42] Hopkins SR, Schoene RB, Henderson WR, et al. Sustained submaximal exercise does not alter the integrity of the lung blood-gas barrier in elite Athletes. J Appl Physiol 1998;84:1185–9.

[43] Schaffartzik W, Arcos JP, Tsukimoto K, et al. Pulmonary interstitial edema in the pig after heavy exercise. J Appl Physiol 1993;75:2535–40.

[44] Schaffartzik W, Poole DC, Derion T, et al. V sub A/Q distribution during heavy exercise and recovery in humans: Implications for pulmonary edema. J Appl Physiol 1992;72:1657–67.

ELSEVIER
SAUNDERS

Clin Chest Med 26 (2005) 415 – 438

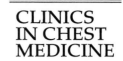

CLINICS
IN CHEST
MEDICINE

The Lung in Space

G. Kim Prisk, PhD, DSc

*Division of Physiology, Department of Medicine, University of California—San Diego, 9500 Gilman Drive, La Jolla,
CA 92093-0931, USA*

The lung is an unusual organ in that it comprises little actual tissue mass in a relatively large volume. It is an expanded network of air spaces and blood vessels designed to bring gas and blood into close proximity to each other to facilitate efficient gas exchange. As a direct consequence of this architecture, the lung is highly compliant and markedly deformed by its own weight.

Although there is little, if any, structural difference between the top and bottom of the normal human lung, there are marked functional differences, caused by the effects of gravity. For example, the alveoli at the top of the lung are overexpanded compared with the bottom of the lung [1–4] because the weight of the dependent portions of the lung stretches the upper portions. As a consequence of this, ventilation, the amount of fresh gas reaching the alveoli is higher at the bottom of the lung, because the initial smaller volume there makes the lung able to expand more readily in response to a given breathing effort. Gravity also causes regional differences in intrapleural pressure [5] and in parenchymal stress [6], both of which result in regional differences in lung function.

There are even larger differences in pulmonary blood flow between the top and bottom of the lung. The pulmonary vascular system operates at a relatively low pressure compared with the systemic circulation and, as a consequence, hydrostatic effects strongly influence the vertical distribution of blood flow in the normal human lung, with greater flows near the bases than the apices [7,8].

Although ventilation and pulmonary perfusion increase toward the lower regions of the lung, the differences in perfusion are larger than those in ventilation. As a result, ventilation-perfusion ratio ($\dot{V}_A/\dot{Q}$) is higher at the top than the bottom of the lung. Because it is the $\dot{V}_A/\dot{Q}$ that determines gas exchange, regional differences in alveolar gas and effluent blood composition occur [9].

Many studies have examined the influence of gravity on the lung, either by using postural change as the alteration in gravity or by using hypergravity as a means of increasing the gravitational effect. These studies point to the conclusion that although much of the unevenness of lung function may be attributable to gravity, some considerable degree may not be. Such conclusions are difficult to be certain of, however, because the extrapolation from the normal and hypergravity environment to zero gravity is a far from obvious step. Over the past 13 years, several studies have been performed providing the first ever comprehensive studies of the lung in the absence of gravity.

The space environment

Making measurements in microgravity

There are only two practical methods of achieving microgravity (μG) suitable for human experimentation, parabolic flight in aircraft and space flight (drop towers and sounding rockets often used by the materials science community are not suitable for humans). Parabolic flight has the advantage of being relatively accessible and (in comparison to space flight) inexpensive. Parabolic flight, however, pro-

---

This work was supported in part by NASA contract NAS9-98124 and NASA cooperative agreement NCC9-168.
   E-mail address: kprisk@ucsd.edu

vides only short periods of μG, and these usually are sandwiched between periods of hypergravity. Space flight provides sustained μG (typically from approximately 1 week to more than 1 year at present) but flight opportunities are infrequent at best.

Parabolic flight is a common means of accessing μG. The United States, Russia, and the European Community all perform parabolic flight campaigns routinely. They essentially are similar, and the choice of carrier makes for only minor technical differences. Typical flights consist of a climb to altitude, followed by a series of parabolic maneuvers. In the case of the NASA KC-135, the aircraft is pitched up at approximately 1.6 to 1.8 Gz until an attitude of approximately 45° nose high is reached. Thrust then is reduced to equal drag and the nose lowered to abolish lift, thus achieving microgavity (or perhaps more correctly in the case of the aircraft, milligravity). The resulting ballistic flight path is maintained for approximately 25 seconds until the aircraft nose is approximately 45° below the horizon, at which point the cycle repeats. A typical flight consists of 40 parabolas, often performed in groups of 10 in so-called "roller-coaster" mode. Other aircraft provide slight differences in the profile, the number of parabolas per flight, and the exact nature of the hypergravity phase of the flight. All aircraft experiments share common characteristics, however, and the problems that stem from those characteristics.

In almost every case, the flight profile required to fly the maneuver mandates a period of hypergravity immediately before the μG phase. Thus, any measurements made in parabolic flight are subject to the effects that may ensue from this period of hypergravity. Other, generally less serious, effects stem from the fact that aircraft cabin pressure is lower than sea level, (in the KC-135, the pressure typically is approximately 600 torr) and can vary during the flight as a result of changes in the engine power settings required to fly the maneuver. In addition, there often are problems associated with motion sickness, especially in less experienced flyers, which at best make for difficult experimental conditions and may contaminate results. For these reasons, this review concentrates on studies performed in sustained μG, except in those areas in which data are not available or where parabolic flight results provide an interesting contrast to those from space flight.

The Space Shuttle and the International Space Station

Space flight provides the only other practical means of performing pulmonary studies in weight-lessness. Although space flight hardly is routine, low earth orbit flights are common and fairly frequent. For more than 10 years, the Russian space station, Mir, was manned permanently, and now the United States–led International Space Station (ISS) provides a more research-friendly environment. Space flight, however, creates a large number of problems that must be overcome to conduct good scientific studies.

Perhaps the largest problem is the inevitably small population available for study. Since 1983, the United States Space Shuttle has, at times, carried the European-built Spacelab in the cargo bay and, subsequently, the commercially built Spacehab. These provided a large increase in the habitable volume of the normally cramped Space Shuttle and provided researchers with a normoxic, normobaric environment in which to conduct research. In a typical flight, however, only four crewmembers were available for operations either as subjects, operators, or both. Thus, in experiments involving human subjects, the design must be such that statistically viable results can be achieved using an n of only 4. Typically, such experiments are designed so that subjects act as their own controls, and extensive preflight and postflight testing is performed on the flight crew to provide baseline and 1 G recovery data. Further, a typical Space Shuttle flight has many experiments on board, so the time available for the crew to participate in any given experiment is limited. Thus, experimenters often are left with a small number of repetitions of any measurement on a small number of subjects.

Space Shuttle flights are limited to short-duration missions (the maximum currently is approximately 17 days) and, therefore, deal necessarily only with acute phases of the adaptation to μG. Longer duration missions now occur on the ISS and, before that, occurred on Mir, Salyut, and Skylab. ISS exacerbates the small n problem, because the crew normally is only three (two in the immediate aftermath of the loss of the Space Shuttle, Columbia), and as a result, there are few studies that make use of the long-term (approximately 6 months and up to approximately 1 year on Mir) μG exposures. In addition, the maintenance requirements are high, so time available for scientific endeavors is limited.

Other problems that have to be faced include the inability of the experimenter to be present during the studies. This is alleviated only partially by transmission of data to the ground in real time in the case of Space Shuttle and ISS experiments. Nevertheless, extensive studies of pulmonary function have been made during Spacelab missions and these are reported in this article.

Early space flight

One unfortunate historical factor, at least for pulmonary function studies, is the atmospheric composition of the earlier spacecraft. Early United States flights (Mercury, Gemini, and Apollo) had a hypobaric, hyperoxic (100% oxygen) environment because of the design of the environmental control systems necessitated by the need for a thin pressure vessel to keep the spacecraft mass low. Skylab provided the first real opportunity to conduct pulmonary function measurements in space [10], but ground simulation studies showed that many of the changes observed may have been at least partly the result of atmospheric conditions (5 psia or approximately 260 mm Hg, 70% oxygen) in the vehicle rather than μG per se [11].

Analogs of microgravity

Over the years, the limited access to actual μG has stimulated the desire to perform ground-based studies using analogs of weightlessness. The two most popular of these, head-down tilt (HDT) (typically 6° head-down, although other angles have been used) and thermoneutral water immersion have been popular for cardiovascular studies, and prolonged bedrest (with and without tilt) has been used for studying muscle and bone function changes. The Russians have used a dry-immersion system with some success for long-term studies on water immersion [12].

HDT is a somewhat useful analog of μG, especially when considering the cardiovascular system and musculoskeletal effects. Although the systemic effects of fluid shifts associated with HDT may in some aspects mimic μG, there still is a large and significant effect of gravity on the lungs and the pulmonary vasculature that cannot be removed by HDT. Further, HDT and immersion result in significant reductions in resting lung volume [13,14], much greater than that seen in μG (see discussion later), and the effects of this larger reduction in lung volume cannot be ignored.

Because neither HDT nor immersion adequately simulates μG in terms of lung function, there is no detailed discussion of them in this article. There is a significant body of work available in the literature that reports measurements performed in actual μG, and the space available is dedicated to a review of that work. There are, however, several reviews of analogs of weightlessness that may prove useful for comparison purposes [12,15].

Studies in microgravity

Lung volumes and chest wall mechanics

Vital capacity

Vital capacity (VC) arguably is the most measured parameter of pulmonary function. Despite that, it was not until Spacelab flights that a clear picture of the behavior of VC in response to μG was obtained. The first detailed study of lung volumes in μG was performed in Skylab in the early 1970s [10]. VC was measured repeatedly during the mission on four subjects and an approximately 10% decrease was observed. Ground controls using the same hypobaric atmosphere, however, also showed a 3% to 5% reduction, confounding the space flight results [11]. Between that time and the flight of Spacelab Life Sciences 1 (SLS-1) in 1991, measurements were restricted to those during parabolic flight. Michels and West [16] showed no consistent differences in VC in μG, except for noting an increase when the initial push to residual volume (RV) was during μG, and the remainder of the inspiration occurred in 1 G. They suggest that this might be the result of a lower RV in μG because of an increase in intrathoracic blood volume. Radiographic measurements also performed in parabolic flight [17] show a nonsignificant decrease in apical-to-basal height and an increase in lung width. Paiva and colleagues [18] show an approxiamately 8% reduction in VC during μG compared with 1 G. Forced vital capacity (FVC) measured in parabolic flight was reduced in most subjects in a carefully conducted study that corrected for changing barometric pressure in the cabin, although the reduction was small (100–200 mL) [19]. This result contradicted that of a previous study of FVC in a KC-135 [20], but the difference seems to be a failure to account for a falling cabin pressure during the μG phase of the flight in the earlier study.

During the 1991 flight of SLS-1, VC was measured in seven subjects over the course of a 9-day flight [21]. Early in flight (flight day 2 [FD-2]), after approximately 24 hours in μG, VC was reduced by approximately 5% compared with that standing in 1 G. By FD-4 the reduction had been abolished, and values from FD-4 and FD-9 were not different to control (Fig. 1). The change seen early in μG was approximately half that seen in the supine position. The suggestion is that an early inflight increase in intrathoracic blood volume was responsible, although other factors cannot be ruled out. A similar pattern in FVC was seen in the same subjects, with a 2.6% reduction on FD-2 and no difference from preflight standing on FD-4 and FD-5 [22]. By FD-9, however,

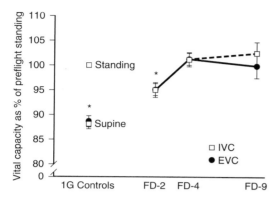

Fig. 1. Inspiratory and expiratory vital capacities (IVC and EVC) for four payload crew members of SLS-1. VC on FD-2 was intermediate between standing and supine values measured in 1 G and was reduced compared with FD-4 and FD-9. Values are means ± SE. *, significantly different from standing ($P \leq 0.05$). (*From* Elliott AR, Prisk GK, Guy HJB, et al. Lung volumes during sustained microgravity on Spacelab SLS-1. J Appl Physiol 1994;77:2008; with permission.)

FVC was significantly higher (4.4%) than that measured preflight. The most plausible explanation for these results is an early inflight increase in intrathoracic blood volume (consistent with an observed increase in cardiac volume) [23] and a subsequent reduction in intrathoracic blood volume as plasma volume is reduced [24].

Functional residual capacity

The functional residual capacity of the lung (FRC) is the lung volume resulting at end expiration of a relaxed breath. It represents the condition in which the opposing forces of the chest wall and lung are in balance. Agostoni and Mead [25] predicted that µG reduces FRC by approximately 10%. This was based on a cranial shift of the diaphragm and abdominal contents as gravity was removed (a potentially large effect that would decrease FRC), an outward move of the rib cage as the weight of the abdomen was removed, and an upward movement of the shoulder girdle (both small effects that would increase FRC). Their prediction was confirmed largely by measurements performed during SLS-1 [21], in which FRC was seen to decrease by approximately 15% in µG compared with that standing in 1 G. As expected, the FRC in µG was intermediate to that measured standing and supine in 1 G. These results were confirmed subsequently by measurements in other flights [26].

The results from sustained µG also are consistent with those from short periods of µG in parabolic

flight. Some early attempts produced conflicting results [27,28] or failed to show a clear change [17]. Carefully performed studies by Paiva and co-workers [18], however, showed a reduction in FRC of approximately 400 mL in µG compared with 1 G in seated subjects, a result consistent with orbital studies. The difficulty of inferring results in sustained µG from changes in FRC during transient accelerations is highlighted in a study of Wilson and Liu [29], in which they attempted to infer the likely changes in FRC in sustained µG by measuring the changes in lung volume in seated subjects in an elevator generating transient accelerations. The predictions of this experiment were opposite to those measured in sustained µG, likely as a result of the inability of the subjects to relax fully during the accelerations.

Residual volume

Residual volume generally is resistant to change. Transitions between upright and supine [21,30,31] and water immersion [32–34] showed no significant decrease in RV. Similarly, central vascular engorgement produced by G-suit inflation does not reduce RV [32]. Residual volume is reduced by chest strapping, which forces the subject to a prolonged period of breathing at a low lung volume, but this is likely the result of an increase in lung-recoil because of changes in surface tension associated with this peculiar situation [35].

In sustained µG, RV was shown to decrease by approximately 18% (310 mL) compared with standing and also was significantly below that measured supine (by approximately 220 mL) [21]. A likely explanation is that in µG, the large apicobasal gradients in regional lung volume present in 1 G, are abolished. The concept is shown in Fig. 2. In 1 G, when lung volume is reduced below FRC, airway closure begins in the more gravitationally dependent lung regions (because of distortion of the lung by its own weight), and this airway closure progresses up the lung until RV is reached [36]. Thus, the regional RV of basal lung units is dependent on airway closure, whereas the regional RV of apical lung units is dependent on the balance of local static forces. The result is a large difference in regional RV between the top and bottom of the lung in 1 G.

In µG, however, the apicobasal gradients in regional lung volume resulting from gravity are abolished. The result is that regional volume of lung units is more uniform throughout the lung at all lung volumes. Upper lung regions are not subject to expansion forces generated by the weight of depen-

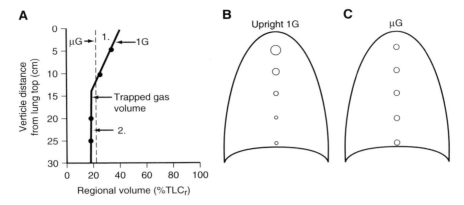

Fig. 2. (*A*) Theoretic model of lung at RV during 1-G conditions and in μG. At RV, alveolar size increases from base of lung to apex in 1 G above the point at which airway closure starts but is uniform in μG. If area 2 is less than area 1, total sum of alveolar volumes may be less at μG than at 1 G (depending on shape of chest wall). TLC_r, regional TLC. (*B, C*) Regional alveolar volumes at different vertical distances during 1 G and μG, respectively. (*From* Elliott AR, Prisk GK, Guy HJB, et al. Lung volumes during sustained microgravity on Spacelab SLS-1. J Appl Physiol 1994;77:2012; with permission.)

dent lung regions. This results in a reduction in the regional RV of upper lung units. The net effect is to reduce the overall RV of the lung. This mechanism depends on the removal of the expanding forces on the upper parts of the lung generated by the weight of the lung tissue beneath. Thus, such an effect is expected either in the upright or supine posture, but only in μG where the weight of the lung is abolished. The recent observation of a lack of change in RV in parabolic flight [37], however, suggests a possible role of changes in intrathoracic blood volume also.

Maximum expiratory flows

Maximum expiratory flow is limited by dynamic compression of the airways. This occurs when airway pressure falls below that outside the airway resulting in the formation of a choke point and, thus, effort-independent expiratory flow limitation. It is reasonable to expect that removal of gravity may result in some alterations in local airway stress and, thus, in expiratory flow limitation. Indeed, Castile and colleagues [38] demonstrated that postural changes and, hence, changes in the gravitational forces on the lung and thorax influence the shape of the effort independent portion of the maximum expiratory flow volume (MEFV) curve. There were changes in the position and magnitude of the sudden changes in flow that characterized an individual's MEFV curve, and these changes were consistent with wave speed theory where changes in local airway stresses could alter the location of airway choke points.

In a carefully conducted study aboard the KC-135, Guy and coworkers [19] observed a reduction in FVC and, at high lung volumes, a reduction in the lung volume at which a given expiratory flow occurred in μG. These effects were consistent with an increase in intrathoracic blood volume, which engorges the lung with blood and increases elastic recoil [39]. At low lung volumes, there was a scooping out of the MEFV curve similar to that seen in recumbency [38] and immersion [39]. This was attributed to vascular engorgement, rather than a more inhomogeneous emptying pattern of the lung, and suggests a degree of optimization of lung function upright in 1 G.

The KC-135 results of Guy and colleagues [19] suffer from the ever-present criticism that the period of hypergravity preceding μG may be influencing the results. Elliott and coworkers [22] measured MEFV curves on the SLS-1 crew using the analysis techniques of Guy and colleagues [19]. They found an early inflight reduction in FVC (see previous discussion) that disappeared by FD-4. In addition, the reduction in lung volume at which a given expiratory flow occurred was seen in the early flight data but this too disappeared later in flight, suggesting that early increases in intrathoracic blood volume may have been responsible. At low lung volumes, however, there were no discernable changes in the shape of the MEFV curve, as seen in the KC-135. There were no significant changes in the forced expiratory flows (FEF) over the effort-independent portion of the MEFV curve in sustained μG ($FEF_{50\%}$ and $FEF_{25\%-75\%}$ were unchanged compared with standing). This suggests little, if any, change in the behavior of the central and peripheral airways, or the respiratory muscles.

In contrast to the effort-independent portion of the MEFV curve, peak expiratory flow rate (PEFR) was reduced significantly on FD-2, FD-4, and FD-5 (although the reduction on FD-5 was much less than earlier in flight), but back to control values on FD-9. These reductions largely were in the absence of parallel changes in lung volumes (eg, FVC), suggesting that the change was not simply a consequence of scaling (as was the case supine). Although the PEFR is effort dependent, it was thought unlikely that the change was the result of alterations in respiratory muscle strength, especially as the PEFR recovered as the flight progressed. Rather, it was suggested that the lack of a firm platform to push against during the maneuver compromised the ability of the subjects to generate maximum flows. In the only other study performed in μG in the KC-135, the subjects were restrained in aircraft seats throughout the course of the study. The recovery later in space flight may be the result of improved subject performance as they adapted to operating in a μG environment.

Shape and movement of chest wall

There are no studies to date that directly measure the mechanical properties of the lung and chest wall in sustained μG. There are a few indirect studies that deal with the chest and abdominal wall motions, most notably those performed by Paiva and coworkers on the Spacelab D-2 mission [40]. The best source of data at present remains studies performed aboard the KC-135.

Perhaps not surprisingly, μG influences chest and abdominal wall shape. In five seated subjects, an inward displacement of the abdominal wall was seen in μG compared with 1 G, causing a reduction in lung volume [18]. There was no corresponding change in the rib cage, consistent with the radiographic observations of Michels and colleagues in parabolic flight [17]. The results are consistent with an increase in abdominal wall compliance, which was confirmed by Edyvean and colleagues [41], who showed an increase in the abdominal contribution to tidal volume from 33% in 1 G to 51% in μG. By measuring gastric pressures, abdominal compliance was shown to increase from 43 to 70 mL/cm H_2O between 1 G and μG. Their data suggest that there may be small residual pleural pressure gradients present in μG as a result of shape changes in the chest wall, which may result in some residual inhomogeneity of ventilation. Although some of the change in rib cage contribution likely results from alterations in the coupling between the abdomen and thorax [42],

there also is a consistent decrease in the EMG activity of the muscles that activate the upper portion of the rib cage [43]. The suggestion is that this is part of the reflex referred to as operational length compensation [44]. As the length of the diaphragm (thus, its ability to generate force) increases, there is a compensatory decrease in the activation of the other inspiratory muscles to keep tidal volume constant [45]. More recent studies in parabolic flight show a decrease in lung recoil pressure in μG, presumably the result of the removal of lung parenchymal distortion caused by gravity [37,46]. These studies show significant nonlinearities in chest wall behavior, highlighting the inability to predict behavior in accurately μG by extrapolating from the hypergravity condition.

In space flight, the measurements have been limited to noninvasive studies of pulmonary mechanics (ie, it has not been possible to measure esophageal or gastric pressures using a nasogastric catheter). In the D-2 and Euromir 95 studies [40], the abdominal contribution to tidal volume was seen to increase from 31% to 58% (that is, the rib cage contribution decreased), consistent with the results from the KC-135.

Pulmonary ventilation

Gravity is known to have marked effects on the distribution of ventilation in the upright human lung. The weight of the lung itself causes the lower zones to be, relatively speaking, compressed and the upper zones expanded. When lung volume increases, the lower regions are on a steeper portion of the pulmonary compliance curve, so, for a given change in overall lung volume, the lower regions expand more than the upper. Thus, ventilation to the lower portions of the lung is greater than to the upper [1–3] and given the smaller resting alveolar volume at the bottom of the lung [4], the ventilation per unit lung volume also is high.

The inhomogeneity of pulmonary ventilation is known to result from two major sources. The first is recognized commonly and termed convective-dependent inhomogeneity (CDI). CDI results from two regions of lung having different amounts of ventilation per unit lung volume (specific ventilation). CDI may result from gravitational and nongravitational effects. The second source is diffusion–convective-dependent inhomogeneity (DCDI). This is a complex interaction between the convective and diffusive transport of gas in the branching structure of the lung [47]. Because it depends on the interaction between convection and diffusion, DCDI is only operative when these two mechanisms are of a similar magnitude. This condition is met when the convective velocity of the inhaled gas decreases to an appropriate level as the total cross-sectional area of the airways increases with each successive generation. In humans, DCDI is only operative at approximately the level of the entry of the acinus. Thus, DCDI can be thought of as small-scale inhomogeneity, whereas CDI necessarily is observed at a scale larger than this (because even if CDI were present within the acinus, diffusive transport abolishes any concentration gradients it establishes). Both of these mechanisms contribute to the sloping alveolar plateau (phase III) seen in single-breath washout (SBW) and multiple-breath washout (MBW) tests.

SBWs have been performed several times in μG. The first was in parabolic flight when Michels and West [16] showed that there were marked reductions in the main markers of inter-regional inhomogeneity, cardiogenic oscillation size, and the terminal rise in nitrogen concentration after a VC inspiration of pure oxygen. Such reductions are consistent with a reduction or removal of top-to-bottom differences in ventilation. Michels and West, however, showed that these markers of inhomogeneity persist in μG. The question that could not be resolved was whether or not the preceding period of hypergravity necessary to fly the parabolic maneuvers resulted in residual inhomogeneities in the μG phase.

During SLS-1, Guy and colleagues [48] performed VC single-breath nitrogen washout tests on the seven-member crew. These tests also contained a small argon bolus inhaled at RV to provide information on airway closure. The results largely confirmed those from parabolic flight, with marked reductions in the height of the terminal rise in nitrogen and in cardiogenic oscillations, but a clear persistence nevertheless, suggesting a strong role of gravity in the normal inhomogeneity of ventilation but with considerable influence as a result of nongravitational factors. Of particular interest is the observation that airway closure, often considered a gravitational phenomenon, still occurred at a similar lung volume in μG, although clearly this was not closure of the gravitationally dependent regions of the lung seen in 1 G. The onset of airway closure occurred at the same absolute lung volume in 1 G and in μG, suggesting that some units reach the point of zero elastic recoil at a similar absolute lung volume regardless of the gravitational distortion of the lung. This concept is consistent with the suggestion of patchy airway closure suggested by Engel and coworkers [49].

The other commonly used means of studying the inhomogenity of pulmonary ventilation is the MBW, where nitrogen is eliminated over a series of breaths. The potential advantage of this is that the breaths used are much smaller than the VC maneuvers used in the SBW tests and more closely approximate those of normal breathing. MBW tests performed during SLS-1 were analyzed in six different ways to assess the degree of change in ventilatory inhomogeneity [50]. There were few significant changes seen between the standing data and those collected in μG, although there were increases in the degree of inhomogeneity seen in the supine position. This surprising result leads to the conclusion that the primary determinants of ventilatory inhomogeneity during tidal breathing in the upright posture were not primarily gravitational in origin.

In analysis of the data collected during rebreathing tests performed on D-2, Verbanck and colleagues [51] show that the degree of gravity-independent inhomogeneity of specific ventilation was at least as large as the gravity-dependent inhomogeneity of specific ventilation. Given the results from SBW and MBW, this result added to the considerable weight of evidence that much of the inhomogeneity of ventilation seen in 1 G likely was the result of differences in the behavior of different regions of the lung, largely independent of the effects of gravity.

SBW performed in SLS-1 [48] also confirmed the previous observation made in parabolic flight [16], namely that phase III slope was reduced only slightly by the removal of gravity. Although CDI effects in conjunction with asynchronous emptying of different lung regions contribute to phase III slope, various studies [52] suggest that approximately only one quarter of the observed phase III slope in normal subjects was the result of CDI. Other studies [53] show that the continued exchange of respiratory gases in the lung made a further approximately 10% contribution to phase III slope, leaving the bulk of the slope the result of DCDI effects. The observations in SLS-1 show that phase III slope for nitrogen in μG was approximately 75% of that seen standing in 1 G [48].

Although there was good reason to suspect that CDI should be subject to considerable alteration in μG, there generally was no consideration that DCDI should be affected. Although approximately 95% of the lung volume is contained in the acini, each acinus is a physically small structure and the effects of gravity on that structure were believed minimal. It is only at this level in the human lung, where a quasistationary concentration front forms as diffusion takes over from convection as the primary gas transport mechanism, that DCDI effects are prominent. DCDI effects can be studied by performing

SBW in which trace quantities of helium and sulfur hexafluoride are included in the test gas used for inspiration. Because of the wide difference in molecular weight (4 versus 146) between these gases, there is a marked difference in gas diffusivity, with helium diffusing approximately six times more readily than sulfur hexafluoride. In 1 G, this difference in diffusivity results in the phase III slope for sulfur hexafluoride considerably steeper than that for helium. There are two causes for this. First, the transport of the more diffusible helium becomes dominated by diffusion at a point in the airways more proximal (central) than does the less diffusible sulfur hexafluoride. Because the structure of the human acinus is such that the more peripheral branch points subtend a more asymmetric structure than the more central [54], and because this greater asymmetry increases the DCDI effect, sulfur hexafluoride exhibits a steeper slope than does helium. Second, the more rapid diffusion of helium serves to abolish concentration gradients established by CDI or DCDI, flattening the helium slope more than the sulfur hexafluoride slope [55].

During D-2 and SLS-2, SBWs were performed in which trace quantities of helium and sulfur hexafluoride were included in the inspiratory gas. In both cases, there was a flattening of the phase III slopes for both gases but, surprisingly, the magnitude of the effect was such that helium and sulfur hexafluoride slope became the same in μG [56,57]. Even more extreme were the results in which a breath hold also was performed, in which case the phase III slope for sulfur hexafluoride actually became flatter than that for helium [56]. The only other known example of the sulfur hexafluoride slope becoming flatter than the helium slope was in heart-lung transplant recipients undergoing acute rejection episodes. In that case, conformational changes near the entrance of the acinus, possibly as a result of acute inflammation, steepened the helium slope [58]. Lung inflammation clearly was not the cause in μG, and the phase III slope difference had returned to preflight values within 6 to 10 hours of the landing of SLS-2. The results from μG suggest that a conformational change in the structure of the acinus was responsible or, perhaps, changes in cardiogenic mixing altering the position or extent of the quasistationary concentration front. No actual mechanism could be identified, however.

One difficulty with the space flight results was that it was not possible to determine if the changes in sulfur hexafluoride–helium slope difference arose from a relative steeping of the helium slope (implying more central changes) or a relative flattening of the

sulfur hexafluoride slope (implying more peripheral changes). Lauzon and coworkers [59] performed the same helium–sulfur hexafluoride SBW tests in parabolic flight in an attempt to shed light on the space flight results. They studied eight subjects, one of whom was a member of the SLS-2 subject pool. In the 25 seconds of μG available in the KC-135, however, the phase III slope difference between sulfur hexafluoride and helium increased, as opposed to the decrease seen in sustained μG (Fig. 3). It was observed, however, that the differences resulted from differences in the behavior of the more diffusible helium, whereas sulfur hexafluoride behaved similarly in space flight and parabolic flight. The implication from these experiments is that the surprising results seen in sustained μG result from changes in peripheral gas mixing in the lung, likely at the level of the entrance of the acinus, where the effects predominate in the behavior of helium. Whatever the cause, it has a time constant greater than approximately half a minute of μG available in parabolic flight, yet less than approximately 6 to 10 hours, by which time the postflight measurements returned to normal [56]. Several attempts to replicate these

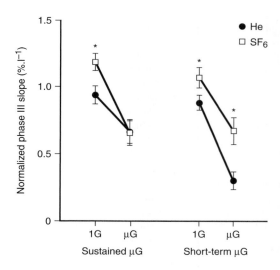

Fig. 3. Normalized phase III slopes of helium (He; ●) and sulfur hexafluoride (SF$_6$; □) from space flight mission, subjects standing in 1 G and during sustained μG, and from short-term μG study, subjects sitting in 1 G and during short-term μG. *, sulfur hexafluoride slope significantly different from that of helium ($P < 0.05$). (*From* Lauzon A-M, Prisk GK, Elliott AR, et al. Paradoxical helium and sulfur hexafluoride single-breath washouts in short-term vs. sustained microgravity. J Appl Physiol 1997;82:861; with permission.)

observations in conditions other than space flight largely have been unsuccessful, but studies point to the importance of the contributions of events near residual volume (presumably associated with airway closure) on phase III slope [60]. Recent observations in steep (60°) HDT suggest a possible role of changes in lung hydration on acinar conformation [61], but these conclusions are preliminary at best.

During SLS-2, MBW using helium and sulfur hexafluoride also were performed [62]. During the SLS-1 MBW, there was a change in absolute lung volume at which the tests were performed, and this confounding effect was eliminated from the SLS-2 study and the results largely confirmed those of the previous study. CDI largely was unaltered between 1 G and μG, in line with the SLS-1 study [50], and the sulfur hexafluoride–helium slope difference was reduced (although in these smaller volume breaths, not abolished), similar to that seen in the SBW study [56]. Of particular note, however, was the partitioning of the rise of phase III slope with breath number. It has previously been shown [63,64] that the effects of CDI and DCDI produce a marked difference in the rise of phase III slope with breath number. This difference allows the relative contributions of CDI and DCDI to overall gas mixing to be determined [65,66]. Although the SLS-2 results were somewhat noisy, such partitioning showed that for nitrogen and sulfur hexafluoride, both of which have relatively distal quasistationary diffusion fronts, there was little difference in the contribution of CDI to overall inhomogeneity between 1 G and μG. For helium, however, with a more proximal front, the CDI contribution was abolished in μG (Fig. 4). This suggests that the CDI seen to persist in μG must be located between units that are sufficiently close such that diffusion of helium, but not of nitrogen or sulfur hexafluoride, is an efficient means of reducing the concentration gradients it produces. Thus, the non-gravitational CDI must exist between acini or between groups of a few acini. This is the first instance where it has been possible to estimate the size of the structures responsible for the inhomogeneity of ventilation in μG.

Cardiac output

Various descriptions of what would happen to overall pulmonary blood flow in μG were postulated. For example, it was proposed that stroke volume would rise (to an unknown degree) in the first 24 hours of flight and then decrease to 15% below ground control values thereafter. Cardiac output would, however, remain unchanged [67].

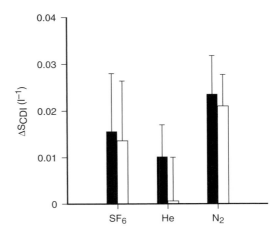

Fig. 4. CDI (ΔS_{cdi}) calculated from the normalized phase III slopes of MBWs of sulfur hexafluoride (SF_6), helium (He), and nitrogen (N_2). Standing position (*filled bars*); μG (*open bars*). (*From* Prisk GK, Elliott AR, Guy HJB, et al. Multiple-breath washin of helium and sulfur hexafluoride in sustained microgravity. J Appl Physiol 1998;84:248; with permission.)

The first direct measurements of pulmonary blood flow using soluble gas rebreathing were made during SLS-1 in 1991. Seven subjects were studied over the course of a 9-day mission. Cardiac output was seen to rise by approximately 35% above preflight standing levels 24 hours after the onset of μG and then decrease over the course of the μG exposure. This was accompanied by a slight bradycardia and, as a result, stroke volume increased by 60% to 70% early in flight and also showed a subsequent decrease [68]. Subsequent measurements on D-2 [26] and on later flights [14] confirmed the SLS-1 measurements. Similar results were obtained using an independent technique of carbon dioxide rebreathing on SLS-1 and SLS-2 and showed an overall 26% increase in cardiac output at rest in μG [69] and a 55% increase in cardiac stroke volume. The data suggest, however, that cardiac output rises after approximately 2 weeks in μG (Fig. 5) [14], resulting from an increase in heart rate in the face of a constant stroke volume. Similar effects were observed in 17 days of HDT, but to date there are no studies of longer duration μG to support these observations. One study of long-duration HDT showed a slight (not significant) reduction in cardiac output after 113 days, but there were no data from early in tilt for comparison [70].

The data measured from soluble gas rebreathing were confirmed by echocardiographic measurements made during SLS-1 [71], which showed increases in cardiac dimensions and stroke volume of a similar

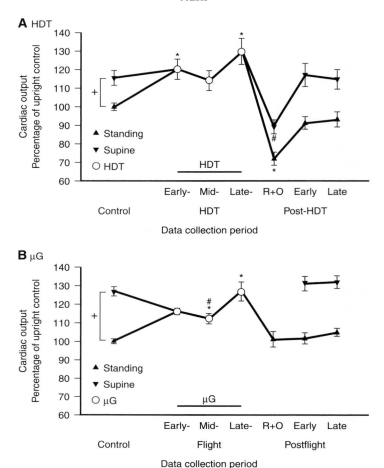

Fig. 5. Cardiac output during 17 days of 6° HDT in 1 G (*A*) and in space flights of 14 to 17 days' duration (*B*). Note the similar response with an initial rise and a subsequent reduction in cardiac output at the mid point (approximately 1 week). There is a subsequent rise in cardiac output resulting from an increase in heart rate (initially depressed in HDT and μG) with no change in stroke volume (stable from the midpoint on). There are no data available for longer duration exposure to μG. (*From* Prisk GK, Fine JM, Elliott AR, et al. Effect of 6° head-down tilt on cardiopulmonary function: comparison with microgravity. Aviat Space Environ Med 2002;73:11; with permission.)

magnitude. It is of particular interest, however, that these increases in cardiac output occurred in the face of significant decreases in cardiac filling pressures inferred from central venous pressure (CVP). Measurements made on SLS-1 and SLS-2 using fluid-filled catheters [72] and independently on D-2 using pressure-tip catheters [73] positioned in the superior vena cava show convincingly that contrary to expectations, CVP falls in μG. A decrease in filling pressure in conjunction with increases in cardiac output necessarily implies a change in cardiac compliance. Because the changes in CVP occur within seconds of the removal of gravity as evidenced by studies in

parabolic flight [74], it seems highly unlikely that there is any change in cardiac muscle performance per se. Thus, the change implies that cardiac transmural pressure must have increased, presumably because of a decrease in extracardiac pressure. The fact that lung volume actually decreases slightly on entry into μG (suggesting an overall increase in pleural pressure) indicates that local pressure changes must be considered when considering cardiac performance [75]. Similar changes in intravascular pressures have been seen in the KC-135 [76], although a clear understanding of the seemingly contradictory results is not yet available.

Diffusing capacity and lung water

Pulmonary diffusing capacity for carbon monoxide (DLCO) measured using the single-breath technique rose substantially (by 28%) on exposure to μG and remained elevated over the course of 9-day flight [68]. This was a result of parallel increase in pulmonary capillary blood volume (Vc), which rose by 28%, and in membrane-diffusing capacity (Dm), which rose by 27%. Qualitatively similar results were obtained on a subsequent mission using a rebreathing technique [26]. In both cases, there was a rapid return to preflight conditions after return to 1 G.

The possibility of pulmonary edema formation in μG caused by a headward shift of fluid, and what was at the time a presumed increase in CVP, is suggested by Permutt [77]. The increases of DLCO and Dm [68], however, with no change in either parameter over the course of a 9-day flight, suggest that pulmonary edema does not occur in μG. If edema had occurred, a decrease in either DLCO or Dm would have been expected early in flight with possible increases later as the edema resolved, but this was not the case.

The changes in DLCO and its components were attributed to the transition of the lung from its zone 1, 2, 3 configuration to a situation in which it was entirely in either zone 2 or zone 3 (see later discussion of pulmonary perfusion) [68]. This results in a more uniform filling of the pulmonary capillary bed with an attendant increase in the surface area available for gas exchange. Studies in parabolic flight to examine the acute transition to μG showed qualitatively similar results. In that circumstance, however, the magnitude of the changes was much greater than those seen in sustained μG with DLCO increasing by 61% and Dm and Vc by 47% and 71%, respectively [78]. Once again, however, the period of hypergravity preceding μG may have affected these results. Nevertheless, it is clear that there is more uniform filling of the pulmonary capillary bed in μG than in 1 G.

Perhaps more compelling in the context of the possibility of the formation of pulmonary edema in μG are the changes in pulmonary tissue volume recorded during D-2 [26]. Pulmonary tissue volume is known to be a parameter sensitive to extravascular fluid in the lungs [79]. Pulmonary tissue volume was unchanged after 24 hours of μG and was 20% to 25% lower after 9 days, despite increases in thoracic blood volume [80–82]. These results are consistent with observations of the low compliance of the pulmonary interstitium [83,84], which, in the presence of a fall in CVP [72,73] is expected to result in a grad-ual reduction in fluid in these tissues. In addition, the reduction in circulating plasma volume as the subjects adapt to μG [24] also may contribute.

Pulmonary perfusion

Gravity long has been known to have a strong influence on the distribution of pulmonary perfusion. In the late 1950s and early 1960s, West and coworkers directly measured the pulmonary blood flow at different heights in the upright human [7,8]. These studies showed that although blood flow was large at the bottom of the lung, under resting conditions, it was virtually absent at the top. This led to the development of the widely used zone 1, 2, 3 model [8]. In this, regional pulmonary blood flow is determined by the relationship between pulmonary vascular pressure and alveolar pressure. At the bottom of the lung, pulmonary arterial and venous pressure exceed alveolar pressure, so blood flow is determined by the difference between the arterial and venous sides. The increase in flow toward the lower portion of this zone is attributed to distension of the pulmonary vessels, resulting from increasing hydrostatic pressure toward the bottom of the lung. This is termed zone 3. In contrast, at the top of the lung, the situation can exist where alveolar pressure exceeds venous and arterial pressures, closing off the vessels and resulting in zero blood flow. This is termed zone 1. Between these is the situation where alveolar pressure exceeds venous pressure, zone 2 conditions. In zone 2, flow is determined by the difference between arterial and alveolar pressure. Because alveolar pressure is uniform throughout the lung, blood flow varies with the hydrostatic gradient in arterial pressure and is strongly gravity dependent. More recently, studies show that, at least in some species, nongravitational factors also are important [85–87] and that there is nongravitational inhomogeneity of pulmonary blood flow in human lungs [88].

There are no direct measurements of the distribution of pulmonary blood flow during space flight, principally because of the technical challenges such measurements entail. The earliest imaging of pulmonary perfusion in μG was performed after parabolic flight in an F-100 jet during which radioactively labeled microaggregated albumen was injected into the subjects during the weightless portion of the flight [89]. These studies showed some increase in apical blood flow in μG compared with the upright position in 1 G. Similar studies in pigs using fluorescent microspheres have been performed in parabolic flight [90], showing a clear influence of gravity, albeit with a considerable degree of anatomic (nongravitational) influence also.

An indirect technique originally used in parabolic flight [16] allowed inferences to be made about the distribution of pulmonary blood flow. Subjects hyperventilated for 20 seconds, reducing the overall P_{CO_2} in the lungs. They then rapidly inhaled to TLC and held their breath for 15 seconds. During this breath-hold period, carbon dioxide evolves into the alveoli at a rate proportional to the blood flow per unit alveolar volume. Because the lung is at TLC, any inter-regional differences in lung volume are minimized, however, so the carbon dioxide level in a lung region becomes a marker of the perfusion of that region. At the end of the breath-hold period, the subject exhales in a controlled fashion to RV. During the exhalation, markers of inter-regional inhomogeneity, such as cardiogenic oscillations and terminal fall in carbon dioxide after the onset of airway closure, provide indications of the degree of inhomogeneity of perfusion.

In 1 G, there were prominent cardiogenic oscillations and a marked fall in carbon dioxide toward the end of exhalation [91]. These observations were consistent with the known vertical gradient of pulmonary blood flow, because the carbon dioxide near the apices of the lung, where the blood flow is lowest, is low. These are the same lung regions that continue to empty after the onset of airway closure in the gravitationally dependent regions of the lung. When the measurements were performed supine in 1 G, the height of the cardiogenic oscillations and the terminal fall were decreased to approximately 60% of that seen standing (Fig. 6). These reductions are consistent with the reduced vertical height of the lung in the supine position.

In parabolic flight, it was found that the size of the cardiogenic oscillations depended strongly on gravity, with the largest oscillation seen in 2 G [16]. The cardiogenic oscillations were not absent, however, in μG and the residual effects of the preceding period of hypergravity could not be eliminated as a possible cause. In sustained μG, the size of the cardiogenic oscillations is decreased to a similar degree to that seen supine, whereas the terminal fall is absent, confirming the observations in parabolic flight. Observations of the distribution of pulmonary ventilation (see previous discussion of pulmonary ventilation) show clearly that airway closure still occurs in μG. Thus the absence of a terminal fall of carbon dioxide means that the carbon dioxide in the regions of lung behind airways that close, and in the regions of lung behind airways that remain open, must be similar. The conclusion was that the blood flow to

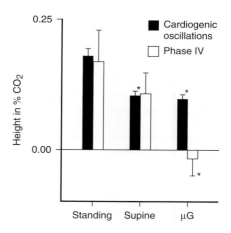

Fig. 6. Relative size of cardiogenic oscillations in carbon dioxide and height of phase IV. Values are means ± SE (n = 4). For purposes of comparison, height of phase IV (negative in 1 G) has been inverted. In μG, height of phase IV becomes disproportionately small compared with 1 G standing and 1 G supine. *, significantly different ($P < 0.05$) compared with standing. (*From* Prisk GK, Guy HJB, Elliott AR, et al. Inhomogeneity of pulmonary perfusion during sustained microgravity on SLS-1. J Appl Physiol 1994; 76:1737; with permission.)

regions that experience airway closure near RV, and regions that do not experience airway closure must be similar [91]. This is consistent with the abolition of the top to bottom gradients in blood flow present in 1 G.

The persistence of cardiogenic oscillations in μG, however, implies that there is persisting inhomogeneity of pulmonary blood flow, although this clearly is not a result of gravitational differences between the top and bottom of the lung. Although μG is expected to abolish apicobasal differences in perfusion, it does not necessarily affect inter-regional mechanisms of inhomogeneity, such as central-to-peripheral differences in blood flow [88] or inter-regional differences in vascular conductance [86], nor does μG necessarily affect the variability in lung compliance within small regions of lung [92] that may contribute to differential gas flows from different areas of the lung during the cardiac cycle. Thus, the data are consistent with the removal of apicobasal gradients in blood flow, whereas other differences, including smaller scale inhomogeneity, persist. The residual inhomogeneity must, however, be on a scale larger than the acinus, because events on that scale are not be seen at the mouth (where the measurements were made) because of different path lengths from different regions of the lung and because of diffusional mixing, which reduces differences in carbon diooxide between closely spaced regions.

The results also are consistent with observations made of pulmonary diffusing capacity and its subdivisions, Dm and Vc [68]. In those studies, the transition from 1 G to μG was associated with large increases in Dm and Vc. In contrast, the standing-to-supine transition results in a large increase in Vc, with virtually no change in Dm. The interpretation drawn from that is that in μG, the lung becomes uniformly perfused with blood, and all the pulmonary vasculature is recruited, raising Dm and Vc. This abolishes the terminal fall in carbon dioxide in the hyperventilation–breath-hold test but does not necessarily alter the presence of cardiogenic oscillations resulting from smaller regions of lung with differing perfusion.

Pulmonary gas exchange and ventilation-perfusion ratio

Measurements made during SLS-1 and SLS-2 show that oxygen consumption per unit time ($\dot{V}O_2$) and carbon dioxide production per unit time ($\dot{V}CO_2$) are unchanged by exposure to μG [93]. There are, however, changes in the parameters associated with gas exchange. Tidal volume decreased by approximately 15%, and there was a compensatory increase in breathing frequency (9%). The increase in frequency does not completely compensate for the change in tidal volume and, total ventilation decreased by approximately 7%. When the reduction in physiologic dead space (from 181 ± 3 mL standing to 137 ± 3 mL in μG), which presumably results from the removal of areas of high $\dot{V}A/\dot{Q}$, was factored in, alveolar ventilation remained unchanged in μG compared with standing in 1 G. The selection of a different combination of tidal volume and breathing frequency seems to result from the removal of the weight of the abdominal contents and shoulder girdle placing the inspiratory muscles in a different configuration. There was no evidence of significant changes in respiratory drive, with the bulk of the change in respiratory frequency accounted for by changes in expiratory time, the passive portion of the respiratory cycle. Inspiratory time (T_I/T_{TOT} [inspiratory time as a fraction of breath length]) was elevated slightly in μG (approximately 3%). Average inspiratory flow rate (V_T/T_I [tidal volume divided by inspiratory time]) was decreased in μG (approximately 10%). The opposite direction of the changes in both primary measures of respiratory drive suggest that any overall change in resting respiratory drive is small in μG.

Because there were no changes in $\dot{V}O_2$ or $\dot{V}CO_2$ in μG, the respiratory exchange ratio also was unaltered. Because the subjects were on stabilized diets for these flights and the associated ground data collection, the constancy of the respiratory exchange ratio is not surprising. Similarly there was no change in the fraction of end-tidal oxygen, but end-tidal PCO_2 ($PETCO_2$) was elevated (approximately 2.0 torr) when the data from the two flights were pooled. This resulted from the combination of no change in $PETCO_2$ in SLS-1, and a 4.5 torr increase in SLS-2. Ground control data revealed no differences in $PETCO_2$ between the two crews either standing or supine. The environmental carbon dioxide levels in the spacecraft on SLS-1 were well controlled and not significantly different from those on the ground. In SLS-2, however, environmental carbon dioxide rose by 1 to 3 torr compared with that on the ground, and this presumably led to the increase in $PETCO_2$.

There are no direct measurements of $\dot{V}A/\dot{Q}$ distribution in μG. No imaging techniques have been shown which would allow such measurements, and techniques such as the multiple inert gas elimination technique [94] are too complex and time consuming for space flight at this time. Even indirect but invasive methods, such as measuring the alveolar-arterial oxygen gradient, have not been performed in μG. There is a report of a large decrease in arterial saturation measured from arterialized capillary blood sample [95], but this is not confirmed and, given the absence of any physiologically significant changes in end-tidal gas concentrations [93], a large change in arterial content seems unlikely.

The subjects studied on SLS-1 and SLS-2 performed a controlled slow exhalation from TLC to RV after a period of air breathing. The resulting exhalation has a slope to the carbon dioxide expirogram, cardiogenic oscillations, and a terminal fall, all of which can be used as markers of inhomogeneity. During the exhalation, the intrabreath respiratory exchange ratio (intrabreath-R) can be calculated, and by comparing this to a mathematic model of gas exchange in comparable lung, the deviation from a perfect lung can be determined [96]. Thus, the range in intrabreath-R can be converted to a range of $\dot{V}A/\dot{Q}$ [97–99], and the slope of a plot of this as a function of expired volume (iV/Q [intrabreath V/Q]) correlates with the degree of $\dot{V}A/\dot{Q}$ inequality determined by the multiple inert gas elimination technique [100].

As was the case with the studies of the distribution of pulmonary perfusion, there were significant cardiogenic oscillations seen in the carbon dioxide expirogram in μG. On the basis of purely gravitational models of the inhomogenity of ventilation and perfusion, these oscillations should be absent in μG. Their continuing presence is strong evidence for continued interregional differences in $\dot{V}A/\dot{Q}$ in μG, because cardiogenic oscillations largely reflect regional differences in gas concentration [101], differences that in this case result from gas exchange.

There was a marked reduction in $\dot{V}A/\dot{Q}$ range over phase IV, consistent with the idea that the top-to-bottom gradient in $\dot{V}A/\dot{Q}$ had been abolished in μG (Fig. 7). This showed a steady progression, with the largest range in $\dot{V}A/\dot{Q}$ seen with standing and the smallest seen in μG with supine intermediate. This is what is predicted from the changes in the vertical height of the lung in the different states (in μG the entire lung is, effectively, at the same "height"). The result also is consistent with the observation that alveolar (physiologic less anatomic) dead space was reduced in μG, presumably because of a reduction in the high $\dot{V}A/\dot{Q}$ regions of the lung.

During phase III of the prolonged expiration, the portion approximating the volume range used during tidal breathing, there was no change in the range of $\dot{V}A/\dot{Q}$ between standing and μG. This result is surprising given the prior observations that μG

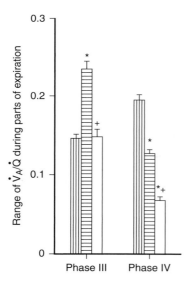

Fig. 7. Range of $\dot{V}A/\dot{Q}$ seen over phase III and phase IV of prolonged exhalations in eight subjects studied standing (*vertically lined bars*), supine (*horizontally lined bars*), and in μG (*open bars*). Values are means ± SE. Significantly different ($P < 0.05$) compared with: standing (*) and supine (+). (*From* Prisk GK, Elliott AR, Guy HJB, et al. Pulmonary gas exchange and its determinants during sustained microgravity on Spacelabs SLS-1 and SLS-2. J Appl Physiol 1995;79:1294; with permission.)

results in reduction in the topographic gradients of ventilation [48] and perfusion [91]. Thus, it seems that at lung volumes above the onset of airway closure, the principal determinants of $\dot{V}A/\dot{Q}$ inequality in normal subjects are not gravitational in origin.

Understanding the apparent paradox between reductions in the inhomogeneity of ventilation and of perfusion, with no change in the range of $\dot{V}A/\dot{Q}$, lies in a closer examination of the details of some of the measurements. Lauzon and colleagues [102] examined the phase relationships that existed between the cardiogenic oscillations in the expired gas signals measured during the SBW tests performed on SLS-2. Because the cardiogenic oscillations largely reflect regional gas concentration differences [101], the phase relationships between different gases must reflect concentration differences between different gases. Consider, for example, a nitrogen SBW test performed in 1 G that includes helium and sulfur hexafluoride in the inspirate. The bases of the lungs are better ventilated than the apices, so more of the inspired gas goes to the bases of the lung, resulting in higher concentrations of helium and sulfur hexafluoride. Because nitrogen is the resident gas and is diluted by the (nitrogen-free) inspirate, the nitrogen concentration is low in the bases of the lung. Thus, when the resulting cardiogenic oscillations are examined, helium and sulfur hexafluoride are in phase with each other, and nitrogen is out of phase with both of them. When Lauzon and coworkers [102] examined the phase relationships between carbon dioxide, a gas that is added to the alveolar space at a rate dependent on the $\dot{V}A/\dot{Q}$, they found a phase change between 1 G and μG. For example, in 1 G, carbon dioxide was in phase with helium (high carbon dioxide was associated with high helium), consistent with the gravitational model where high ventilation (the bases of the lungs) is associated with low $\dot{V}A/\dot{Q}$ (resulting in high carbon dioxide, also in the bases of the lungs). In μG, however, this phase relationship was reversed and high ventilation associated with high $\dot{V}A/\dot{Q}$.

In 1 G, gravity results in topographic gradients in $\dot{V}$ and $\dot{Q}$, but because areas of high $\dot{V}$ are associated with areas of high $\dot{Q}$, the resulting range of $\dot{V}A/\dot{Q}$ is kept to a minimum. In μG, however, the results of Lauzon and colleagues [102] show that areas of high $\dot{V}$ are associated with areas of low $\dot{Q}$ and vice versa. Thus, although the topographic gradients in $\dot{V}$ and $\dot{Q}$ are separately reduced in μG, the lack of spatial correlation between $\dot{V}$ and $\dot{Q}$ results in a wider distribution of $\dot{V}A/\dot{Q}$ than otherwise expected. Thus, it seems that gravity may impose some degree of matching of ventilation to perfusion in the normal lung.

Exercise

The ventilatory response to exercise largely is unaffected by μG. The first data come from three subjects on Skylab in the 1970s [103], although in that circumstance there were questions that arose because of the hypobaric, hyperoxic environment of Skylab [11]. When studies were performed on SLS-1 and SLS-2 [69] and on the German Spacelab flight D-2 [104], the results confirmed those found earlier and showed an essentially similar ventilatory response to exercise as that measured in 1 G. Maximum oxygen consumption seems to be maintained in short-duration flights (9–14 days), suggesting that there is no pulmonary limitation to exercise occasioned by μG [105]. This is in agreement with the improvements in DLCO seen in μG [68] and further argues against any development of pulmonary edema in μG.

Although peak $\dot{V}O_2$ is maintained in short-term μG, there is an abrupt reduction on return to 1 G of approximately 22% [69,105]. After the longer duration missions in Skylab, there were even more substantial reductions [106]. $\dot{V}O_2$ shows a return to preflight levels within 6 to 9 days of return from short-duration space flight [69,105], with the recovery in the first 2 days extremely rapid. This suggests that adjustments to the circulating blood volume of the subjects after return are a major factor.

Although the ventilatory response to exercise is similar between μG and 1 G [69,103,105], the cardiac response is not. When cardiac output and stroke volume were measured during exercise, the increases seen were less than those measured in ground control data [69]. Fig. 8 shows that during flights of 9 to 14 days duration, the cardiac output increase with increasing $\dot{V}O_2$ is substantially lower that that measured upright or supine on the ground preflight. No such data exist for long-duration space flight. This behavior is in contrast to the changes in the cardiac output response to exercise in hypergravity, where an essentially parallel shift to the right (similar to the difference between supine and standing in Fig. 8) is observed [107], highlighting the difficulty of extrapolating data from the hypergravity condition to μG. The cause for these changes is unknown, although several possibilities exist. It may be that if it is oxygen delivery that is controlled in response to exercise, as opposed to cardiac output, then the lower circulating blood volume in μG [24] and associated increase in Hb may allow maintenance of the same oxygen delivery at lower flows [69]. An alternative idea is that extra sequestration of circulatory blood volume in a more evenly filled pulmonary circulation is a factor, although the modest changes in VC [21] argue against this idea. There also may be changes in the efficiency of the muscle pump returning blood to the thorax, which may contribute [108].

Ventilatory control

In studies performed on Neurolab, a Spacelab flight focusing on neurosciences in 1998, the crew

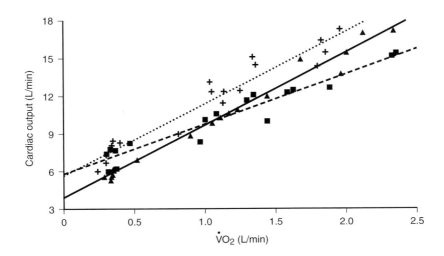

Fig. 8. Cardiac output as a function of $\dot{V}O_2$: preflight erect (*triangles* and *solid lines*); preflight supine (+ and *dotted line*); and μG (*squares* and *dashed line*). Substantial decrease in cardiac output increase in response to exercise in μG. (*Redrawn from* Shykoff BE, Farhi LE, Olszowka AJ, et al. Cardiovascular response to submaximal exercise in sustained microgravity. J Appl Physiol 1996;81:28; with permission.)

performed hypercapnic and hypoxic ventilatory challenges. µG resulted in substantial changes in the ventilatory response to hypoxia, but left the ventilatory response to carbon dioxide essentially unchanged [109].

The hypercapnic tests were performed using the rebreathing technique of Read [110] in which the subject rebreathed from a bag filled with a hyperoxic gas mixture (60% oxygen) to ensure compete abolition of any hypoxic drive. The gas in the bag had a carbon dioxide content approximating that of the mixed venous blood. As the rebreathing continues, the carbon dioxide in the bag rises as a result of metabolic production, and the resulting rise in arterial carbon dioxide stimulates the chemoreceptors. The typical response is biphasic, with little change in ventilation, as carbon dioxide rises until a break point is reached beyond which there is a brisk and essentially linear rise in ventilation as carbon dioxide levels rise. The results from Neurolab showed minor changes in the slope of the rise in ventilation with carbon dioxide (it rose by approximately 21% in µG) but other changes in the response combined to leave ventilation at a PCO_2 of 60 mm Hg unchanged (a nonsignificant rise of 0.6%). Similarly, post flight, the hypercapnic ventilatory response was unchanged compared with preflight [109].

The hypoxic ventilatory response was measured in a similar fashion using the technique of Rebuck and Campbell [111]. Subjects rebreathed from a bag initially containing a slightly hypoxic gas mixture (17% oxygen), and a carbon dioxide level approximating that of mixed-venous blood. As the rebreathing continued, the oxygen in the bag fell resulting from metabolic consumption, but the carbon dioxide was held constant by recirculation of part of the bag volume though a carbon dioxide absorber, using a computer to fix end-tidal carbon dioxide at approximately 46 mm Hg. Rebreathing continued to an inspired oxygen of 43 mm Hg. The hypoxic ventilatory response is curvilinear when plotted against PO_2, but linear when plotted against arterial oxygen saturation. Unlike the hypercapnic ventilatory response, µG approximately halved the hypoxic drive (Fig. 9). The measurements were performed 4 times preflight, 4 times inflight, and 6 times postflight. There was no adaptive component that could be seen in the data suggesting the response likely was the result of a strictly mechanical change as opposed to a slower adaptation to µG (as for example with cardiac output [see Fig. 5]). The decrease in the hypoxic response in µG was similar to that seen in the same subjects when they were placed acutely into the supine position (see Fig. 9).

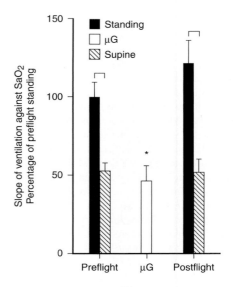

Fig. 9. Slope of the ventilatory response to hypoxia. Data collected multiple times standing and supine in 1 G and in µG. Data normalized to each subject's individual preflight control value in the standing position. Bars indicate $P < 0.05$ and * indicates $P < 0.05$ compared with preflight standing. (*From* Prisk GK, Elliott AR, West JB. Sustained microgravity reduces the human ventilatory response to hypoxia but not hypercapnia. J Appl Physiol 2000;88:1424; with permission.)

The pressure measured 100 ms after the unexpected occlusion of the inspiratory path (P_{100}) provides a good measure of ventilatory drive [112]. Simultaneous measures of inspiratory drive assessed by inspiratory occlusion pressures essentially mirrored the combined results of the hypercapnic and hypoxic responses. The similarity of the P_{100} measurements with those of the ventilatory responses, combined with lack of change in the hypercapnic response data, suggests that the changes observed were in fact the result of changes in the response, not the result of changes in the mechanical configuration of the respiratory system limiting ventilation.

The likely cause of the change in the hypoxic response is an increase in blood pressure at the level of the carotid bodies. Overall, systemic blood pressure is changed little either by the supine position or by µG [113]. In the upright position in 1 G, however, blood pressure at the carotid bodies is lower than at heart level because of the hydrostatic pressure difference. This difference is abolished in the supine position and in µG. In dogs, it is established that stimulation of the carotic baroreceptors results in an inhibition of the carotid chemoreceptor output [114]. This occurs via a central nervous system path, as

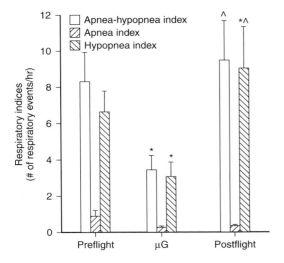

Fig. 10. Indices of sleep-disordered breathing in five subjects. *, $P < 0.05$ compared with preflight. ^, $P < 0.05$ compared with inflight. (*From* Elliott AR, Shea SA, Dijk D-J, et al. Microgravity reduces sleep-disordered breathing in normal humans. Am J Respir Crit Care Med 2001; 164:480; with permission.)

isolated studies in animals show changes in chemo-receptor output on the contralateral side of a preparation in which the pressure change was unilateral [115,116]. This effect largely has been ignored in humans, although there are some limited studies [117,118]. Given the magnitude of the reduction in hypoxic response in μG and supine (see Fig. 9), it is interesting to speculate on the possible role this may have in some hypoventilation syndromes and their postural components.

Sleep

There are reports of poor sleep in space flight [119–121], although the reasons for this remain unclear. There is a high use of hypnotics on the part of Space Shuttle crews [122], indicating poor sleep performance. As part of the Neurolab mission, comprehensive sleep recordings were made, extending previous studies of sleep in space flight [123]. One of the reasons for the studies of ventilatory control (discussed previously) is that change in ventilatory control might contribute to a greater degree of wakefulness in space flight. Discussion of why sleep is poor during space flight is beyond the scope of this review but, based on these studies, it seems that disruption to circadian rhythms by the timelines associated with short-duration flights (in which

orbital mechanics can result in "days" of more or less than 24 hours), disrupted light-dark cycles, shortened sleep periods as a result of the inflight timeline, and environmental factors all contribute [123,124]. The question of whether or not μG per se contributes to sleep disruption remains unclear.

The record is clearer with respect to respiratory-related disruptions to sleep. Full polysomnography was performed on the Neurolab crew and on one subject on a subsequent Spacehab mission (STS-95). Each subject had between 13 and 16 polysomnographic recordings, four of which were in μG [125]. Although the crew as a group was normal in terms of sleep-disordered breathing, they all experienced a small number of apneas and hypopneas. During flight, there was a significant reduction in the apnea-hypopnea index from 8.3 per hour preflight to 3.4 per hour inflight (Fig. 10). One subject who showed mild sleep-disordered breathing preflight had a reduction in apnea-hypopnea index from 22.7 per hour to 9.7 per hour inflight. There were concomitant reductions in the amount of time spent snoring.

The other striking result from these studies is in the number of electroencephalogram-based arousals from sleep. Preflight there were on average 18 arousals per hour, of which 5.5 arousals per hour could be attributed to respiratory events occurring in the 15 seconds preceding the arousal. Inflight, the number of arousals fell to 13.4 per hour almost entirely as a consequence of a 70% reduction in the number of respiratory-related arousals, which fell to only 1.8 arousals per hour (Fig. 11). Postflight arousals were reduced, but this likely is a conse-

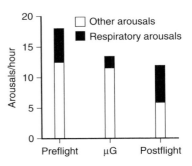

Fig. 11. Electroencephalogram-based arousals from sleep resulting from respiratory related events and all other causes. Note that the reduction in the total number of arousals in μG almost entirely is a consequence of the large reduction in the number of respiratory-related arousals. (*From* Elliott AR, Shea SA, Dijk D-J, et al. Microgravity reduces sleep-disordered breathing in normal humans. Am J Respir Crit Care Med 2001;164:481; with permission.)

quence of the altered sleep pattern of the crew caused by tiredness, as evidenced by the electroencephalogram record [124,125].

The conclusion drawn from these studies is that μG reduced sleep disordered breathing significantly, likely through the elimination of the tendency of the soft tissues of the pharynx to fall back, causing an obstructive event. Although it generally is accepted that obstructive sleep apnea has a strong gravitational component, this is first direct demonstration of that. The marked similarity of the ventilatory responses in μG to those supine in 1 G and the reduction in respiratory-related disruptions to sleep indicate that the cause of poor sleep in space flight is not related to the respiratory system.

Inhaled aerosols

It now is recognized that the deposition of aerosols from the environment in the lung is a health risk, at least in some subjects. These aerosols (often referred to as particulate matter) are the subject of recent more stringent regulation in their generation and are implicated as a risk factor in various pulmonary diseases [126] and in myocardial infarction [127]. Long-term space flight probably represents a situation in which aerosol deposition may be an important health consideration. In the spacecraft environment, the potential for significant airborne particle loads is high, because the environment is closed, and no sedimentation occurs. Some of these particles probably are contaminated and include hair, food, paint chips, synthetic fibers, and so forth. Fires aboard the spacecraft (for example, those that occurred on the Mir space station and on Salyut 7) [128] also produce large amounts of airborne particles. Similarly, μG provides for potentially high particle concentrations in the periphery of the lung, because particles that normally sediment are not removed from the airways, leaving them potentially available for transport to the alveolar regions. Thus, there may be long-term health implications to astronauts exposed to these high concentrations of particulates. In the context of future exploration missions to the moon and Mars, aerosols may be an important factor. The dust on the surface of Mars is oxidative as a result of to the ultraviolet environment and reacts in the presence of water [129]. This, combined with the low gravity environments (approximately one-sixth G on the moon and approximately one-third G on Mars), may result in a disproportionate response of the pulmonary system to such dust.

The only studies of aerosol deposition performed in μG are during parabolic flight. Hoffman and Billingham [130] studied the deposition of 2.0 μm particles during parabolic flights in parabolic flight. They saw an almost linear increase in deposition with G level over the range 0 to 2 G. They showed a lower deposition than that suggested by Beeckmans [131,132], who predicted a reduction in total deposition but an increase in deposition in the alveolar region in μG as a result of greater penetration of the particles into the lung. Muir [133] made similar predictions.

In retrospect, it seems that the predictable nature of the results of Hoffman and Billingham [130] were a result of their choice of particle size (2.0 μm). Darquenne and colleagues [134] studied the total deposition of 0.5-, 1-, 2-, and 3-μm particles in a series of KC-135 flights, making measurements at 0, 1, and approximately 1.6 G. They compared their results to predictions from existing models [135]. For measurements made in 1 or 1.6 G the results correlated closely with model predictions, with a tendency for the models to overestimate total deposition slightly. In μG, however, total deposition significantly exceeded predictions in all particles below 3 μm. The effect was greatest for 1-μm particles, where total deposition in μG was more than twice that predicted (Fig. 12). Because for 0.5- and 1-μm particles, deposition by impaction is negligible, and because in μG there is no sedimentation, only diffusion is left to account for the deposition. The conclusion drawn is that some form of "enhanced diffusion," likely the result of nonreversibilities of flow in the branching airway structure, must play a role. Importantly, there is nothing to suggest that this process is exclusively related to μG and that the hypothesized effect likely was operating in 1 G also.

Subsequently, Darquenne and colleagues [136–138] performed a series of bolus deposition studies in 0, 1, and 1.6 G. They injected approximately 70-mL boluses of aerosol particles into controlled breaths and measured the deposition of those particles and the dispersion of the bolus (a measure of convective mixing) when the boluses were inhaled to penetration volumes between 200 and 1500 mL. They found a strong dependence of deposition on gravity and on penetration volume. Importantly, dispersion continued to increase with penetration volume in μG, showing that gravity is not the only mechanism responsible for dispersion in the human lung. It seems likely that the previously hypothesized nonreversibility of flow plays a significant role in this process.

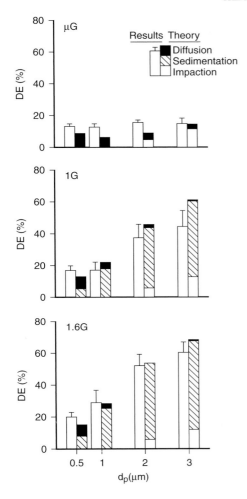

Fig. 12. Comparison between experimental data of aerosol deposition in short periods of μG in 1 G and in 1.6 G. Numeric data obtained within a 1-dimensional model. For each particle size, left bar of each pair represents experimental value and right bar of each pair represents numeric value with contribution of each mechanism of deposition: deposition by diffusion (*solid segments*); deposition by sedimentation (*hatched segments*); and deposition by impaction (*open segments*). (*From* Darquenne C, Paiva M, West JB, et al. Effect of microgravity and hypergravity on deposition of 0.5- to 3-μm-diameter aerosol in the human lung. J Appl Physiol 1997;83:2033; with permission.)

Extravehicular activity

The Space Shuttle and the ISS have a 14.7 psia (760 mm Hg) breathing air environment. Because of the need for mobility, space suits operate at a much lower pressure with a 100% oxygen environment. Therefore a denitrogenation procedure must be performed before an extravehicular activity (EVA) in the current 4.3-psia (approximately 220 mm Hg) United States space suit or the slightly higher-pressure Russian Orlon suits (5.9 psia, approximately 290 mm Hg). A direct transition from cabin pressure to suit pressure would result in decompression sickness (DCS). Risk mitigation strategies to prevent DCS in the EVA environment are prebreathing 100% oxygen for 4.0 hours while resting in the space suit; undergoing a staged decompression to 10.2 psia for 12 or more hours while breathing 26.5% oxygen, followed by a shorter prebreathe; or exercising during the initial part of an even-shorter 2-hour prebreathe [139]. In all cases, the goal of these procedures is to reduce the amount of nitrogen in the tissues before the final decompression to suit pressure.

To date, no astronaut formally has reported DCS during EVA [140,141], although at least one astronaut has reported informally symptoms in the knee on two occasions, during Gemini X and Apollo 11. This was after depressurization to a 5.0-psia cabin pressure and after several hours of prelaunch prebreathe [142,143]; it is unclear whether or not this was a case of DCS. Chamber studies on earth report at least three cases of type I DCS during EVA suit development at Johnson Space Center. Research subjects during prebreathe validation tests report DCS in substantial numbers [144]. There are many reasons why DCS may not have been reported in EVA, including the routine use of aspirin before EVA, masking of joint symptoms when working in uncomfortable space suits, repressurization at the completion of the EVA, and underreporting by the flight crew [145].

Whether or not frank DCS occurs in EVA, it is almost certain that venous gas emboli are present. In a study of prebreathes and decompressions comparable to those used during EVA, more than 50% of the participants had detectable bubbles, as indicated by Doppler ultrasound [146]. Venous gas emboli are a common finding in virtually all circumstances involving significant decompressions, and as virtually all of the venous blood passes through the lungs, the lungs act a filter for the bubbles. During ascents from deep saturation dives, these bubbles are shown to alter the range of $\dot{V}A/\dot{Q}$ in the lung significantly, as evidenced by the intrabreath measurements of iV/Q [147], presumably as a result of their embolic effects.

In a recent study performed on the ISS, astronauts performing EVA measured iV/Q before and on the day after EVA (it was impractical to perform the measurements immediately after the EVA because of the large number of other activities that had to be performed on those days). Although the results are preliminary, there was no significant change in the degree of $\dot{V}_A/\dot{Q}$ inequality in the lungs of the crew-members 24 hours after EVA, suggesting that the current denitrogenation protocols are sufficiently protective to not cause lasting harm to the lungs of the EVA crew [148]. Whether or not there is an acute effect of venous gas emboli resulting from EVA remains unknown.

Summary

Comprehensive studies of the respiratory system in μG over the past 2 decades show that although the respiratory system clearly is affected greatly by gravity, it continues to function well and in some cases, better than in 1 G. Studies to date suggest that respiratory consequences of μG are by and large benign and that the respiratory system is unlikely to limit human ability to venture beyond the near-earth environment. From a scientific standpoint, the studies are useful in elucidating the effects of gravity on the lung in the earth-bound populace.

Acknowledgments

The author thanks Manuel Paiva, Sylvia Verbanck, Chantal Darquenne, and John West for critical reading of the manuscript.

References

[1] Milic-Emili J, Henderson JAM, Dolovich MB, et al. Regional distribution of inspired gas in the lung. J Appl Physiol 1966;21:749–59.

[2] Bryan AC, Milic-Emili J, Pengelly D. Effect of gravity on the distribution of pulmonary ventilation. J Appl Physiol 1966;21:778–84.

[3] Kaneko K, Milic-Emili J, Dolovich MB, et al. Regional distribution of ventilation and perfusion as a function of body positon. J Appl Physiol 1966;21:767–77.

[4] Glazier JB, Hughes JMB, Maloney JE, et al. Vertical gradient of alveolar size in lungs of dogs frozen intact. J Appl Physiol 1967;23:694–705.

[5] Hoppin FG, Green ID, Mead J. Distribution of pleural surface pressure in dogs. J Appl Physiol 1969;27:863–73.

[6] West JB, Matthews FL. Stresses, strains, surface pressures in the lung caused by its weight. J Appl Physiol 1972;31:332–45.

[7] West JB, Dollery CT. Distribution of blood flow and ventilation-perfusion ratio in the lung, measured with radioactive CO_2. J Appl Physiol 1960;15:405–10.

[8] West JB, Dollery CT, Naimark A. Distribution of bloodflow in isolated lung: relation to vascular and alveolar pressures. J Appl Physiol 1964;19:713–24.

[9] West JB. Regional differences in gas exchange in the lung of erect man. J Appl Physiol 1962;17:893–8.

[10] Sawin CF, Nicogossian AE, Rummel JA, et al. Pulmonary function evaluation during the Skylab and Apollo-Soyuz Missions. Aviat Space Environ Med 1976;47:168–72.

[11] Robertson WG, McRae GL. Study of man during a 56-day exposure to an oxygen-helium atmosphere at 258 mm Hg total pressure. VII. Respiratory function. Aerosp Med 1966;37:453–6.

[12] Nicogossian AE. Microgravity simulations and analogues. In: Nicogossian AE, Huntoon CL, Pool SL, editors. Space physiology and medicine. Philadelphia: Lea & Febiger; 1994. p. 363–71.

[13] Derion T, Guy HJB, Tsukimoto K, et al. Ventilation-perfusion relationships in the lung during head-out water immersion. J Appl Physiol 1992;72:64–72.

[14] Prisk GK, Fine JM, Elliott AR, et al. Effect of 6° head-down tilt on cardiopulmonary function: comparison with microgravity. Aviat Space Environ Med 2002;73:8–16.

[15] Greenleaf JE. Physiological responses to prolonged bed rest and fluid immersion in humans. J Appl Physiol 1984;57:619–33.

[16] Michels DB, West JB. Distribution of pulmonary ventilation and perfusion during short periods of weightlessness. J Appl Physiol 1978;45:987–98.

[17] Michels DB, Friedman PJ, West JB. Radiographic comparison of human lung shape during normal gravity and weightlessness. J Appl Physiol 1979;47:851–7.

[18] Paiva M, Estenne M, Engel LA. Lung volumes, chest wall configuration, and pattern of breathing in microgravity. J Appl Physiol 1989;67:1542–50.

[19] Guy HJB, Prisk GK, Elliott AR, et al. Maximum expiratory flow-volume curves during short periods of microgravity. J Appl Physiol 1991;70:2587–96.

[20] Foley MF, Tomashefski JF. Pulmonary function during zero-gravity maneuvers. Aerosp Med 1969;40:655–7.

[21] Elliott AR, Prisk GK, Guy HJB, et al. Lung volumes during sustained microgravity on Spacelab SLS-1. J Appl Physiol 1994;77:2005–14.

[22] Elliott AR, Prisk GK, Guy HJB, et al. Forced expirations and maximum expiratory flow-volume curves during sustained microgravity on SLS-1. J Appl Physiol 1996;81:33–43.

[23] Buckey JC, Gaffney FA, Lane LD, et al. Central venous pressure in space. N Engl J Med 1993;328:1853–4.

[24] Alfrey CP, Udden MM, Leach-Huntoon C, et al. Control of red blood cell mass in spaceflight. J Appl Physiol 1996;81:98–104.

[25] Agostoni E, Mead J. Statics of the respiratory system. In: Fenn WO, Rahn H, editors. Handbook of physiology, section 3: respiration, volume 1. Wash-

ington (DC): American Physiological Society; 1964. p. 387–428.

[26] Verbanck S, Larsson H, Linnarsson D, et al. Pulmonary tissue volume, cardiac output, and diffusing capacity in sustained microgravity. J Appl Physiol 1997;83:810–6.

[27] von Baumgarten RJ, Baldrighi G, Vogel H, et al. Physiological response to hyper- and hypogravity during rollercoaster flight. Aviat Space Environ Med 1980;51:145–54.

[28] Wetzig J, Von Baumgarten R. Respiratory parameters aboard an aircraft performing parabolic flights. Proc Third Eur Symp Life Sci Res Space 1987;271: 47–50.

[29] Wilson TA, Liu S. Effect of acceleration on the chest wall. J Appl Physiol 1994;76:1242–6.

[30] Agostoni E, Gurtner G, Torri G, et al. Respiratory mechanics during submersion and negative-pressure breathing. J Appl Physiol 1966;21:251–8.

[31] Tenney SM. Fluid volume redistribution and thoracic volume changes during recumbency. J Appl Physiol 1959;14:129–32.

[32] Buono MJ. Effect of central vascular engorgement and immersion on various lung volumes. J Appl Physiol 1983;54:1094–6.

[33] Burki NK. Effects of immersion to water and changes in intrathoracic blood volume on lung function in man. Clin Sci Mol Med 1976;51:303–11.

[34] Robertson Jr CH, Engle CM, Bradley ME. Lung volumes in man immersed to the neck: dilution and plethysmographic techniques. J Appl Physiol 1978; 44:679–81.

[35] Sybrecht GW, Garrett L, Anthonisen NR. Effect of chest strapping on regional lung function. J Appl Physiol 1975;39:707–13.

[36] Milic-Emili J. Static distribution of lung volumes. Handbook of physiology. The respiratory system. Mechanics of breathing, section 3, volume III, part 2. Bethesda (MD): American Physiological Society; 1986.

[37] Bettinelli D, Kays C, Bailliart O, et al. Effect of gravity and posture on lung mechanics. J Appl Physiol 2002;93:2044–52.

[38] Castile R, Mead J, Jackson A, et al. Effects of posture and on flow-volume curve configuration in normal humans. J Appl Physiol 1982;53:1175–83.

[39] Prefaut C, Lupi HE, Anthonisen NR. Human lung mechanics during water immersion. J Appl Physiol 1976;40:320–3.

[40] Wantier M, Estenne M, Verbanck S, et al. Chest wall mechanics in sustained microgravity. J Appl Physiol 1998;84:2060–5.

[41] Edyvean J, Estenne M, Paiva M, et al. Lung and chest wall mechanics in microgravity. J Appl Physiol 1991; 71:1956–66.

[42] de Troyer A. Respiratory muscles. In: Crystal RG, West JB, editors. The lung, volume 1. New York: Raven Press; 1991. p. 869–83.

[43] Estenne M, Gorini M, Van Muylem A, et al. Rib cage shape and motion in microgravity. J Appl Physiol 1992;73:946–54.

[44] Green M, Mead J, Sears TA. Muscle activity during chest wall restriction and positive pressure breathing in man. Respir Physiol 1978;35:283–300.

[45] Estenne M. Lung volumes and chest wall mechanics. In: Prisk GK, Paiva M, West JB, editors. Gravity and the lung: lessons from microgravity. New York: Marcel Dekker; 2001. p. 75–92.

[46] Bettinelli D, Kays C, Bailliart O, et al. Effect of gravity on chest wall mechanics. J Appl Physiol 2002;92:709–16.

[47] Paiva M, Engel LA. The anatomical basis for the sloping N_2 alveolar plateau. Respir Physiol 1981;44: 325–37.

[48] Guy HJB, Prisk GK, Elliott AR, et al. Inhomogeneity of pulmonary ventilation during sustained microgravity as determined by single-breath washouts. J Appl Physiol 1994;76:1719–29.

[49] Engel LA, Grassino A, Anthonisen NR. Demonstration of airway closure in man. J Appl Physiol 1975; 38:1117–25.

[50] Prisk GK, Guy HJB, Elliott AR, et al. Ventilatory inhomogeneity determined from multiple-breath washouts during sustained microgravity on Spacelab SLS-1. J Appl Physiol 1995;78:597–607.

[51] Verbanck S, Linnarsson D, Prisk GK, et al. Specific ventilation distribution in microgravity. J Appl Physiol 1996;80:1458–65.

[52] Crawford ABH, Makowska M, Paiva M, et al. Convection-and diffusion-dependent ventilation maldistribution in normal subjects. J Appl Physiol 1985;59:838–46.

[53] Cormier Y, Bélanger J. Quantification of the effect of gas exchange on the slope of phase III. Bull Eur Physiopathol Respir 1983;19:13–6.

[54] Haefeli-Bleuer B, Weibel ER. Morphometry of the human pulmonary acinus. Anat Rec 1988;220:401–14.

[55] Verbanck S, Weibel ER, Paiva M. Simulations of washout experiments in postmortem rat lung. J Appl Physiol 1993;75:441–51.

[56] Prisk GK, Lauzon A-M, Verbanck S, et al. Anomalous behavior of helium and sulfur hexafluoride during single-breath tests in sustained microgravity. J Appl Physiol 1996;80:1126–32.

[57] Verbanck S, Prisk GK, Guy HJB, et al. Ventilation distribution and chest wall mechanics in microgravity AR-RMS3. In: Sahm PR, Keller MH, Schiewe B, editors. Proceedings of the Norderney Symposium on Scientific Results of the German Spacelab Mission D-2. DLR Koln (Germany): WPF; 1995. p. 754–9.

[58] Van Muylem A, DeVuyst P, Yernault J-C, et al. Inert gas single-breath washout and structural alteration of respiratory bronchioles. Am Rev Respir Dis 1992; 146:1167–72.

[59] Lauzon A-M, Prisk GK, Elliott AR, et al. Paradoxical helium and sulfur hexafluoride single-breath washouts in short-term vs. sustained microgravity. J Appl Physiol 1997;82:859–65.

[60] Dutrieue B, Lauzon A-M, Verbanck S, et al. Helium and sulfur hexafluoride bolus washin in short-term microgravity. J Appl Physiol 1999;86:1594–602.

[61] Olfert IM, Prisk GK. Effect of 60 degrees head-down tilt on peripheral gas mixing in the human lung. J Appl Physiol 2004;97(3):827–34.

[62] Prisk GK, Elliott AR, Guy HJB, et al. Multiple-breath washin of helium and sulfur hexafluoride in sustained microgravity. J Appl Physiol 1998;84: 244–52.

[63] Crawford ABH, Kelly S, Makowska M, et al. Functional localisation of ventilation inhomogeneity during tidal breathing [abstract]. Am Rev Respir Dis 1985;131:310.

[64] Crawford ABH, Makowska M, Engel LA. Effect of atropine on static mechanical properties of the lung and ventilation distribution. J Appl Physiol 1987;63: 2278–85.

[65] Verbanck S, Schuermans D, Van Muylem A, et al. Conductive and acinar lung-zone contributions to ventilation inhomogeneity in COPD. Am J Respir Crit Care Med 1998;157(5 Pt 1):1573–7.

[66] Verbanck S, Schuermans D, Noppen M, et al. Evidence of acinar airway improvement in asthma. Am J Respir Crit Care Med 1999;159:1545–50.

[67] Nicogossian A. Overall physiological response to space flight. In: Nicogossian A, editor. Space physiology and medicine. Philadelphia: Lea and Febiger; 1989. p. 213–27.

[68] Prisk GK, Guy HJB, Elliott AR, et al. Pulmonary diffusing capacity, capillary blood volume and cardiac output during sustained microgravity. J Appl Physiol 1993;75:15–26.

[69] Shykoff BE, Farhi LE, Olszowka AJ, et al. Cardio-vascular response to submaximal exercise in sustained microgravity. J Appl Physiol 1996;81:26–32.

[70] Montmerle S, Spaak J, Linnarsson D. Lung function during and after prolonged head-down bed rest. J Appl Physiol 2002;92:75–83.

[71] Buckey Jr JC, Lane LD, Levine BD, et al. Orthostatic intolerance after spaceflight. J Appl Physiol 1996;81: 7–18.

[72] Buckey Jr JC, Gaffney FA, Lane LD, et al. Central venous pressure in space. J Appl Physiol 1996;81: 19–25.

[73] Foldager N, Andersen TAE, Jessen FB, et al. Central venous pressure during microgravity. In: Wissen-schaftliche Projectführung D-2, editor. German Spacelab Mission D-2 results. Cologne (Germany): German Aerospace Research Establishment (DLR); 1994. p. 695–6.

[74] Videbaek R, Norsk P. Atrial distension in humans during microgravity induced by parabolic flights. J Appl Physiol 1997;83:1862–6.

[75] West JB, Prisk GK. Chest volume and shape and intrapleural pressure in microgravity [letter]. J Appl Physiol 1999;87:1240–1.

[76] Latham RD, Fenton JW, Vernalis MN, et al. Central circulatory hemodynamics in non human primates during microgravity induced by parabolic flight. Adv Space Res 1994;14:349–58.

[77] Permutt S. Pulmonary circulation and the distribution of blood and gas in the lungs. Physiology in the space environment. Washington (DC): NAS NRC 1485B; 1967.

[78] Vaida P, Kays C, Rivière D, et al. Pulmonary diffusing capacity and pulmonary capillary blood volume during parabolic flights. J Appl Physiol 1997; 82:1091–7.

[79] Petrini MF, Peterson BT, Hyde RW. Lung tissue volume and blood flow by rebreathing: theory. J Appl Physiol 1978;44:795–802.

[80] Baisch FJ. Fluid distribution in man in space and effect of lower body negative pressure treatment. Clin Investig 1993;71:690–9.

[81] Kirsch KA, Baartz FJ, Gunga HC, et al. Fluid shifts into and out of superficial tissues under microgravity and terrestrial conditions. Clin Investig 1993;71: 687–9.

[82] Norsk P, Epstein M. Manned space flight and the kidney. Am J Nephrol 1991;11:81–97.

[83] Miserocchi G, Negrini D, Del Fabbro M, et al. Pulmonary interstitial pressure in intact in situ lung: transition to interstitial edema. J Appl Physiol 1993;74:1171–7.

[84] Negrini D, Miserocchi G. Pulmonary interstitial fluid balance. In: Prisk GK, Paiva M, West JB, editors. Gravity and the lung: lessons from microgravity. New York: Marcel Dekker; 2001. p. 255–70.

[85] Glenny RW, Robertson HT. Fractal properties of pulmonary blood flow: characterization of spatial heterogeneity. J Appl Physiol 1990;69:532–45.

[86] Beck KC, Rehder K. Differences in regional vascular conductances in isolated dog lung. J Appl Physiol 1986;61:530–8.

[87] Wagner PD, McRae J, Read J. Stratified distribution of blood flow in secondary lobule of the rat lung. J Appl Physiol 1967;22:1115–23.

[88] Hakim TS, Lisbona R, Dean GW. Gravity-independent inequality of pulmonary blood flow in humans. J Appl Physiol 1987;63:1114–21.

[89] Stone HL, Warren BH, Wager H. The distribution of pulmonary blood flow in human subjects during zero-G. AGARD Conf Proc 1965;2:129–48.

[90] Glenny RW, Lamm WJE, Bernard SL, et al. Redistribution of pulmonary perfusion during weightlessness and increased gravity. J Appl Physiol 2000;89:1239–48.

[91] Prisk GK, Guy HJB, Elliott AR, et al. Inhomogeneity of pulmonary perfusion during sustained microgravity on SLS-1. J Appl Physiol 1994;76:1730–8.

[92] Olson LE, Rodarte JR. Regional differences in expansion in excised dog lung lobes. J Appl Physiol 1984;57:1710–4.

[93] Prisk GK, Elliott AR, Guy HJB, et al. Pulmonary gas exchange and its determinants during sustained microgravity on Spacelabs SLS-1 and SLS-2. J Appl Physiol 1995;79:1290–8.

[94] Wagner PD, Saltzman HA, West JB. Measurement of continuous distributions of ventilation-perfusion ratios: theory. J Appl Physiol 1974;36:588–99.

[95] Haase H, Baranov VM, Asyamolova NM, et al. First results of PO_2 examinations in the capillary blood of cosmonauts during a long-term flight in the space station "MIR". Presented at the 41st Congress of the International Astronautical Federation. Dresden (Germany), October 6–12, 1990.

[96] Guy HJ, Gaines RA, Hill PM, et al. Computerized noninvasive tests of lung function. A flexible approach using mass spectrometry. Am Rev Respir Dis 1976;113:737–44.

[97] Meade F, Pearl N, Saunders MJ. Distribution of lung function (V_A/Q) in normal subjects deduced from changes in alveolar gas tensions during expiration. Scand J Respir Dis 1967;48:354–65.

[98] Reed JW, Guy HJB, Hammond MD, et al. Measurement of ventilation-perfusion inequality: Comparison of inert gas elimination and intrabreath respiratory exchange ratio [abstract]. Physiologist 1986;29:93.

[99] West JB, Fowler KT, Hugh-Jones P, et al. Measurement of the ventilation-perfusion ratio inequality in the lung by the analysis of a single expirate. Clin Sci 1957;16:529–47.

[100] Prisk GK, Guy HJB, West JB, et al. Validation of measurements of ventilation-to-perfusion ratio inequality in the lung from expired gas. J Appl Physiol 2003;94:1186–92.

[101] Engel LA. Dynamic distribution of gas flow. In: Macklem PT, Mead J, editors. Handbook of physiology. The respiratory system. Bethesda (MD): American Physiological Society; 1986. p. 575–93.

[102] Lauzon A-M, Elliott AR, Paiva M, et al. Cardiogenic oscillation phase relationships during single-breath tests performed in microgravity. J Appl Physiol 1998;84:661–8.

[103] Michel EL, Rummel JA, Sawin CF, et al. Results from Skylab medical experiment M 171 - metabolic activity. In: Johnston RS, Dietlein LF, editors. Biomedical results from Skylab SP-377. Washington (DC): NASA; 1977. p. 284–312.

[104] Stegemann J, Hoffman U, Erdmann R, et al. Exercise capacity during and after spaceflight. Aviat Space Environ Med 1997;68:812–7.

[105] Levine BD, Lane LD, Watenpaugh DE, et al. Maximal exercise performance after adaption to microgravity. J Appl Physiol 1996;81:686–94.

[106] Buderer MC, Rummel JA, Michel EL, et al. Exercise cardiac output following Skylab missions: the second manned Skylab mission. Aviat Space Environ Med 1976;47:365–72.

[107] Rosenhamer G. Influence of increased gravitational stress on the adaptation of cardiovascular and pulmonary function to exercise. Acta Physiol Scand 1967;276(Suppl):1–61.

[108] Linnarsson D. Exercise and gas exchange. In: Prisk GK, Paiva M, West JB, editors. Gravity and the lung: lessons from microgravity. New York: Marcel Dekker; 2001. p. 207–24.

[109] Prisk GK, Elliott AR, West JB. Sustained microgravity reduces the human ventilatory response to hypoxia but not hypercapnia. J Appl Physiol 2000; 88:1421–30.

[110] Read DJC. A clinical method for assessing the ventilatory response to carbon dioxide. Aust Ann Med 1967;16:20–32.

[111] Rebuck AS, Campbell EJM. A clinical method for assessing the ventilatory response to hypoxia. Am Rev Respir Dis 1974;109:345–50.

[112] Whitelaw WA, Derenne J-P, Milic-Emili J. Occlusion pressure as a measure of respiratory center output in conscious man. Respir Physiol 1975;23: 181–99.

[113] Fritsch-Yelle JM, Charles JB, Jones MM, et al. Microgravity decreases heart rate and arterial pressure in humans. J Appl Physiol 1996;80:910–4.

[114] Heymans C. The part played by vascular presso- and chemo-receptors in respiratory control. Nobel lectures—physiology or medicine (1922–1941). Amsterdam: Elsevier; 1965. p. 460–81.

[115] Heistad D, Abboud F, Mark AL, et al. Interaction of baroreceptor and chemoreceptor reflexes. J Clin Invest 1974;53:1226–36.

[116] Heistad D, Abboud FM, Mark AL, et al. Effect of baroreceptor activity on ventilatory response to chemoreceptor stimulation. J Appl Physiol 1975;39: 411–6.

[117] Somers VK, Mark AL, Abboud FM. Interaction of baroreceptor and chemoreceptor reflex control of sympathetic nerve activity in normal humans. J Clin Invest 1991;87:1953–7.

[118] Serebrovskaya T, Karaban I, Mankovskaya I, et al. Hypoxic ventilatory responses and gas exchange in patients with Parkinson's disease. Respiration (Herrlisheim) 1998;65(1):28–33.

[119] Frost JD, Shumante WH, Salamy JG, et al. Sleep monitoring: the second manned Skylab mission. Aviat Space Environ Med 1976;47:372–82.

[120] Santy PA. Analysis of sleep on shuttle missions. Aviat Space Environ Med 1988;59:1094–7.

[121] Gundel A, Polyakov VV, Zulley J. The alteration of human sleep and circadian rhythms during space flight. J Sleep Res 1997;6:1–8.

[122] Putcha L, Berens KL, Marshburn TH, et al. Pharmaceutical use by US astronauts on space shuttle missions. Aviat Space Environ Med 1999;70:705–8.

[123] Monk TH, Buysse DJ, Billy BD, et al. Sleep and circadian rhythms in four orbiting astronauts. J Biol Rhythms 1998;13:188–201.

[124] Dijk D-J, Neri DF, Wyatt JK, et al. Sleep, performance, circadian rhythms, and light-dark cycles during two space shuttle flights. Am J Physiol Regul Integr Comp Physiol 2001;281:R1647–64.

[125] Elliott AR, Shea SA, Dijk D-J, et al. Microgravity reduces sleep-disordered breathing in normal humans. Am J Respir Crit Care Med 2001;164:478–85.

[126] Dockery DW, Pope III CA, Xu X, et al. An association between air pollution and mortality in six US cities. N Engl J Med 1993;329:1753–9.

[127] Peters A, Dockery DW, Muller JE, et al. Increased particulate air pollution and the triggering of myocardial infarction. Circulation 2001;103:2810–5.

[128] Burrough B. Dragonfly, NASA and the crisis aboard Mir. New York: HarperCollins; 1998.

[129] Klein HP. The Viking biological investigations: review and status. Orig Life 1978;9:157–60.

[130] Hoffman RA, Billingham J. Effect of altered G levels on deposition of particulates in the human respiratory tract. J Appl Physiol 1975;38:955–60.

[131] Beeckmans JM. The deposition of aerosols in the respiratory tract I. Mathematical analysis and comparison with experimental data. Can J Physiol Pharmacol 1965;43:157–72.

[132] Beeckmans JM. Alveolar deposition of aerosols on the moon and in outer space. Nature 1966;211:208.

[133] Muir DCF. Influence of gravitational changes on the deposition of aerosols in the lungs of man. Aerosp Med 1967;38:159–61.

[134] Darquenne C, Paiva M, West JB, et al. Effect of microgravity and hypergravity on deposition of 0.5- to 3-μm-diameter aerosol in the human lung. J Appl Physiol 1997;83:2029–36.

[135] Darquenne C, Paiva M. One-dimensional simulation of aerosol transport and deposition in the human lung. J Appl Physiol 1994;77:2889–98.

[136] Darquenne C, West JB, Prisk GK. Deposition and dispersion of 1 μm aerosol boluses in the human lung: effect of micro- and hypergravity. J Appl Physiol 1998;85:1252–9.

[137] Darquenne C, West JB, Prisk GK. Dispersion of 0.5–2 μm aerosol in micro- and hypergravity as a probe of convective inhomogeneity in the human lung. J Appl Physiol 1999;86:1402–9.

[138] Darquenne C, Paiva M, Prisk GK. Effect of gravity on aerosol dispersion and deposition in the human lung after periods of breath-holding. J Appl Physiol 2000;89:1787–92.

[139] Webb JT, Fisher MD, Heaps C, et al. Prebreathe enhancement with dual-cycle ergometry may increase decompression sickness protection. Aviat Space Environ Med 1996;67:624.

[140] Conkin J, Powell MR. Lower body adynamia as a factor to reduce the risk of hypobaric decompression sickness. Aviat Space Environ Med 2001;72:202–14.

[141] Powell MR, Waligora JM, Norfleet WT. Decompression in simulated microgravity: bedrest and its influence on stress-assisted nucleation. Undersea Biomed Res 1992;19(S):54.

[142] Nicogossian AE, Huntoon CL, Pool SL. Space physiology and medicine. 2nd edition. Washington (DC): National Aeronautics and Space Administration; 1987.

[143] Collins M. Carrying the fire. An astronaut's journey. Toronto (Canada): Doubleday; 1974.

[144] Conkin J, Klein JS, Acock KE. Description of 103 cases of hypobaric decompression sickness from NASA-sponsored research (1982–1999). NASA technical publication 2003–212052. Houston (TX): Johnson Space Center; 2003.

[145] Bendrick G, Ainscough MJ, Pilmanis AA, et al. Prevalence of decompression sickness among U2 pilots. Aviat Space Environ Med 1996;67:199–205.

[146] Waligora JM, Horrigan Jr D, Conkin J, et al. Verification of an altitude decompression sickness prevention protocol for shuttle operations utilizing a 10.2-psi pressure stage. NASA technical memorandum 58259. Houston (TX): NASA; 1984.

[147] Thorsen E, Risberg J, Segadal K, et al. Effects of venous gas microemboli on pulmonary gas transfer function. Undersea Hyperb Med 1995;22:347–53.

[148] Prisk GK, Fine JM, Cooper TK, et al. Ventilation-perfusion ratio inequality in the lung is only slightly increased one day following extravehicular activity. Aviat Space Environ Med 2004;75:B95.

Clin Chest Med 26 (2005) 439 – 457

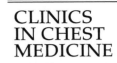

CLINICS
IN CHEST
MEDICINE

Responses and Limitations of the Respiratory System to Exercise

Andrew T. Lovering, PhD[a],*, Hans C. Haverkamp, PhD[b],
Marlowe W. Eldridge, MD[a,c]

[a]*The John Rankin Laboratory of Pulmonary Medicine, Department of Population Health Sciences,
University of Wisconsin at Madison, Madison, WI, USA*
[b]*Vermont Lung Center, University of Vermont, Burlington, VT, USA*
[c]*Department of Pediatrics, Critical Care Medicine, and Biomedical Engineering, University of Wisconsin School of Medicine,
Madison, WI, USA*

The normal healthy respiratory system must adapt to the conditions imposed on it by extreme environments and conditions. There are unique (or extreme) circumstances in which the respiratory system is unable to accommodate appropriately (or adequately) these impositions. This article discusses how the respiratory system in healthy untrained individuals readily accommodates the demands of exercise. Then, several unique cases and their associated consequences are presented in which the respiratory system was unable to accommodate successfully these exercise-induced demands.

Response of the respiratory system to exercise: healthy untrained normal subjects

The primary purpose of the lung is to maintain the arterial partial pressure of oxygen (PaO_2) and carbon dioxide ($PaCO_2$) near normal resting levels.

This article was supported by National Institutes of Health grants HL15469-33 and T32 HL 07654-16.

* Corresponding author. The John Rankin Laboratory of Pulmonary Medicine, Department of Population Health Sciences, University of Wisconsin School of Medicine, Rm 4245 MSC, 1300 University Avenue, Madison, WI 53706-1532.

E-mail address: atlovering@wisc.edu (A.T. Lovering).

During exercise, this is challenged because (1) oxygenation of the mixed venous blood delivered to the lungs is reduced greatly; (2) a fourfold increase in cardiac output causes a reduction in pulmonary capillary transit time, thus decreased time, for complete equilibration of oxygen between alveoli and pulmonary capillaries; (3) the lung receives all of the cardiac output, so it has to adapt to maintain low vascular pressures and protect against exudation of plasma water into the alveoli; and (4) there is a 20-fold increase in minute ventilation ($\dot{V}_E$) to meet the increased metabolic demand (increased carbon dioxide production [$\dot{V}CO_2$]), which necessitates a need for efficiency in breathing. In healthy untrained young adults who have a maximal oxygen consumption ($\dot{V}O_{2max}$) in the normal range (40–50 mL · kg^{-1} · min^{-1}), the respiratory system is able to meet these demands imposed on it during maximal exercise by implementing several key mechanisms (discussed later).

Exercise hyperventilation

With mild-to-moderate exercise, it is evident from the alveolar gas equations (Fig. 1A) that as oxygen consumption and carbon dioxide production ($\dot{V}O_2$ and $\dot{V}CO_2$) rise, alveolar ventilation ($\dot{V}_A$) must increase proportionally to maintain homeostasis of alveolar gases. Above 75% to 80% $\dot{V}O_{2\ max}$, $\dot{V}_A$, however, increases out of proportion to $\dot{V}CO_2$ and $PaCO_2$

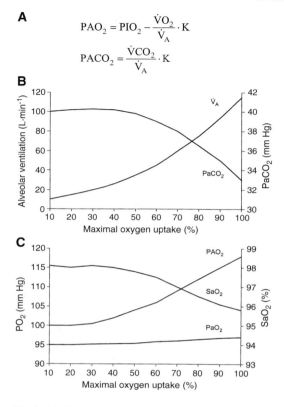

A

$$PAO_2 = PIO_2 - \frac{\dot{V}O_2}{\dot{V}_A} \cdot K$$

$$PACO_2 = \frac{\dot{V}CO_2}{\dot{V}_A} \cdot K$$

Fig. 1. (*A*) Alveolar gas equations. (*B*) Alveolar ventilation ($\dot{V}_A$) and arterial PCO_2 ($PaCO_2$) during progressive exercise to maximal in a healthy young adult. $\dot{V}_A$ increases out of proportion to $\dot{V}CO_2$ resulting in a fall in $PaCO_2$ as exercise approaches maximal intensity. (*C*) Alveolar PO_2 (PAO_2), arterial PO_2 (PaO_2), and saturation of hemoglobin with oxygen (SaO_2) during progressive exercise to maximal in a healthy young adult. Despite a progressively widened $PAO_2 - PaO_2$, PaO_2 is maintained near resting levels at all exercise intensities. SaO_2 falls primarily because of temperature and pH-mediated effects on the oxyhemoglobin dissociation curve. (*Data from* authors' laboratory.)

decreases (see Fig. 1B). This hyperventilatory response to heavy exercise is important for two reasons. First, the resultant respiratory alkalosis minimizes the metabolic acidosis resulting from the accumulation of lactic acid generated by the working muscle. Second, hyperventilation increases alveolar oxygen tension, and thus PaO_2, guarding against the development of arterial hypoxemia.

Minimization of the work of breathing

The increased metabolic demand during exercise requires a 20-fold increase in ventilation to maintain

alveolar and ultimately arterial blood gases at near resting levels. This increase in ventilation results in an oxygen cost of breathing of approximately 10% of the $\dot{V}O_2$ during maximal exercise. Several aspects of the respiratory system (breathing pattern, respiratory muscles, and airways) are configured to allow for efficient breathing during exercise.

First, exercise hyperventilation is achieved by a combination of increased frequency of breathing and tidal volume (V_T), with V_T increasing to approximately 50% of vital capacity. This breathing pattern minimizes lung stretch and allows the lung to operate on the linear portion of the pressure-volume relationship, minimizing the elastic work of breathing [1].

Second, expiratory muscles are activated at mild levels of exercise, which reduces end-expiratory lung volume [2]. This lengthens inspiratory muscles to more optimal levels for force generation and the expiratory effort stores energy in the chest wall that is released at the onset of inspiration, thus sparing the work of the inspiratory muscles. Furthermore, diaphragm fatigue is observed only when heavy exhaustive exercise intensities (>85% $\dot{V}O_{2max}$) are maintained until the limit of tolerance [3]. Thus, the mechanical work of breathing is optimized during exercise.

Lastly, despite tenfold increases in inspiratory flow rates during exercise, airway resistance is maintained near resting levels secondary to the contraction of abductor skeletal muscles regulating upper-airway diameter (extrathoracic) and by bronchodilation in the lower airways (intrathoracic). This exercise-induced bronchodilation results from (1) a reduced parasympathetic tone [4], resulting in bronchial smooth muscle relaxation and (2) airway tethering to lung parenchyma, which acts to increase airway diameter at the greater operating lung volumes during exercise [5]. In addition, airway stretch may modulate cross-bridge formation of bronchial smooth muscle. Fredberg and colleagues find that sinusoidal stretches (within the range of V_T excursions) of isolated, tracheal smooth muscle result in a decrease in tracheal smooth muscle force and stiffness [6]. Thus, airway stretch also may result in a relaxation of airway smooth muscle. So, although ventilation is increased significantly during exercise, the breathing pattern, respiratory muscle function, and airway responses all are suited to avoid flow limitation and reduce the resistive and elastic work of breathing.

Maximizing gas exchange efficiency

Pulmonary gas-exchange efficiency for oxygen is defined and quantified as the difference between the

PAO_2 and the PaO_2 and is known as the alveolar-arterial difference in partial pressure of oxygen (PAO_2 − PaO_2). Fig. 1C shows that the normal PAO_2 − PaO_2 in young, healthy individuals increases from 5 to 10 mm Hg at rest to 15 to 25 mm Hg at maximal exercise with PAO_2 rising and PaO_2 remaining relatively constant [7,8]. Approximately one third to one half of the PAO_2 − PaO_2 during exercise is caused by $\dot{V}_A$/perfusion ($\dot{Q}$) mismatch [9–11]. The remainder can be caused by extrapulmonary shunt, diffusion limitation [10], or, possibly, intrapulmonary shunt [12]. Significant diffusion limitation is unlikely, however, in normal adults because there are several key mechanisms that help to ensure alveolar end-capillary equilibrium for oxygen during exercise. First, increased pulmonary blood flow causes capillary recruitment, resulting in an increased surface area for diffusion. Second, the increased PAO_2 that results from hyperventilation increases the diffusion gradient. Lastly, pulmonary capillary volume expands up to threefold greater than at rest, which minimizes the reduction in transit time (transit time = pulmonary capillary blood volume/pulmonary blood flow).

Increased cardiac output (pulmonary blood flow)

As a result of the increased pulmonary blood flow that occurs with exercise, hydrostatic pressures potentially can increase enough to result in plasma exudation and, thus, alveolar edema. Pulmonary arterioles, however, are distensible and maintain pulmonary vascular resistance at or below normal values during exercise and, therefore, minimize increases in pulmonary capillary (hydrostatic) pressure. Nevertheless, plasma exudation into the interstitial space increases as the alveolar capillary diffusion surface expands. Fortunately, there are sufficient mechanisms that prevent intravascular fluid accumulation in the alveolar space, including the osmotic pressure gradient and increased lymphatic drainage, which both act to oppose edema formation [13]. Consequently, through increased $\dot{V}_A$, increased cardiac output (and, thus, pulmonary blood flow), decreased pulmonary vascular resistance, and ample thoracic lymphatic drainage, the respiratory system is able to maintain arterial blood gas homeostasis during exercise in healthy adults.

Based on the previous discussion, it seems that under the circumstances, the respiratory system is well suited to handle the increased demands of exercise in healthy, untrained young adults by maximizing gas exchange efficiency and concomitantly minimizing the negative consequences of the increased cardiac output and decreased $P\bar{v}O_2$ while minimizing the work of breathing. The following examples illustrate several situations, however, in which the respiratory system fails to accommodate appropriately the demands placed on it by whole-body exercise.

Response of the respiratory system to exercise: pulmonary vascular limitations

Shunting in normal healthy untrained subjects

Blood flow entering the systemic arterial circulation without traveling through ventilated areas of the lung is defined as shunt. In healthy individuals who do not have cardiac anomalies, the only sources of shunt are intra- and extrapulmonary. Because shunted blood is deoxygenated and becomes more so with exercise as oxygen extraction increases, only a small fraction of the cardiac output as shunt is necessary to worsen gas exchange by widening the PAO_2 − PaO_2 significantly. For example, at maximal exercise in healthy untrained adults who have a maximal $\dot{V}O_2 = 4.0$ L · min^{-1} and a cardiac output ($\dot{Q}_T$) equal to approximately 25 L · min^{-1}, the PAO_2 − PaO_2 equals approximately 25 mm Hg. At maximal exercise, PAO_2 equals approximately 120 mm Hg, and because there is $\dot{V}_A/\dot{Q}$ mismatch, pulmonary end-capillary PO_2 equals approximately 113 mm Hg ($Cc'O_2 = 20.6$ mL O_2 · 100 mL^{-1}). Thus, $\dot{V}_A/\dot{Q}$ mismatch accounts for approximately one third of the PAO_2 − PaO_2. Therefore, using the shunt equation with an assumed $P\bar{v}O_2 = 20$ mm Hg and resulting mixed venous oxygen content ($C\bar{v}O_2$) = 5.6 mL O_2 · 100 mL^{-1} at maximal exercise, the contribution of a 2% shunt ($\dot{Q}_S$) to the PAO_2 − PaO_2 can be calculated as follows:

$$CaO_2 = \frac{\dot{Q}_S \cdot C\bar{v}O_2 + (\dot{Q}_T - \dot{Q}_S) \cdot Cc'O_2}{\dot{Q}_T}$$

$$CaO_2 = \frac{0.5 \cdot 5.6 + (25 - 0.5) \cdot 20.6}{25}$$

$$CaO_2 = 20.3 \text{ mL } O_2 \cdot 100 \text{ mL}^{-1}$$

The resulting arterial oxygen content (CaO_2) of 20.3 mL O_2 · 100 mL^{-1} is equivalent to a PaO_2 of 95 mm Hg, thus a PAO_2 − $PaO_2 = 25$ mm Hg at maximal exercise. Thus, $\dot{V}_A/\dot{Q}$ mismatch accounts for one third of the PAO_2 − PaO_2, and a shunt of only 2% of the $\dot{Q}_T$ can account for the remaining two thirds of the $PAO_2 - PaO_2$.

Extrapulmonary shunt results from blood flow from the thebesian circulation, which empties directly into the left heart, and the bronchial vein flow into the pulmonary vein, although in humans the oxygen content of the bronchial venous blood remains unknown. The contribution of these shunts to arterial oxygenation is expected to increase with increasing exercise intensities resulting from increased myocardial oxygen extraction [14] and increased thebesian drainage. Although the total contribution of extrapulmonary shunt is assumed to be approximately 1% of the cardiac output [15–21], it should be considered a minor but significant (see previous calculations) contributor to the gas exchange inefficiency that occurs during exercise.

Intrapulmonary shunt can be caused by either extreme $\dot{V}_A/\dot{Q}$ mismatch (zero $\dot{V}_A/\dot{Q}$ units caused by atelectasis or alveolar flooding) or direct anastomoses (anatomic) between the pulmonary artery and pulmonary vein. The importance of intrapulmonary arteriovenous shunts during exercise has been discounted previously [22,23]. Using the 100% oxygen technique, Wagner and colleagues determined shunt fractions of approximately 2%, which have been interpreted to reflect extrapulmonary shunts, because the multiple inert gas elimination technique (MIGET) did not detect intrapulmonary shunts [22,23]. The validity of these standard tests (MIGET and 100% oxygen) for detecting shunting is questionable, however, because it is now known that significant prepulmonary capillary gas exchange occurs [24], and its magnitude is critically dependent on the concentration gradient of the gas. MIGET may underestimate intrapulmonary shunting because the detection of shunting is dependent on the retention of sulfur hexafluoride, an inert gas with a low solubility (and therefore a reduced retention) in blood [25]. Accordingly, the low solubility and large concentration gradient may allow for precapillary elimination of sulfur hexafluoride. Precapillary gas exchange likely occurs also with the 100% oxygen technique, thus underestimating shunting. Furthermore, in the case of the 100% oxygen technique, measurements of blood oxygen tension are not sufficiently accurate to distinguish shunts less than 10% of the cardiac output resulting from machine error [26]. Consequently, current techniques used to detect shunt may underestimate intrapulmonary shunting.

Studies of pulmonary vascular morphology provide anatomic evidence for direct vascular conduits

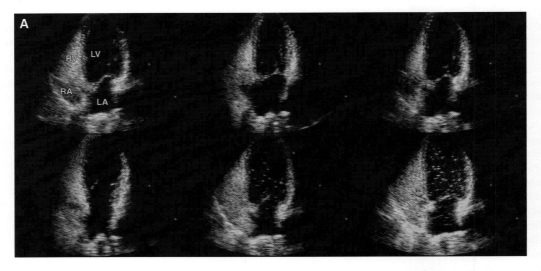

Fig. 2. (*A*) Contrast echocardiograms from a 28-year-old female during exercise at 100 W (40% $\dot{V}O_{2max}$) showing the delayed appearance of contrast bubbles in the left heart. Each sequential image (*left-to-right, top-to-bottom*) is separated in time by 1 second. The first evidence of shunting is in the fifth image, which is eight cardiac cycles after contrast appears in the right atrium. (*B*) Exercise contrast echocardiograms at 100, 230, and 260 W in one subject. At 100 W, there is no evidence of intracardiac or intrapulmonary shunting, because the left heart is free of contrast bubbles. The first evidence of intrapulmonary shunting is seen at 230 W (85% $\dot{V}O_{2max}$). Note the delayed appearance (>5 cycles) of contrast bubbles in the left heart. The same pattern is seen at 260 W. All images are apical four-chamber views. LA, left atrium; LV, left ventricle; RA, right atrium; RV, right ventricle. (*From* Eldridge MW, Dempsey JA, Haverkamp HC, et al. Exercise-induced intrapulmonary arteriovenous shunting in healthy humans. J Appl Physiol 2004;97(3):797–805; with permission.)

between pulmonary arteries and veins in dogs [27–29] and humans [30–32]. In several of these studies, the investigators report that synthetic beads with diameters ranging from 50 to 200 μm were able to pass through the pulmonary circulation of human infants [32] and dogs [30,31]. Although the vessels responsible for intrapulmonary shunting of these synthetic beads remain unidentified, Tobin identified vessels in 47% of the lobules of human lungs, which had secondary glomus-like vessels that branched from the parent arterioles at right angles [30]. Tobin suggested that these vessels might act as intrapulmonary shunts. In addition, Elliott and Reid describe small muscular arteries in humans that, like those vessels described by Tobin, branch from the conventional pulmonary arteries at right angles and, because they do not accompany airways, are referred to as supernumerary arteries [33]. These supernumerary arteries have a muscular baffle at their origin, which seems to regulate blood flow [34].

Contrast echocardiography is a standard clinical method for detecting cardiac and intrapulmonary shunting at rest. To detect shunt, sterile saline is agi-

tated to create microbubbles that are injected into a peripheral vein. If individuals have shunting at the cardiac level resulting from a patent foramen ovale, contrast bubbles appear in the left heart immediately. If contrast bubbles appear in the left heart, however, after a delay ($\geq$ 3 cardiac cycles), this is diagnostic of intrapulmonary shunting. Recent work using contrast echocardiography provides indirect evidence that intrapulmonary shunting occurs during exercise in healthy individuals who have a wide range of fitness (predicted $\dot{V}O_{2max}$ ranging from 70% to 200%) [12]. In this study, subjects who did not have cardiac anomalies and did not have arteriovenous malformations showed no shunting at rest. During progressive cycle ergometer exercise, however, approximately 90% of the subjects showed shunting of contrast bubbles at submaximal oxygen consumptions. For example, in a 28-year-old female subject, shunting began at a workload of 100 W. In this subject, after injection of contrast bubbles into the median basilic vein, contrast bubbles filled the right heart rapidly (Fig. 2A). Then, after a delay (in this case, 8 cardiac cycles/4 seconds), contrast bubbles began to appear

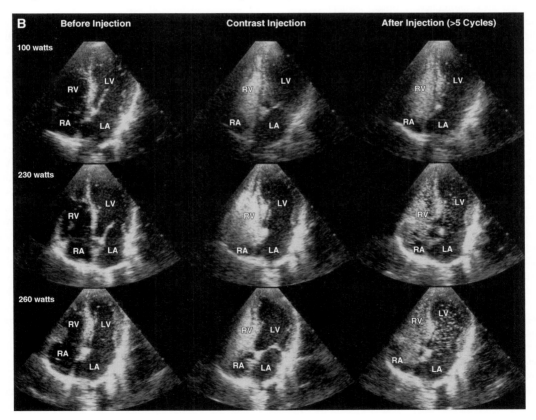

Fig. 2 (*continued*).

in the left heart, indicative of intrapulmonary shunting. Once shunting occurred, it continued at all subsequent workloads (see Fig. 2B). The magnitude of this anatomic shunt has yet to be quantified, so its contribution to gas exchange inefficiency can only be estimated. As discussed previously, a shunt of approximately 2% of the cardiac output could account for the all of the $PaO_2 - PaO_2$ not explained by $\dot{V}_A/\dot{Q}$ mismatch at moderate and high-intensity exercise [9,12].

Is contrast echocardiography a valid method for detecting intrapulmonary shunting? To answer this question, the limitations of contrast echocardiography (including pulmonary vascular morphology considerations and bubble dynamics in vivo) should be examined in detail. First, pulmonary capillaries are small, approximately 7 to 10 μm in diameter at rest [35,36]. Although it is unknown how much they distend during exercise, Reeves and colleagues estimate that the distensibility coefficient (percent change in capillary diameter per unit change in pressure) of human pulmonary microcirculation is 1.35% [37]. Thus, at peak exercise with an estimated mean pulmonary capillary distending pressure of 36 mm Hg in zone III, pulmonary capillary distention does not exceed 20 μm. The second consideration is microbubble size. The injected contrast microbubbles have a wide spectrum of sizes. Small bubbles, less than 10 μm, collapse rapidly [38–41], whereas larger microbubbles are filtered and eliminated by the pulmonary vasculature [27,39, 40,42]. Microbubble survival time in static blood is predicted to be 200 ms for a bubble with a diameter of 8 μm. Because the mean pulmonary capillary transit time at rest is 750 ms and does not fall below 450 ms in well-trained athletes [43], microbubbles with diameters small enough to traverse the pulmonary microcirculation collapse before they are able to traverse the pulmonary microcirculation and be detected in the left heart. Nevertheless, contrast echocardiography can detect only anatomic intrapulmonary shunts and cannot detect physiologic intrapulmonary shunt caused by atelectasis or alveolar flooding.

In summary, shunting occurs in normal healthy individuals during exercise. The contributors to this shunting include extrapulmonary (thebesian and bronchial venous drainage) and possibly intrapulmonary (anatomical conduits) shunts. Although the total contribution of these shunts to the $PaO_2 - PaO_2$ remains unknown, small shunt fractions of approximately 2% can play a significant role in the worsening of gas exchange efficiency in healthy humans during maximal exercise.

Exercise tolerance in individuals who have large intrapulmonary arteriovenous shunts

An extreme example of intrapulmonary right-to-left shunting occurs in individuals who have pulmonary arteriovenous malformations (PAVM). These unique pulmonary lesions are believed to be relatively uncommon. The true prevalence is not known, however, because the clinical manifestations of small lesions may go unnoticed. Approximately 70% of the cases of PAVM are congenital and associated with hereditary hemorrhagic telangiectasia [44].

Individuals who have PAVM have reduced exercise tolerance. The exercise capacity often is remarkably well maintained, however, relative to the large shunt fractions and resting hypoxemia. Indeed, individuals who have similar degrees of resting hypoxemia from other causes, including cyanotic congenital heart disease, pulmonary hypertension, or interstitial lung disease, have considerably less tolerance to exercise. Chilvers and coworkers performed incremental exercise tests in 15 patients who had PAVM and reported a fall in arterial oxygen saturation (SaO_2) from 86% at rest to 73% at peak exercise [45]. Despite the impressive desaturation, exercise capacity was well preserved, with 11 of 15 patients achieving a predicted maximal work rate greater than 70%.

Whyte and colleagues examined the cardiopulmonary responses to exercise in seven individuals who had PAVM and resting intrapulmonary shunt fractions ranging from 11% to 57% and SaO_2 ranging from 65% to 91% [46]. Despite the large shunt fractions and marked desaturations, these patients had mean maximal power outputs of 80% predicted. $\dot{V}_E$ during exercise was excessively high relative to the power output. The ventilatory equivalent for oxygen ($\dot{V}_E/\dot{V}O_2$) and carbon dioxide ($\dot{V}_E/\dot{V}CO_2$) were significantly greater than predicted. Fig. 3 shows the individual maximal $\dot{V}_E/\dot{V}O_2$ and percent predicted $\dot{V}_E/\dot{V}O_2$ plotted against the right-to-left shunt fraction. As seen in Fig. 3, there is a strong relationship between shunt fraction and excessive ventilatory drive. The finding of this excessive ventilatory drive with exercise is not surprising and likely the result of the combined effects of shunt-induced hypoxemia and relative hypercapnia compared to rest.

Furthermore, these patients who had PAVM displayed a remarkable ability to maintain normal pulmonary capillary blood flow and tissue oxygen delivery during exercise. Chilvers and colleagues suggest that exercise tolerance was relatively well maintained because of a low pulmonary vascular resistance that allows generation of high cardiac out-

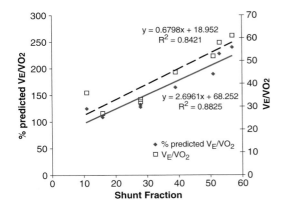

Fig. 3. Measured ventilatory equivalent ($\dot{V}_E/\dot{V}O_2$ [*solid line*]) and percent predicted (*dashed line*) plotted against right-to-left shunt fraction (percent cardiac output) during exercise measured with radiolabeled microspheres. (*Data from* Whyte MK, Hughes JM, Jackson JE, et al. Cardiopulmonary response to exercise in patients with intrapulmonary vascular shunts. J Appl Physiol 1993;75:321–8.)

puts. These patients also were polycythemic (mean hemoglobin concentration >17 g · dL^{-1}); thus, despite a low SaO_2 (mean 74%), with exercise, the mean CaO_2 was 17.8 mL O_2 · 100 mL^{-1} blood (mean, 90% predicted). In combination, the high cardiac outputs (mean, 142% predicted) and near-normal CaO_2 resulted in systemic oxygen delivery slightly higher than predicted. Apparently, individuals who have large PAVM can have well preserved exercise tolerance despite impressive intrapulmonary arteriovenous shunting and hypoxemia. This is because they can achieve large increases in cardiac output and oxygen delivery in response to exercise.

Pulmonary vascular response to exercise in high-altitude pulmonary edema–prone individuals

High-altitude pulmonary edema (HAPE) is the result of a unique form of reversible pulmonary capillary leak that develops in individuals ascending rapidly to high altitude and often is associated with heavy exercise [47,48]. A postulated mechanism is capillary stress failure resulting from nonhomogeneous distribution of pulmonary blood flow in response to hypoxia and exercise. The pulmonary capillaries that must accommodate the high pressures and flow are disrupted and allow leakage of large proteins and red blood cells into the alveolar space. People who develop HAPE are more susceptible to future episodes than the general population [47]. HAPE-prone individuals have been studied extensively and reported to have an augmented pulmonary

vascular reactivity to hypoxic stress [47,49]. It is unclear if the hyper-reactivity of the pulmonary vascular bed is an inherit abnormality or if it develops subsequent to the initial HAPE episode.

The pulmonary vascular response to exercise seems to be an important factor in determining HAPE susceptibility. Kawashima and coworkers [50] find HAPE-prone subjects to have increased pulmonary arterial pressures and pulmonary vascular resistance in response to low-level exercise. Eldridge and coworkers [51] studied several aspects of pulmonary vascular reactivity in HAPE-prone individuals and in healthy control subjects during normoxic and hypoxic exercise. They showed that with exercise, HAPE-prone individuals have a greater increase in pulmonary arterial pressures with increasing pulmonary blood flow than HAPE-resistant controls (Fig. 4A, B). Thus, HAPE-prone individuals have an increased pulmonary vascular reactivity and a steeper pressure-flow relationship to exercise than the control subjects. Furthermore, HAPE-prone individuals showed a dramatic increase in pulmonary arterial occlusion pressure as exercise intensity increased (see Fig. 4A, B). In combination, high pulmonary artery and wedge pressures, which can exceed mean values of 40 and 20 torr, respectively, during heavy exercise, increase the likelihood of transcapillary fluid movement into the interstitial tissue. HAPE-prone subjects have a greater exercise-induced $\dot{V}_A/\dot{Q}$ mismatch, as determined by MIGET, than HAPE-resistant controls [52]. With high pulmonary vascular pressures, estimated pulmonary capillary pressure may exceed 35 torr in dependent regions of the lung, potentially causing capillary stress failure and, thus, regional flooding of alveolar space with fluid, protein, and red blood cells [53,54].

The cause for the higher pulmonary vascular reactivity in response to exercise in HAPE-prone individuals is not clear. A variety of mechanisms is suggested, however, including pulmonary vascular endothelial dysfunction with reduced nitric oxide synthesis. There is some support for this hypothesis, as HAPE-prone individuals have lower exhaled nitric oxide levels [55,56]. Furthermore, nitric oxide inhalation reduces pulmonary vascular pressures and improves the clinical status of individuals suffering acutely from HAPE [56].

Several reports document that HAPE-prone individuals have an approximately 10% smaller vital capacity [51,52,57,58] than HAPE-resistant cohorts, leading some investigators to speculate that this might indicate a smaller pulmonary capillary capacity in subjects prone to HAPE [51]. Smaller lungs and a reduced total pulmonary capillary cross-sectional area

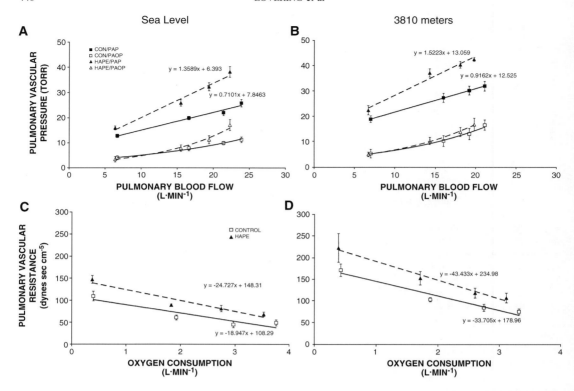

Fig. 4. Relationship between cardiac output and mean pulmonary vascular pressure at sea level (*A*) and an altitude (*B*) of 3810 meters. Pulmonary arterial pressures (PAP, *filled symbols*); pulmonary arterial occlusion pressure (PAOP, *open symbols*); control (CON, *solid lines*); high-altitude pulmonary edema (HAPE)–susceptible (*dashed lines*). Relationship between oxygen consumption and mean pulmonary vascular resistance at sea level (*C*) and an altitude (*D*) of 3810 meters. CON [*open symbols, solid lines*]; HAPE (*filled symbols, dashed lines*). Data are means ± SE. (*Adapted from* Eldridge MW, Podolsky A, Richardson RS, et al. Pulmonary hemodynamic response to exercise in subjects with prior high-altitude pulmonary edema. J Appl Physiol 1996;81:911–21; with permission.)

may be one determinant of the augmented pressure-flow relationship seen during exercise in HAPE-prone individuals [51]. In support of this hypothesis, Steinacker and coworkers [59] show that HAPE-prone individuals have lower diffusing capacity for carbon monoxide, cardiac output, and stroke volumes during exercise than matched HAPE-resistant controls. Similar findings are reported with direct Fick measurements and calculations of lower diffusing capacity for oxygen [52].

HAPE-prone individuals seem to have a unique pulmonary vascular response to exercise, with an exaggerated pulmonary vascular reactivity and higher pulmonary vascular resistances (see Fig. 4C, D). The pathophysiologic basis for this unique pulmonary vascular response to exercise remains undefined. Structural and functional causes are possible. Further work is needed to better define endothelial function in these susceptible individuals. In addition, the potential protective role of recently identified arteriovenous

intrapulmonary shunts [12] needs to be investigated. Approximately 10% of the subjects studied do not open intrapulmonary shunts during exercise. Are these subjects prone to pulmonary microvascular injury during exercise and hypoxic stress because they do not have or fail to recruit intrapulmonary shunts? Indeed, local recruitment of intrapulmonary shunts as regional pulmonary vascular pressures and flow increases should help to divert the potentially damaging hydraulic energy away from vulnerable alveolar capillaries.

Response of the respiratory system to exercise: extrathoracic airway limitations

Exercise-induced extrathoracic obstruction

In recent years it has become clear that severe flow limitation caused by narrowing of the extrathoracic airway (as opposed to intrathoracic or bronchial airway narrowing) can occur during high-intensity exercise or emotionally stressful moments during exercise in otherwise healthy people [60,61]. In theory, the differential diagnosis between upper airway dysfunction during exercise and exercise-induced bronchospasm (EIB) should be straightforward. EIB is characterized by decreases in forced expiratory flow rates between 5 and 15 minutes after exercise [62], whereas postexercise pulmonary function is not different from pre-exercise values in exercise-induced upper airway dysfunction. Unfortunately, patients often are incorrectly diagnosed with EIB, when in fact the wheezing and severe dyspnea are the result of a marked narrowing of the glottis [60,61]. Obstructions arise as a result of either collapse of supraglottic structures into the glottis during inspiration or an abnormal abduction of the vocal folds into the airway lumen during inspiration [60], expiration, or both phases of the breathing cycle [61]. Obstructions are characterized by a sudden onset, a loud stridor, and extreme dyspnea that invariably force subjects to discontinue exercise, with a rapid resolution of stridorous breathing and obstruction after exercise cessation.

Fig. 5 contains breath-by-breath ventilatory and arterial blood data obtained during the final 75 seconds of cycle exercise to exhaustion at $\dot{V}O_{2max}$ in a 22-year-old competitive female cyclist. The vertical line indicates the appearance of a loud stridor and severe dyspnea. $\dot{V}_E$ was reduced immediately by 25 L · min^{-1} as a consequence of decreases in inspiratory and expiratory flow rates. Breath-by-breath tidal flow-volume loops analyzed before and after the onset of the stridor also revealed a clear decrease in flow rates. The subject was able to continue exercising, and because metabolic rate had not changed, hypercapnia (PaCO$_2$ increase, 34.6 to 44.4 mm Hg) and arterial hypoxemia (PaO$_2$ decrease, 90.2 to 76.5 mm Hg) ensued. The stridor and dyspnea subsided within approximately 45 seconds after exercise cessation and postexercise pulmonary function was not different from pre-exercise values. This finding eliminates EIB as the cause of the flow limitation and insufficient ventilation during the exercise, because the airflow limitation caused by EIB always is evident after exercise during the recovery period. This does not preclude the development of a small amount of airway narrowing during an exercise bout, which has been shown before [63], but the major increase in airway resistance becomes apparent after exercise in EIB.

The prevalence of exercise-induced upper airway dysfunction is unknown, but the fact that it often is diagnosed incorrectly as EIB suggests that it is more common than believed previously. Furthermore, it is traditionally believed that upper airway dysfunction during exercise can be diagnosed only with flexible fiberoptic laryngoscopy, a somewhat uncomfortable and invasive procedure. Extrathoracic obstructions also are easily identifiable, however, via analysis of the tidal flow-volume loops during exercise. That is, a sudden and significant decrease in expiratory or inspiratory flow rates during exercise is strong evidence of a narrowed upper airway. Extrathoracic obstruction during exercise always has been reported to be exercise limiting. There may be individuals, however, who develop a less profound, tolerable, and non–exercise limiting narrowing of the glottis during exercise. Even a small amount of extrathoracic airway narrowing is accompanied by an increased resistive work of breathing and a potentially less vigorous hyperventilatory response to the exercise, thus predisposing to or worsening any existing exercise-induced arterial hypoxemia (EIAH). Although speculative, this may in part explain the large intrasubject variability in the magnitude of the hyperventilatory response to exercise in trained individuals [64].

Response of the respiratory system to exercise: intrathoracic airway limitations

Asthma

Asthma is a disease characterized by a variable amount of airflow limitation, bronchial smooth muscle hyperreactivity to a variety of specific (eg, methacholine or histamine) and nonspecific (eg, exercise or hypertonic aerosols) stimuli, and airway inflammation typically defined by the presence of inflammatory cells and mediators in sputum, bronchoalveolar lavage, or bronchial biopsy specimens [65]. Asthma is a heterogeneous disease with multiple phenotypes and, as such, recently has become known as a syndrome rather than a distinct disease with a single set of pathophysiologic findings and clinical symptoms.

There are several reasons to suspect that asthmatics are more likely than healthy people to experience excessive gas exchange disturbance during exercise and deviate from the usual maintenance of PaO$_2$ and SaO$_2$. For example, airflow limitation is a common finding in asthmatics and is the result of variable contributions from bronchial smooth muscle contraction and increases in airway wall thickness (as a consequence of inflammatory mediated airway remodeling) [65]. Thus, the expiratory limb of the maximal volitional flow-volume envelope often is

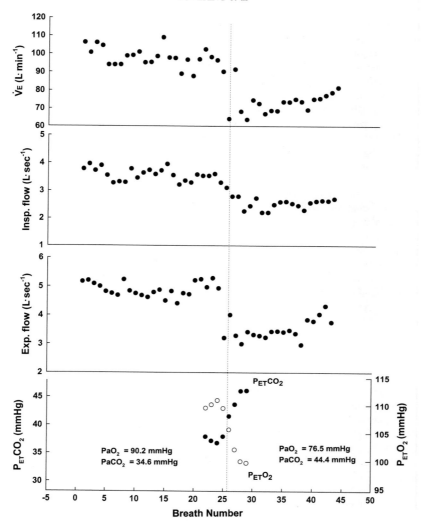

Fig. 5. Breath-by-breath analysis of $\dot{V}_E$, peak inspiratory flow, peak expiratory flow, and partial pressures of end-tidal oxygen ($P_{ET}O_2$) and end-tidal carbon dioxide ($P_{ET}CO_2$) during cycling exercise to exhaustion (total time = 75 seconds) at $\dot{V}O_{2max}$. Dashed vertical line indicates the breath at which a loud stridor and severe dyspnea developed secondary to a sudden and severe extrathoracic airway narrowing. PaO_2 and $PaCO_2$ before and after the obstruction are included. Immediately after the obstruction, $\dot{V}_E$ and inspiratory and expiratory flows decreased substantially and carbon dioxide retention and arterial hypoxemia occurred.

scooped, with diminished flow rates across all lung volumes. Narrowed, high-resistance airways presumably lead to an increase in the flow-resistive work of breathing during exercise. Airway obstruction caused by luminal mucus and fluid accumulation or excessive bronchial smooth muscle contraction also may be present in asthmatics. All these changes in the airways likely predispose asthmatics to greater amounts of gas exchange disturbance during exercise.

Fig. 6 illustrates results from an exercise study in a 37-year-old male triathlete ($\dot{V}O_{2max} = 39$ mL ·

$kg^{-1} \cdot min^{-1}$) who had asthma. Data are shown at rest, during steady-state exercise at 60% and 75% of $\dot{V}O_{2max}$, and during heavy constant workload exercise performed to exhaustion. The expiratory limb of the maximal volitional flow-volume loop reveals substantially narrowed airways that restrict expiratory flow to low levels at all lung volumes. As a consequence, the subject developed expiratory flow limitation at moderate levels of $\dot{V}_E$ during the exercise. Overlap of tidal expiratory flow during spontaneous breathing with the maximal voli-

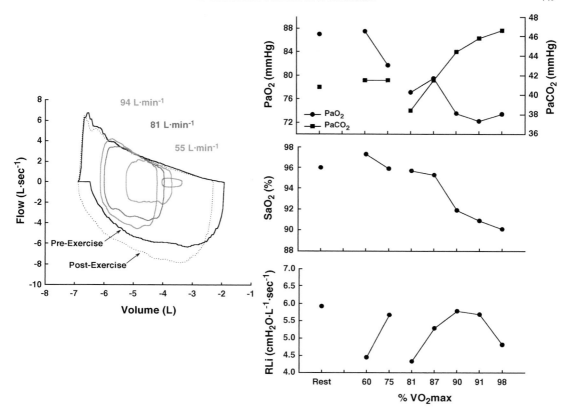

Fig. 6. Ventilatory and arterial blood data at rest, during treadmill exercise at two submaximal workloads, and during constant load exercise to exhaustion at approximately 90% $\dot{V}_{O_{2max}}$ in a 37-year-old male triathlete competitor with bronchial asthma. (*Left panel*) Exercise tidal flow-volume loops during submaximal exercise (60% $\dot{V}_{O_{2max}}$) and at several time points during exercise performed to exhaustion. The exercise loops are plotted within the maximal volitional flow-volume loops obtained before and immediately after (within 60 seconds of) exercise. Also labeled is the $\dot{V}_E$ associated with each exercise flow-volume loop. (*Right panel*) PaO_2 and $PaCO_2$, SaO_2, and pulmonary resistance (RLi) during two submaximal workloads and exercise to exhaustion. In this subject, substantial carbon dioxide retention and arterial hypoxemia occur during exercise at modest ventilation and metabolic rates. This is because of the limited capacity for expiratory flow due to narrowed airways and the lack of a bronchodilatory response to the exercise.

tional expiratory flow limb are not seen in young healthy men until a $\dot{V}_E$ of greater than approximately 120 L $\cdot$ min^{-1} is reached [66]. The expiratory flow limitation instigated a marked dynamic hyperinflation and increase in end-expiratory lung volume to 0.84 L above resting functional residual capacity.

Healthy humans exhibit a decreased airway resistance during exercise [4]. A decrease in airway resistance during exercise also is shown in asthmatics [67,68], but the robustness of the response may be more variable as a result of the degree and causes of any baseline airflow limitation present before the exercise. In the case of the 37-year-old triathelete (Fig. 6), pulmonary resistance (measured with an esophageal balloon tipped catheter) was

high at rest and did not exhibit any major changes during exercise (normal value is between 1 and 2 cm $H_2O \cdot L^{-1} \cdot sec^{-1}$ at rest and does not change during exercise). There also was no improvement in the maximal volitional flow-volume loop immediately after exercise. These findings suggest the presence of a fixed airway narrowing in this subject, perhaps as a result of thickened (ie, remodeled) airway walls. The mechanical limitation provided by the airways and the high-resistive and elastic work of breathing (as a consequence of dynamic hyperinflation) resulted in a clearly inadequate ventilatory response, seen by the rise in $PaCO_2$ to 46 mm Hg by the end of exercise. The insufficient ventilatory response caused a marked decrease in SaO_2 via two separate mechanisms: (1) by causing a reduced $\dot{V}_A/\dot{V}O_2$ (and also PAO_2, by definition) and, therefore, a reduced PaO_2; and (2) an insufficient ventilatory compensation for the metabolic acidosis caused by the exercise, thus, a more pronounced Bohr effect. Finally, the decreases in PaO_2 and SaO_2 are substantial given the metabolic rate the subject was working at (39 mL $\cdot$ kg^{-1} $\cdot$ min^{-1} at the end of exercise); EIAH of this magnitude is rare and does not occur in healthy men until maximal aerobic capacities of 150% to 200% of predicted normal (approximately 65 mL $\cdot$ kg^{-1} $\cdot$ min^{-1}) can be attained [69].

How representative is the case of the 37-year-old triathelete of the responses in asthmatics during exercise? Previous studies evaluating gas exchange during exercise in asthmatics generally report an adequate hyperventilatory response to the exercise [67,70,71]. These studies, however, are difficult to interpret because of poor characterization of the subjects' asthma, small sample sizes, low exercise workloads that do not stress the respiratory system's capacity for generating airflow and gas exchange, the interpretive confounder of often extremely low resting $PaCO_2$ values (eg, approximately 30 mm Hg), and a lack of any integrative studies examining the gas exchange and breathing mechanics responses to exercise. Alternatively, the ventilatory responses to exercise in asthmatics likely depend on a complex interaction between many factors including: (1) the level of baseline airflow limitation and obstruction; (2) the amount of fixed (ie, nonimprovable) airway narrowing; (3) the robustness of the exercise-induced bronchodilatory response; and (4) the $\dot{V}_E$ required to maintain normal arterial blood gas tensions, which is dictated by metabolic rate and, thus, exercise workload and fitness level. In any case, the phenotypic heterogeneity of the disease might preclude a generalizable description of a typical or usual gas exchange response to exercise in asthmatics. Thus, the response likely varies on a case-by-case basis in concert with the particular characteristics of individuals' asthma.

Respiratory system limitations to exercise in habitually active, highly fit elderly subjects

The normal healthy aging process, beginning as early as the third decade of life in humans, includes structural and functional changes that exert a significant influence on the age-dependant reduction in exercise performance capacity. These changes include age-dependant reductions in muscle myofibrillar protein, fiber cross-sectional area, and muscle

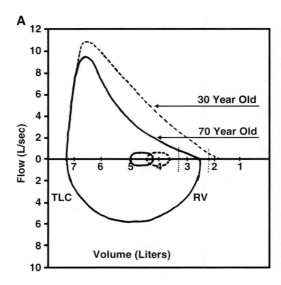

Fig. 7. (*A*) Maximal flow-volume loops at rest, residual volume (RV), closing volume in 30-year-old and in 70-year-old men. Note the scooping in the flow-volume loop, the higher closing volume (3.2 L, *vertical dashed line*) and end expiratory lung volume for expiratory flow in the 70-year-old subjects. These changes result from the reduced lung elastic recoil in older subjects, causing reduced maximal expiratory flow rates and lower expiratory pressures and higher lung volumes at which airways are compressed dynamically and flow rate becomes independent of effort. Total lung capacity (TLC). (*B*) This is a 70-year-old highly fit subject with $\dot{V}O_{2max}$ 200% of age-predicted and lung function 100% to 150% of age predicted. Note the relatively small maximal volitional flow-volume loop. With progressive exercise, mechanical limits to ventilation are reached during heavy submaximal and at maximal exercise and end-expiratory lung volume rises. Maximal effective expiratory pressures were exceeded and the capacity for inspiratory pressure development (P_{capl}) was reached at maximal exercise. The oxygen cost of breathing was estimated at 23% of total $\dot{V}O_{2max}$ in this subject. PaO_2 fell to 59 mm Hg from a normal resting level and $PaCO_2$ rose throughout the final workload to approximate resting values. (*C*) This shows the effects of exercise in a 70-year-old subject but in contrast to the subject shown in (*B*), this subject has a substantially lower $\dot{V}O_{2max}$ (100% of age-predicted) and a drastically reduced maximal flow-volume envelope (forced expiratory flow at 50% of vital capacity = 35% age predicted). This subject also reached flow limitation at low $\dot{V}_E$ and achieved maximal inspiratory and expiratory pressures, although at a significantly reduced ventilation and metabolic demand during exercise compared with the subject in Fig. 7B. (*See* Refs. [82,83].)

strength; and reduced maximal heart rate, cardiac output, and arterial vessel compliance [72]. Exercise training (aerobic and strength training)—even in the seventh and eighth decades of life—has a positive effect on slowing many of these aging effects and of increasing $\dot{V}O_{2max}$ at any given age. The lung also ages, showing two major structural changes and to similar extents in trained and untrained healthy subjects: (1) loss of elastic recoil, most likely the result of a gradual change in the spatial arrangement in cross-linking of the lungs' elastin and collagen

fiber network and (2) alveoli increase in size, whereas the number of alveoli and total gas exchange surface area falls markedly with age [73]. The loss of elastic recoil, combined with a reduced number of attachments of supporting alveoli to small airways, results in excessive airway narrowing during a forced expiration. Thus, normal age-dependant reductions in forced expiratory volume in 1 second occur over a lifetime and rival those attributable to habitual smoking. The increased tendency for small airways to close also causes an increased functional residual

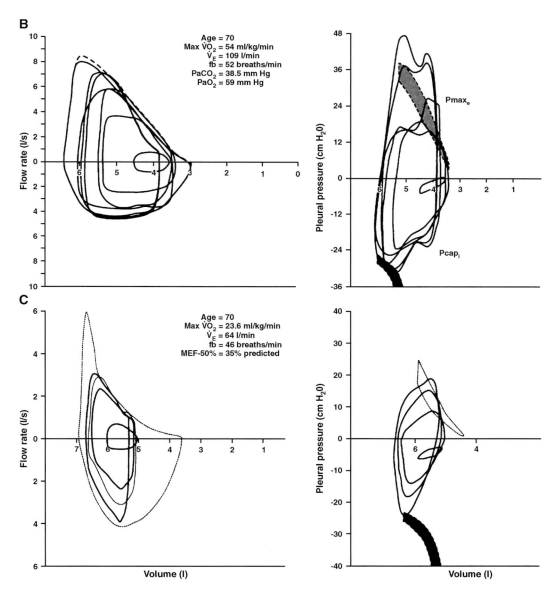

Fig. 7 (*continued*).

capacity with age, as does the airway closing volume (ie, the lung volume that small airways close) (Fig. 7A). Other relevant age-dependant changes to pulmonary system structures include: (1) a reduced chest wall compliance secondary to costal cartilage calcification; (2) a narrowing of intervertebral distances and an increase in the anterior-posterior diameter of the chest; and (3) a reduced compliance of pulmonary arterioles and an increase in pulmonary vascular resistance [74,75].

These age-induced changes in lung structure are manifested most clearly in response to the increased demands for gas exchange, ventilation, and cardiac output during exercise, especially in elderly, healthy, habitually active subjects who maintain a relatively high $\dot{V}O_{2max}$. The most consistent age-dependant effect shown in these subjects during exercise is expiratory flow limitation, which occurs during moderately heavy through maximal exercise intensities. This is shown in two subjects in Fig. 7B and C, representing two extremes of the aging effect on $\dot{V}O_{2max}$. The elderly subjects' propensity for expiratory flow limitation during exercise occurs because of the convergence of two aging factors: (1) the reduced maximal volitional flow-volume loop; and (2) the increased ratio of dead space to $\dot{V}_T$ at rest and during exercise, which requires a greater overall ventilatory response to maintain $PaCO_2$ throughout exercise. These responses translate into substantially increased mechanical work, thus, increased energy costs of breathing, during exercise in the elderly (see Fig. 7B, C), because expiratory muscle work is increased and, more importantly, the expiratory flow limitation prevents an exercise-induced reduction in end-expiratory lung volume. This means that older subjects must breathe at the upper, stiffer portion of their pressure-volume relationship, thereby increasing the elastic work of inspiration. The inspiratory muscles also are shortened by this lung hyperinflation, causing a reduction in maximal force generation by these muscles. Accordingly, the inspiratory muscles in these subjects are working near capacity for pressure generation during heavy exercise (see Fig. 7B, C), requiring high-energy expenditures and muscle blood flows by the respiratory musculature. Significant dyspneic sensations also result from the increased sensory input to the brainstem and higher central nervous system and raised respiratory motor output associated with the increased work of breathing.

The $PAO_2 - PaO_2$ during exercise tends to be increased at any given $\dot{V}O_2$ in older subjects compared with younger counterparts. In approximately three quarters of fit subjects tested to date, however, the hyperventilatory response to heavy exercise intensities is sufficient to raise PAO_2 to prevent significant reductions in PaO_2 [76]. The majority of fit elderly subjects who show significant EIAH (SaO_2, 93% to 86%) do so for the same reasons as their younger highly fit counterparts (ie, combining an excessive $PAO_2 - PaO_2$ [>25 mm Hg at $\dot{V}O_{2max}$] with a mechanically limited hyperventilatory response). The major difference between younger and older fit subjects in this regard is that the older persons experience EIAH at metabolic rates (40–55 mL $O_2 \cdot$ $kg^{-1} \cdot min^{-1}$) that are considerably less than in the younger subjects (>60 mL $O_2 \cdot kg^{-1} \cdot min^{-1}$).

It is reasonable to speculate from available data that in untrained sedentary subjects who have average age-dependant reductions in lung elastic-recoil, the respiratory system does not play any significantly greater role in limiting peak or endurance exercise performance than it does in the younger sedentary counterparts. Even though the lung and airways age substantially, and most noticeably, throughout the sixth through eighth decades, $\dot{V}O_{2max}$ also is reduced markedly and nearly in parallel to the declines in lung function. Accordingly, the concomitant fall in $\dot{V}O_{2max}$ reduces the demand on the lung and chest wall for oxygen transport (ie, ventilation and gas exchange). The structural and functional cardiovascular determinants of $\dot{V}O_{2max}$ that are important as limiting factors to $\dot{V}O_{2max}$ in young adults (discussed previously) decline with age and thus remain major determinants of a declining $\dot{V}O_{2max}$. Alternatively, the relatively overbuilt respiratory system in the young also undergoes approximately equal decrements in capacity (to their cardiovascular counterparts) with normal aging, so its capacity continues to exceed the declining maximal metabolic demand. Exceptions to this generalization occur with the extremes of age-dependant loss of lung elastic recoil, where even relatively modest increases in $\dot{V}_E$ during exercise cause flow limitation and its sequellae (see Fig. 7B). In untrained, very sedentary elderly, it also is likely that a reduced metabolic capacity of locomotor muscles—as opposed to oxygen delivery—becomes an important determinant of $\dot{V}O_{2max}$.

The authors believe that it is only in habitually active elderly subjects who attain relatively high $\dot{V}O_{2max}$ with commensurate high demands for ventilation and gas exchange that there is a significant prevalence of respiratory system limitations to exercise performance. The importance of the respiratory system as a limiting factor to exercise, especially in active fit elderly subjects, is exacerbated by the ineffectiveness of physical training to alter the aging effect on respiratory system structure, as opposed to highly significant beneficial effects of exercise training on cardiovascular system and locomotor muscle structure and function [72]. A significant but small proportion of fit elderly subjects experience EIAH. Accordingly, it is expected that this arterial oxygen desaturation limits—as in their younger counterparts—their maximal arteriovenous oxygen content difference and, therefore, their $\dot{V}O_{2max}$ by approximately 5% to 15% [77]. Expiratory flow limitation leading to increased elastic and flow-resistive work of breathing in heavy exercise seems to occur more consistently than does EIAH in the fit elderly. Based on the effects of respiratory muscle unloading studies in the young [78], the increased loads on the respiratory muscles in elderly subjects are expected to enhance the probability of occurrence of exercise-induced diaphragm fatigue and redistribution of blood flow from the working locomotor muscles—along with enhanced progression of perceptions of breathlessness and limb discomfort. These experiments have not yet been applied to the fit elderly. Finally, there are the exceptional extremely fit elderly subjects (see Fig. 7B) whose lungs have undergone near-normal aging effects and whose $\dot{V}O_{2max}$ is more than twice age-predicted normal. The normally aged airways and alveolar-capillary diffusion surface do not support these supranormal metabolic and ventilatory demands. Accordingly, severe EIAH and excessive respiratory muscle work occur in these subjects, and the respiratory system presents a major limitation to $\dot{V}O_{2max}$ and endurance exercise performance.

Response of the respiratory system to exercise: pulmonary vascular and airway limitations

The equine thoroughbred athlete: an extreme case of the underbuilt lung!

Thoroughbreds are remarkable middle-distance runners. For example, their average $\dot{V}O_{2max}$ (approximately 160 mL $\cdot$ kg^{-1} $\cdot$ min^{-1}) exceeds that of the fittest humans by more than twofold, and in competition they complete the mile in less than 2 minutes and maintain an average velocity of running over the entire distance (approximately 950 m $\cdot$ min^{-1}), which approximates what the world's fastest human sprinters achieve over 100 meters. In these animals, evidence points consistently to a predominant limitation of $\dot{V}O_{2max}$ by the lung (Fig. 8A, B). The human-like arterial blood gases are normal at rest, but as exercise progresses to levels of moderate intensity, $PAO_2 - PaO_2$ widens abnormally, $PaCO_2$ begins to

rise, and PaO_2 falls. Unlike in human athletes, this EIAH occurs in all thoroughbred horses studied to date. Why the $PAO_2 - PaO_2$ widens abnormally—even at submaximal exercise—is not known, although an exercise-induced opening of intrapulmonary shunt pathways (see previous discussion) is a possibility in these animals. Also, given the apparent limited capability of the pulmonary vasculature to accommodate their high cardiac output (see discussion later), a drastically reduced red cell transit time and diffusion limitation in the lung likely occurs, at least near maximal exercise intensities [79].

Exercise-induced carbon dioxide retention with $PaCO_2$ rising to 10 mm Hg or greater than at rest is unique to thoroughbreds. Why does this frank respiratory failure occur? During galloping exercise, respiratory rate must entrain with the footplant in these animals and the resultant high breathing frequency and short inspiratory time limit $\dot{V}_T$ and, therefore, $\dot{V}_A$. Marked carbon dioxide retention, however, also occurs at high $\dot{V}CO_2$, somewhat independent of stride frequency [80]. Given the high airflow rates required at high metabolic demands in this species, mechanical limits to expiratory flow and to ventilation are implicated but not proved [80]. Remarkably (and inexplicably), prolonging exercise at peak work rates by 1 or 2 minutes, and at a time when $\dot{V}O_2$ and $\dot{V}CO_2$ are beginning to fall significantly, results in an increase in V_T and $\dot{V}_A$ and, therefore, a reduction in $PaCO_2$ back to within the range of resting values. Prevention of EIAH in thoroughbreds using an increased fraction of inspired oxygen increases the $\dot{V}O_{2max}$ by 25% to 30% [69].

Thoroughbred pulmonary vasculature seems to be especially vulnerable to the high cardiac outputs achieved during maximal exercise in these animals. Mean pulmonary arterial pressures rise to greater than 100 mm Hg (or 4 to 5 times that of the human athlete). Bronchoscopy studies conducted immediately after even moderate intensity exercise in thoroughbreds show red cells accumulating in the airways, secondary to disruption (or fracture) of the alveolar-capillary barrier [54]. It is unclear whether or not the alveolar capillary fracture is related causally to the exercise $PAO_2 - PaO_2$ and EIAH in this species.

Thoroughbred horses trace their lineage back several centuries to a handful of animals with middle-east origins. Respiratory physiologists view the "underbuilt" structure of the thoroughbred lung to be a case of misdirected human genetic engineering. Other equines, such as ponies, whose average $\dot{V}O_{2max}$ is approximately 25% less than thoroughbreds', hyperventilate progressively with increasing exercise

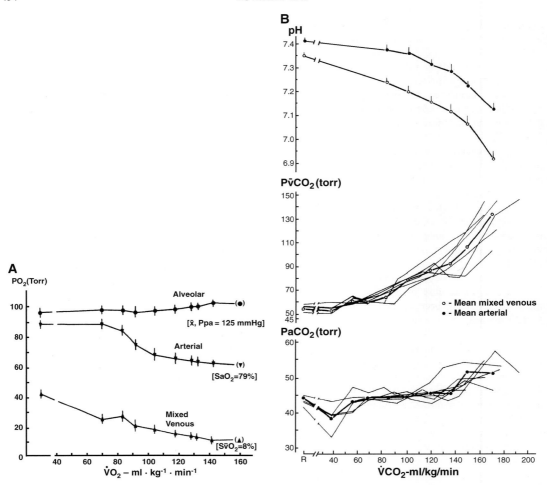

Fig. 8. The effects of progressive exercise to maximal in thoroughbred horses running on a treadmill at increasing speeds (individual and mean values in six horses). (*A*) Fall in venous PO_2 as oxygen extraction by the muscle increases with progressive increases in exercise intensity. (*B*) Fall in arterial pH; marked increases in mixed venous PCO_2 ($P\bar{v}CO_2$) as $\dot{V}CO_2$ of the contracting muscle increases. Excessive widening of the $PAO_2 - PaO_2$ (>40 mm Hg), carbon dioxide retention, and arterial hypoxemia begin to develop at submaximal exercise and worsen with further increases in exercise intensity. (*From* Bayly WM, Hodgson DR, Schulz DA, et al. Exercise-induced hypercapnia in the horse. J Appl Physiol 1989;67:1958–66; with permission.)

intensities and do not experience EIAH or severe pulmonary hypertension during exercise, even when comparisons between ponies and thoroughbreds are made at equivalent exercise $\dot{V}O_2$ [80,81]. Thoroughbreds having locomotor muscles capable of developing high force and velocity of shortening, and large metabolic energy production when coupled with the herculean capability of the cardiovascular system for cardiac output, have evolved to greatly exceed the capability of the pulmonary vasculature to accept this high cardiac output without incurring severe pulmonary hypertension and its sequelae.

Summary

Details in this article support the idea that the respiratory system of healthy untrained normal human subjects is able to accommodate all the demands of exercise virtually without compromise. Thus, exercise performance in these individuals is uncompromised, because the respiratory system in healthy individuals has been engineered biologically throughout evolutionary history via natural selection to meet or exceed the demands of exercise. Nevertheless, data also support the idea that there are some circumstances that either do not allow for or undermine the appropriate respiratory responses. In these cases, exercise tolerance and performance are limited by a respiratory system that is unable to accommodate the demands of exercise despite an evolutionary history presumably similar to the healthy untrained normal human subject. Why then is exercise performance limited by the respiratory system in some individuals and not others? In circumstances, such as those of aged individuals, this is explained readily by the naturally occurring ageing processes. This also is the case in thoroughbred horses, because artificial (rather than natural) selection of a specific "important" trait (running speed), without regard to other "unimportant" traits (respiratory system), resulted in a breed of animal with a respiratory system unable to cope with animals' physical performance. Other cases are not addressed as easily. For instance, why some individuals develop asthma or are susceptible to high-altitude pulmonary edema still is not understood entirely. Also, because of the random nature of genetic heritability, random variations in genotype, and ultimately phenotype, contribute to some limitations in exercise performance, such as the case of individuals who have extrathoracic airway obstruction during exercise. Hopefully, future research will integrate modern molecular techniques with whole-body physiologic techniques for a better understanding of how and why the respiratory system sometimes fails under extreme environments or conditions.

Acknowledgments

We thank Dr. Jerome A. Dempsey for consultation and critical review of this manuscript and Mr. Mark C. Reiner for assistance with the preparation of this work.

References

[1] Hey EN, Lloyd BB, Cunningham DJ, et al. Effects of various respiratory stimuli on the depth and frequency of breathing in man. Respir Physiol 1966;1:193–205.

[2] Ainsworth DM, Smith CA, Eicker SW, et al. The effects of chemical versus locomotory stimuli on respiratory muscle activity in the awake dog. Respir Physiol 1989;78:163–76.

[3] Johnson BD, Babcock MA, Suman OE, et al. Exercise-induced diaphragmatic fatigue in healthy humans. J Physiol 1993;460:385–405.

[4] Warren JB, Jennings SJ, Clark TJ. Effect of adrenergic and vagal blockade on the normal human airway response to exercise. Clin Sci (Lond) 1984;66:79–85.

[5] Haverkamp HC, Dempsey JA, Miller JD, et al. Physiologic response to exercise. In: Hamid Q, Shannon J, Martin J, editors. Physiologic basis of respiratory disease. Hamilton (Canada): BC Decker Inc.; in press.

[6] Fredberg JJ, Inouye D, Miller B, et al. Airway smooth muscle, tidal stretches, and dynamically determined contractile states. Am J Respir Crit Care Med 1997; 156:1752–9.

[7] Assmussen E, Nielsen M. Alveolo-arterial gas exchange at rest and during work at different O_2 tensions. Acta Physiol Scand 1960;50:153–66.

[8] Whipp BJ, Wasserman K. Alveolar-arterial gas tension differences during graded exercise. J Appl Physiol 1969;27:361–5.

[9] Gledhill N, Frosese AB, Dempsey JA. Ventilation to perfusion distribution during exercise in health. In: Dempsey JA, Reed CE, editors. Muscular exercise and the lung. Madison (WI): University of Wisconsin Press; 1977. p. 325–44.

[10] Torre-Bueno JR, Wagner PD, Saltzman HA, et al. Diffusion limitation in normal humans during exercise at sea level and simulated altitude. J Appl Physiol 1985;58:989–95.

[11] Wagner PD, Laravuso RB, Uhl RR, et al. Continuous distributions of ventilation-perfusion ratios in normal subjects breathing air and 100 per cent O_2. J Clin Invest 1974;54:54–68.

[12] Eldridge MW, Dempsey JA, Haverkamp HC, et al. Exercise-induced intrapulmonary arteriovenous shunting in healthy humans. J Appl Physiol 2004;97(3): 797–805.

[13] Coates G, O'Brodovich H, Jefferies AL, et al. Effects of exercise on lung lymph flow in sheep and goats during normoxia and hypoxia. J Clin Invest 1984;74: 133–41.

[14] Kitamura K, Jorgensen CR, Gobel FL, et al. Hemodynamic correlates of myocardial oxygen consumption during upright exercise. J Appl Physiol 1972;32: 516–22.

[15] Aviado DM, Daly MD, Lee CY, et al. The contribution of the bronchial circulation to the venous admixture in pulmonary venous blood. J Physiol 1961;155:602–22.

[16] Bachofen H, Hobi HJ, Scherrer M. Alveolar-arterial N_2 gradients at rest and during exercise in healthy men of different ages. J Appl Physiol 1973;34:137–42.

[17] Freedman ME, Snider GL, Brostoff P, et al. Effect of training on response of cardiac output to muscular exercise in athletes. J Appl Physiol 1955;8:37–47.

[18] Fritts HW, Harris P, Chidsey CAI, et al. Estimation of flow through bronchial-pulmonary vascular anastomoses with use of T-1824 dye. Circulation 1961;23: 390–8.

[19] Lenfant C. Measurement of factors impairing gas exchange in man with hyperbaric pressure. J Appl Physiol 1964;19:189–94.

[20] Mellemgaard K, Lassen NA, Georg J. Right-to-left shunt in normal man determined by the use of tritium and krypton 85. J Appl Physiol 1962;15:778–82.

[21] Ravin M, Epstein RM, Malm JR. Contribution of

thebesian veins to the physiologic shunt in anesthetized man. J Appl Physiol 1965;20:1148–52.

[22] Hammond MD, Gale GE, Kapitan KS, et al. Pulmonary gas exchange in humans during exercise at sea level. J Appl Physiol 1986;60:1590–8.

[23] Wagner PD, Gale GE, Moon RE, et al. Pulmonary gas exchange in humans exercising at sea level and simulated altitude. J Appl Physiol 1986;61:260–70.

[24] Conhaim RL, Staub NC. Reflection spectrophotometric measurement of O_2 uptake in pulmonary arterioles of cats. J Appl Physiol 1980;48:848–56.

[25] Hlastala MP. Multiple inert gas elimination technique. J Appl Physiol 1984;56:1–7.

[26] Reines HD, Civetta JM. The inaccuracy of using 100% oxygen to determine intrapulmonary shunts in spite of PEEP. Crit Care Med 1979;7:301–3.

[27] Butler BD, Hills BA. The lung as a filter for microbubbles. J Appl Physiol 1979;47:537–43.

[28] Prinzmetal M, Ornitz ME, Simkin B, et al. Arteriovenous anastomoses in liver, spleen and lungs. Am J Physiol 1948;152:48–52.

[29] Rahn H, Stroud RC, Tobin CE. Visualization of arterio-venous shunts by cinefluorography in the lungs of normal dogs. Proc Soc Exp Biol Med 1952;80:239–41.

[30] Tobin CE. Arteriovenous shunts in the peripheral pulmonary circulation in the human lung. Thorax 1966;21:197–204.

[31] Tobin CE, Zariquiey MO. Arteriovenous shunts in the human lung. Proc Soc Exp Biol Med 1950;75:827–9.

[32] Wilkinson MJ, Fagan DG. Postmortem demonstration of intrapulmonary arteriovenous shunting. Arch Dis Child 1990;65:435–7.

[33] Elliott FM, Reid L. Some new facts about the pulmonary artery and its branching pattern. Clin Radiol 1965;16:193–8.

[34] Shaw AM, Bunton DC, Fisher A, et al. V-shaped cushion at the origin of bovine pulmonary supernumerary arteries: structure and putative function. J Appl Physiol 1999;87:2348–56.

[35] Weibel ER. [Morphometric analysis of the number, volume and surface of the alveoli and capillaries of the human lung]. Z Zellforsch Mikrosk Anat 1962;57:648–66.

[36] Weibel ER. Morphometrics of the lung. In: Fenn WO, Rahn H, editors. Handbook of physiology section 3: respiration. Washington, DC: American Physiological Society; 1964. p. 285–307.

[37] Reeves JT, Taylor AE. Pulmonary hemodynamics and fluid exchange in the lung during exercise. In: Rowell LB, Shephard JT, editors. Handbook of physiology: section 12: exercise: regulation and integration of multiple systems. New York: Oxford University Press; 1996. p. 594–5.

[38] Meerbaum S. Principles of echo contrast. In: Nanda N, Schlief R, editors. Advances in echo imaging using contrast enhancement. Netherlands: Kluwer; 1993. p. 9–42.

[39] Meltzer RS, Klig V, Teichholz LE. Generating precision microbubbles for use as an echocardiographic contrast agent. J Am Coll Cardiol 1985;5:978–82.

[40] Meltzer RS, Tickner EG, Popp RL. Why do the lungs clear ultrasonic contrast? Ultrasound Med Biol 1980;6:263–9.

[41] Raisinghani A, DeMaria AN. Physical principles of microbubble ultrasound contrast agents. Am J Cardiol 2002;90(Suppl):3J–7J.

[42] Roelandt J. Contrast echocardiography. Ultrasound Med Biol 1982;8:471–92.

[43] Warren GL, Cureton KJ, Middendorf WF, et al. Red blood cell pulmonary capillary transit time during exercise in athletes. Med Sci Sports Exerc 1991;23:1353–61.

[44] Gossage JR, Kanj G. Pulmonary arteriovenous malformations. A state of the art review. Am J Respir Crit Care Med 1998;158:643–61.

[45] Chilvers ER, Whyte MK, Jackson JE, et al. Effect of percutaneous transcatheter embolization on pulmonary function, right-to-left shunt, and arterial oxygenation in patients with pulmonary arteriovenous malformations. Am Rev Respir Dis 1990;142:420–5.

[46] Whyte MK, Hughes JM, Jackson JE, et al. Cardiopulmonary response to exercise in patients with intrapulmonary vascular shunts. J Appl Physiol 1993;75:321–8.

[47] Hultgren HN. High-altitude pulmonary edema: current concepts. Annu Rev Med 1996;47:267–84.

[48] Schoene RB, Swenson ER, Pizzo CJ, et al. The lung at high altitude: bronchoalveolar lavage in acute mountain sickness and pulmonary edema. J Appl Physiol 1988;64:2605–13.

[49] Gibbs JSR, Schirlo C, Pavlicek V, et al. High altitude pulmonary edema:differences in pulmonary artery pressure between susceptible and non-susceptible subjects in normoxia and hypoxia. Circulation 1997;96(Suppl):I426–7.

[50] Kawashima A, Kubo K, Kobayashi T, et al. Hemodynamic responses to acute hypoxia, hypobaria, and exercise in subjects susceptible to high-altitude pulmonary edema. J Appl Physiol 1989;67:1982–9.

[51] Eldridge MW, Podolsky A, Richardson RS, et al. Pulmonary hemodynamic response to exercise in subjects with prior high-altitude pulmonary edema. J Appl Physiol 1996;81:911–21.

[52] Podolsky A, Eldridge MW, Richardson RS, et al. Exercise-induced VA/Q inequality in subjects with prior high-altitude pulmonary edema. J Appl Physiol 1996;81:922–32.

[53] West JB. Left ventricular filling pressures during exercise: a cardiological blind spot? Chest 1998;113:1695–7.

[54] West JB. Invited review: pulmonary capillary stress failure. J Appl Physiol 2000;89:2483–9.

[55] Duplain H, Sartori C, Lepori M, et al. Exhaled nitric oxide in high-altitude pulmonary edema: role in the regulation of pulmonary vascular tone and evidence for a role against inflammation. Am J Respir Crit Care Med 2000;162:221–4.

[56] Scherrer U, Vollenweider L, Delabays A, et al. Inhaled nitric oxide for high-altitude pulmonary edema. N Engl J Med 1996;334:624–9.

[57] Hohenhaus E, Paul A, McCullough RE, et al. Ventilatory and pulmonary vascular response to hypoxia and susceptibility to high altitude pulmonary oedema. Eur Respir J 1995;8:1825–33.

[58] Viswanathan R, Jain SK, Subramanian S, et al. Pulmonary edema of high altitude. II. Clinical, aerohemodynamic, and biochemical studies in a group with history of pulmonary edema of high altitude. Am Rev Respir Dis 1969;100:334–41.

[59] Steinacker JM, Tobias P, Menold E, et al. Lung diffusing capacity and exercise in subjects with previous high altitude pulmonary oedema. Eur Respir J 1998;11:643–50.

[60] Bittleman DB, Smith RJ, Weiler JM. Abnormal movement of the arytenoid region during exercise presenting as exercise-induced asthma in an adolescent athlete. Chest 1994;106:615–6.

[61] McFadden Jr ER, Zawadski DK. Vocal cord dysfunction masquerading as exercise-induced asthma. a physiologic cause for "choking" during athletic activities. Am J Respir Crit Care Med 1996;153:942–7.

[62] Anderson SD, Holzer K. Exercise-induced asthma: is it the right diagnosis in elite athletes? J Allergy Clin Immunol 2000;106:419–28.

[63] Suman OE, Babcock MA, Pegelow DF, et al. Airway obstruction during exercise in asthma. Am J Respir Crit Care Med 1995;152:24–31.

[64] Harms CA, McClaran SR, Nickele GA, et al. Exercise-induced arterial hypoxaemia in healthy young women. J Physiol 1998;507(Pt 2):619–28.

[65] Bousquet J, Jeffery PK, Busse WW, et al. Asthma. From bronchoconstriction to airways inflammation and remodeling. Am J Respir Crit Care Med 2000;161:1720–45.

[66] Johnson BD, Saupe KW, Dempsey JA. Mechanical constraints on exercise hyperpnea in endurance athletes. J Appl Physiol 1992;73:874–86.

[67] Anderson SD, Silverman M, Walker SR. Metabolic and ventilatory changes in asthmatic patients during and after exercise. Thorax 1972;27:718–25.

[68] Crimi E, Pellegrino R, Smeraldi A, et al. Exercise-induced bronchodilation in natural and induced asthma: effects on ventilatory response and performance. J Appl Physiol 2002;92:2353–60.

[69] Dempsey JA, Wagner PD. Exercise-induced arterial hypoxemia. J Appl Physiol 1999;87:1997–2006.

[70] Feisal KA, Fuleihan FJ. Pulmonary gas exchange during exercise in young asthmatic patients. Thorax 1979;34:393–6.

[71] Graff-Lonnevig V, Bevegard S, Eriksson BO. Ventilation and pulmonary gas exchange at rest and during exercise in boys with bronchial asthma. Eur J Respir Dis 1980;61:357–66.

[72] Dempsey JA, Seals DR. Aging, exercise and cardiopulmonary function. In: Lamb DR, Gisolfi CV, Nadel E, editors. Perspectives in exercise science and sports medicine: exercise in older adults. Carmel (IN): Cooper Publishing Group; 1995. p. 237–304.

[73] Thurlbeck WM. Morphology of the aging lung. In: Crystal RG, West JB, editors. The lung. New York: Raven Press; 1991. p. 1743–8.

[74] Janssens JP, Pache JC, Nicod LP. Physiological changes in respiratory function associated with ageing. Eur Respir J 1999;13:197–205.

[75] Reeves JT, Dempsey JA, Grover RF. Pulmonary circulation during exercise. In: Weir EK, Reeves JT, editors. Pulmonary vascular physiology and pathophysiology. New York: Marcel Dekker; 1989. p. 107–33.

[76] Miller JD, Dempsey JA. Pulmonary limitations to exercise performance: the effects of healthy aging and COPD. In: Massaro DJ, Massaro GD, Chambon P, editors. Lung development and regeneration. New York: Marcel Dekker; 2004. p. 483–524.

[77] Harms CA, McClaran SR, Nickele GA, et al. Effect of exercise-induced arterial O_2 desaturation on VO_2max in women. Med Sci Sports Exerc 2000;32:1101–8.

[78] Harms CA, Wetter TJ, St Croix CM, et al. Effects of respiratory muscle work on exercise performance. J Appl Physiol 2000;89:131–8.

[79] Wagner PD, Gillespie JR, Landgren GL, et al. Mechanism of exercise-induced hypoxemia in horses. J Appl Physiol 1989;66:1227–33.

[80] Bayly WM, Hodgson DR, Schulz DA, et al. Exercise-induced hypercapnia in the horse. J Appl Physiol 1989;67:1958–66.

[81] Parks CM, Manohar M. Blood-gas tensions and acid-base status in ponies during treadmill exercise. Am J Vet Res 1984;45:15–9.

[82] Johnson BD, Reddan WG, Pegelow DF, et al. Flow limitation and regulation of functional residual capacity during exercise in a physically active aging population. Am Rev Respir Dis 1991;143:960–7.

[83] Johnson BD, Reddan WG, Seow KC, et al. Mechanical constraints on exercise hyperpnea in a fit aging population. Am Rev Respir Dis 1991;143:968–77.

ELSEVIER
SAUNDERS

CLINICS
IN CHEST
MEDICINE

Clin Chest Med 26 (2005) 459–468

The Lung at Maximal Exercise: Insights from Comparative Physiology

Susan R. Hopkins, MD, PhD

*Division of Physiology, Department of Medicine, University of California — San Diego, 9500 Gilman Drive,
La Jolla, CA 92093, USA*

Well, it is all right, this running business, but I hope it doesn't distract you from your work as a medical student. [1][1]

Although the first Olympic games were recorded in 776 BC, the intense focus on training for human athletic events is relatively recent; the time spent in preparation for athletic events was minimal by today's standards. The British miler, Joe Binks (4:16.8-mile, circa 1902), described his training regime as follows: "I trained only one evening per week, winter and summer, spending some 30 minutes on each workout. My training was always light. I would run 5 or 6 times 60 to 110-yard burst of speed and finish with a fast 220 or 300 yards" [2]. It was not until Finish runners, particularly Hannes Kolehmainen, adopted systematic approaches to training in the 1910s, and Finish distance runners so dominated distance running at the Olympic games in the ensuing years, that prolonged training for performance enhancement became popular. Paavo Nurmi, the flying Finn, trained as many as 3 times a day, often over distance, and set world records at 1500, 5000, and 10,000 m and 1, 3, 6, and 10 miles in the 1920s. Even so, Sir Roger Bannister, who ran the first sub–4-minute mile in 1954, devoted only 30 minutes a day to training, despite his world record performance.

By contrast, competitive racing of horses is one of the oldest sports and dates to approximately 4500 BC. Professional horse racing, as it is known today, began early in the 1700s, and by 1750 the Jockey Club was formed at Newmarket, England. With this, breeding of racehorses became highly regulated, and the *Introduction to the General Stud Book* was published, tracing the pedigree of all horses racing in England [3]. That book is updated continuously with the lineage of every foal born to racehorses, and only those animals recorded in this record are called Thoroughbreds and allowed to race. The effect of this selective breeding is that all Thoroughbred horses can trace their descent to one of three sires: the Byerley Turk (circa 1679), the Darley Arabian (circa 1700), and the Godolphin Arabian (circa 1742).

In Table 1, the physiology of a Thoroughbred horse is compared with an elite human athlete at rest and during maximal exercise. The human data in this table were reported for Miguel Indurain, a five-time winner of the Tour de France. From rest to maximal exercise, humans are capable of increasing mass-specific oxygen consumption ~20-fold (this refers to elite athletes; untrained humans are capable of approximately one half this increase), a feat matched by horses. On a mass-specific basis, the oxygen consumption of horses is approximately double that of humans, an astonishingly high 140 mL/kg/min. This is more remarkable when the allometric scaling relationships for maximum oxygen consumption ($\dot{V}O_{2max}$) are considered [4]. Generally, $\dot{V}O_{2max}$

This work was supported by National Institutes of Health grant HL-17731.

E-mail address: shopkins@ucsd.edu

[1] Sir Roger Bannister (relating his mother's feeling about his athletic endeavors).

Table 1
The exercise physiology of a horse versus an elite human athlete

Variables	Miguel Indurain (80 kg)		Thoroughbred horse (450 kg)	
	Rest	Maximal exercise	Rest	Maximal exercise
Heart rate (beats/min)	28	195	28	220–230
Cardiac output (L/min)	5	50	25	322
Ventilation (L/min)	10	200	80	1600
$\dot{V}O_2$ (L/min)	0.3	6.8	3	63
$\dot{V}O_2$ (mL/kg/min)	4	88	6	140

Selected cardiopulmonary function variables compared between the human and the horse.

scales as a function of body mass$^{0.75}$; thus, a simple mass-specific comparison underestimates the differences between humans and horses, because larger animals in general are expected to have a lower mass-specific $\dot{V}O_{2max}$.

Pulmonary function and exercise responses

Human and equine athletes experience similar responses to exercise. Oxygen uptake and cardiac output increase linearly with increasing exercise intensity until $\dot{V}O_{2max}$ is reached. There are several important differences between human and equine athletes, however. In Fig. 1, selected variables related to exercise performance in horses [5–7] are divided by body mass and expressed as a percentage of human values [8–12] for elite athletes. Those adapta-

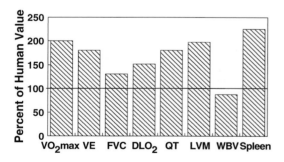

Fig. 1. Selected equine physiologic data expressed as a percentage of human data. All data are expressed relative to body mass. The large mass-specific $\dot{V}O_{2max}$, DLO_2, and cardiac output in horses are surprising when allometric scaling is taken into account [4] and likely reflect some effect of selective breeding for these traits in horses. DLO_2, diffusing capacity of lung for oxygen measured with the multiple inert gas elimination technique (mL/min/mm HG/kg); FVC, forced vital capacity (L/kg); LVM, left ventricular mass (g/kg); QT, maximal cardiac output (L/min); Spleen, splenic weight (g/kg); VE, maximal exercise ventilation (L/min/kg); WBV, whole blood volume (L/kg).

tions in cardiac output, pulmonary ventilation (both ~175% of human), and oxygen diffusing capacity (150% of human) are contributors to the high aerobic performance of horses. Unlike humans, who increase hematocrit only 2% to 5% at maximal exercise, a large spleen and vigorous splenic contraction act to double a horse's hematocrit during exercise, increasing oxygen delivery. Given these high rates of convective oxygen transport, it is surprising that such an aerobic athlete might have pulmonary limitations to exercise performance. These are well described in this animal, however [13]. Many organ systems adapt to training. In particular, the effects of training on the cardiovascular and musculoskeletal systems are well known. It only is in the past 20 years or so, however, that pulmonary limits to human exercise performance have begun to be appreciated. As time is spent devoted to exercise training increased and as performance levels improve, it is possible that pulmonary limits may become more manifest. In this review, human athletes and horses are compared during maximal exercise. Potential pulmonary limitations related to gas exchange and the development of exercise-induced arterial hypoxemia (EIAH), stress failure of pulmonary capillaries, exercise-induced pulmonary hemorrhage (EIPH), and interstitial pulmonary edema are explored.

Exercise-induced arterial hypoxemia

EIAH is characterized by a decrease in the PaO_2 sufficient to impair oxygen transport and a marked increase in the alveolar-arterial difference in partial pressure of oxygen pressure ($PAO_2 - PaO_2$), with little accompanying alveolar hyperventilation. Readers are referred to a review [13] of the potential causes of EIAH, which provides a framework for classification of the severity of hypoxemia. Hypoxemia can be considered from the perspective of oxygen delivery, with arterial oxygen saturation the primary variable of interest. When discussing pulmonary gas exchange, however, $PAO_2 - PaO_2$ and $PaCO_2$ are of primary importance. A $PAO_2 - PaO_2$ of greater than 25 mm HG can be considered as representing a mild gas exchange limitation, with values greater than 35 mm HG representing a severe gas exchange limitation [13]. Similarly, because in normal nonathletic humans, $PaCO_2$ is 30 to 35 mm HG at maximal exercise, a $PaCO_2$ of 35 to 38 mm HG represents borderline hyperventilation, whereas a $PaCO_2$ greater than 38 mm HG at maximal exercise suggests an inadequate hyperventilatory response. A consequence of EIAH is that it may have a significant detrimental effect on limiting oxygen transport and use during maximal exercise [14,15].

Fig. 2 shows arterial blood gas data at $\dot{V}O_{2max}$ for healthy young human subjects of varying degrees of

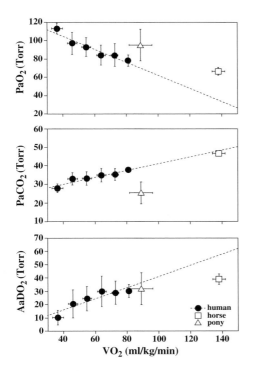

Fig. 2. Arterial blood gases obtained during exercise at 90% to 100% of $\dot{V}O_{2max}$ versus $\dot{V}O_{2max}$ in humans of differing aerobic fitness, compared with horses and ponies. In humans, pulmonary gas exchange worsens as aerobic fitness increases and EIAH is well described in human athletes. Alveolar ventilation during maximal exercise is reduced in subjects of greater fitness. The horse also shows alveolar hypoventilation and gas exchange impairment, which is not observed in the pony. The gas exchange abnormalities in horses, however, are less than expected from humans of comparable aerobic capacity.

aerobic fitness [16], ponies [4], and horses [17]. EIAH is virtually universal in horses [18] exercising at $\dot{V}O_{2max}$. Horses and the ponies experience inadequate gas exchange evidenced by a $PAO_2 - PaO_2$ of ~30 mm HG during heavy and maximal exercise [17,18]. The effect of inefficient gas exchange on PaO_2, however, is less in ponies [19] than in horses, largely because of marked alveolar hyperventilation, which is not seen in horses. As discussed later, the reduction in gas exchange efficiency in horses is compounded by frank hypoventilation during heavy exercise. Fig. 2 suggests that the extent of gas exchange limitations in horses is less than expected from human athletes of comparable fitness.

In healthy humans, gas exchange was long believed not to be a limiting factor to exercise performance. EIAH has been the focus of several research studies, however, especially after Dempsey and colleagues [20] reported arterial blood gases in 16 male athletes during treadmill running. In this study, 12 subjects developed changes in arterial blood gases consistent with EIAH. There is little doubt that EIAH is more common in humans capable of a high level of aerobic work. As seen in Fig. 2, the average PaO_2 at $\dot{V}O_{2max}$ falls with increasing $\dot{V}O_{2max}$, and the $PAO_2 - PaO_2$ shows a corresponding increase with increasing aerobic fitness. The variability in individual response is striking, however, and the $PAO_2 - PaO_2$ varies almost tenfold (~5–50 mm HG) at any given level of oxygen consumption per unit time ($\dot{V}O_2$) [16]. It is suggested that EIAH affects as many as 50% of highly trained human athletes [21]; however, large collated data sets [16] indicate that in subjects who have an aerobic fitness greater than 55 mL/kg/min, ~67% have a $PAO_2 - PaO_2$ greater than 25 mm HG, indicating a mild gas exchange limitation during maximal exercise. Of this population, 28% have severe gas exchange limitations, evidenced by a $PAO_2 - PaO_2$ greater than 35 mm HG.

Although EIAH often is most pronounced at maximal exercise, there is a trend in some human subjects toward developing a reduction in PaO_2 even during moderate exercise [22]. In addition, the gas exchange response to different exercise types varies, even among the same subjects exercising at the same absolute and relative oxygen consumption [23,24]. For example, there is ~10% lower PaO_2 during treadmill running than during cycling exercise [23]. Although it might be tempting to attribute the reduction in PaO_2 with running exercise to differences in alveolar ventilation (and indeed $PaCO_2$ was greater during running than cycling), the efficiency of gas exchange also differs between the two exercise types and the $PAO_2 - PaO_2$ is greater during running than cycling [23]. The reasons for this discrepancy are unknown.

There is considerable interest in defining sex differences in the gas exchange response to exercise (recently reviewed in [16]). Women have significantly smaller lung volumes and a lower resting diffusing capacity for carbon monoxide than males, even when corrected for body size and lower hemoglobin levels [25–27]. Thus, these differences in pulmonary structure may manifest themselves functionally as EIAH, although the area is one of active investigation.

Mechanisms of exercise-induced arterial hypoxemia

Potential mechanisms of an increased $PAO_2 - PaO_2$ with exercise include intrapulmonary or extrapulmonary shunting, ventilation-perfusion ($\dot{V}A/\dot{Q}$) inequality, and failure of end-capillary diffusion equilibrium for oxygen. A brisk hyperventilatory response can, in part, mitigate the effect of gas exchange efficiency on arterial oxygenation. Conversely, inadequate hyperventilation exacerbates the effect of an increased $PAO_2 - PaO_2$ on PaO_2.

Ventilation-perfusion inequality

The cause of the increase in $\dot{V}A/\dot{Q}$ inequality with exercise is not established but may relate to the development of interstitial pulmonary edema (discussed later). Horses are remarkable for uniform $\dot{V}A/\dot{Q}$ matching at rest [18,28]. During exercise, the extent of $\dot{V}A/\dot{Q}$ inequality increases, approximately doubling, but even with the increase associated with exercise, $\dot{V}A/\dot{Q}$ inequality is within the limits of normal for resting humans. However, approximately 30% of the increased $PAO_2 - PaO_2$ is related to the mild degree of $\dot{V}A/\dot{Q}$ inequality in these animals [29]. In humans, $\dot{V}A/\dot{Q}$ inequality contributes a variable amount to the $PAO_2 - PaO_2$ observed during heavy exercise. The effects of $\dot{V}A/\dot{Q}$ inequality may be mitigated in part during exercise, because increasing alveolar ventilation relative to perfusion results in increased ventilation of regions of high $\dot{V}A/\dot{Q}$ ratio, which does not contribute to a widened $PAO_2 - PaO_2$. Thus, the effects on the $PAO_2 - PaO_2$ are less than otherwise expected. Although the amount of $\dot{V}A/\dot{Q}$ inequality in an individual generally increases with increasing exercise intensity, there does not seem to be a significant relationship between the development of $\dot{V}A/\dot{Q}$ inequality and aerobic fitness [16]. $\dot{V}A/\dot{Q}$ inequality varies, however, with study population and may account for the majority of the $PAO_2 - PaO_2$ [10] in some subjects. In fit cyclists selected for

presence or absence of EIAH [30], there was no significant effect of exercise on $\dot{V}A/\dot{Q}$ matching, and the contribution of $\dot{V}A/\dot{Q}$ inequality to the overall $PAO_2 - PaO_2$ was less than 40% of the total $PAO_2 - PaO_2$ in these subjects.

Diffusion limitation

The extent of diffusion limitation to pulmonary oxygen transport can be estimated indirectly using the multiple inert gas elimination technique, which measures the portion of $PAO_2 - PaO_2$ caused by $\dot{V}A/\dot{Q}$ inequality and intrapulmonary shunt. The portion of the $PAO_2 - PaO_2$ remaining is attributed to pulmonary diffusion limitation. The cause of the pulmonary diffusion impairment of oxygen transport is unknown. It is likely because of rapid pulmonary capillary transit resulting in a failure of end-capillary diffusion equilibration for oxygen [9], although this is not established definitively. During maximal exercise, ~70% of the $PAO_2 - PaO_2$ in horses can be attributed to pulmonary diffusion limitation [29], which is greater than in most humans, except those who have marked EIAH [30]. The completeness of end-capillary diffusion equilibrium may be related to the ratio of diffusional to perfusional conductance in the lung [31,32]. Thus, although the mass-specific diffusing capacity for oxygen in horses is ~150% of human values, the very large mass-specific cardiac output (175% of human) may explain the greater extent of diffusion limitation in horses.

In humans, the amount of pulmonary–end-capillary diffusion limitation also varies between individuals [9] and is increased with increasing exercise intensity. The extent of pulmonary diffusion limitation is greater in subjects who have greater aerobic fitness [16] and in those who experience EIAH [30]. Thus, pulmonary diffusion limitation likely is an important feature of EIAH.

Shunt

Although theoretic arguments suggest they are not of primary importance, extrapulmonary noncardiac shunts cannot be ruled out as a cause of an increase in the $PAO_2 - PaO_2$ during exercise. Intrapulmonary shunting can be detected easily using the multiple inert gas elimination technique and has never been demonstrated to any great extent in healthy normal humans or horses, even in those who have marked gas exchange limitations during exercise [10,18,30, 33–35]. Small extrapulmonary shunts from bronchial and thebesian veins in the 1% range of cardiac output could account for almost a 10–mm HG reduction in PaO_2 during exercise and have not been well investigated as a possible contributor to the $PAO_2 - PaO_2$.

Alveolar ventilation

Inadequate hyperventilation during high-intensity exercise also has been implicated as a significant contributor to EIAH [20,36–38] and in horses, unlike in humans, there is insufficient compensatory hyperventilation to avoid hypercapnia [6,29]. Although mass-specific exercise ventilation is increased in horses compared with humans (see Fig. 1), horses are an obligate nasal breather and upper airway obstruction is well described in racehorses [39]. Horses experience a 1:1 ratio of entrainment of ventilation to stride frequency during galloping [40], which is not observed in human athletes [41]. Despite this, airflow resistance increases less with increasing exercise ventilation in horses than humans [42] and may account in part for the extraordinarily high ventilations these animals can achieve. As seen in Fig. 2, alveolar hypoventilation during maximal exercise is not a feature of all equines, because ponies hyperventilate markedly during exercise. Measurements of ventilation and pulmonary function present technical problems in horses, because the levels of exercise ventilation are so high that virtually all mask and valve systems partially obstruct ventilation [5,17] and make it difficult to establish the cause of the lack of compensatory hyperventilation. Inadequate ventilation is believed in part to result from the entrainment of stride frequency to respiratory frequency during galloping [43]; however, blunted chemoreceptor sensitivity also may play a role [5].

Several mechanisms for the failure of some human subjects to lower $PaCO_2$ below 35 mm HG during exercise are possible, including a decreased peripheral chemoreceptor function [38], respiratory muscle fatigue [31,32], and mechanical constraints imposed on inspiratory and expiratory flow [36,44]. In young fit subjects, almost all of the maximal expiratory flow volume curve may be approached during exercise [44], and even when helium-oxygen mixtures are used to mitigate expiratory flow limitation, EIAH is not prevented completely [36].

Interstitial pulmonary edema

The issue of whether or not interstitial pulmonary edema develops during exercise is unresolved, although indirect evidence suggests that it may be important in some human athletes. Diffusing capacity for carbon monoxide [45] and vital capacity are decreased post exercise, without a corresponding reduction in expiratory flow rates, although the change in diffusing capacity for carbon monoxide is explained in part by redistribution of pulmonary blood flow and a reduction in pulmonary capillary blood volume [46]. Interstitial pulmonary edema is expected to affect gas exchange in the lung by reducing the compliance of alveoli and by compressing small blood vessels, resulting in nonuniform airflow and blood-flow distribution in the lung. In support of this idea, $\dot{V}A/\dot{Q}$ inequality persists into recovery from heavy exercise, after ventilation and cardiac output have returned to normal [47], and subjects who have suffered previously from high-altitude pulmonary edema have higher pulmonary arterial pressures and greater $\dot{V}A/\dot{Q}$ inequality during sea-level exercise than control subjects [47,48]. Pig lungs show an increase in perivascular edema on histologic examination [49] in exercised animals compared with resting controls. Direct evidence of interstitial edema as a result of exercise, however, remains to be demonstrated conclusively.

Ventilation-perfusion inequality and pulmonary edema

$\dot{V}A/\dot{Q}$ inequality is increased by exercise (in some individuals) [50] and hypobaric hypoxia [51] and improves with 100% oxygen breathing [35], which alters pulmonary arterial pressure and the driving pressure for fluid flux. This suggests that the cause of increased $\dot{V}A/\dot{Q}$ inequality observed during exercise may be interstitial pulmonary edema. Possible alternate mechanisms include heterogeneity of hypoxic pulmonary vasoconstriction [52], reduction of gas mixing in large airways [53], and heterogeneity resulting from increased ventilation alone. If interstitial pulmonary edema is the cause of the increased $\dot{V}A/\dot{Q}$ inequality with exercise, prolonged exercise is expected to increase the $\dot{V}A/\dot{Q}$ inequality by increasing the duration of the exposure of the pulmonary vascular bed to increased pulmonary vascular pressures. This is expected to result in increased filtration of fluid across the capillary. Unlike in humans (discussed later), $\dot{V}A/\dot{Q}$ inequality does not change with prolonged exercise to exhaustion in horses [28]. Thus, it is possible that horses do not develop interstitial edema with sustained exercise. This idea is supported by recent measurement of intravascular lung water after exercise under normal conditions [54] and suggests that increases in pulmonary arterial pressure and increased transcapillary fluid flux are not important causes of exercise-induced $\dot{V}A/\dot{Q}$ inequality in this species. Alternatively, this difference may argue against interstitial pulmonary edema causing $\dot{V}A/\dot{Q}$ inequality in either humans or horses, since the fluid flux through the lungs of horses, where cardiac output is as high as 300 l/min, is enormous. However, hyperhydration of horses is associated with a deterioration of pulmonary gas exchange [55], and although the effect of this manipulation on $\dot{V}A/\dot{Q}$ heterogeneity has yet to be established, a potential relationship cannot be discounted. In human athletes, 1 hour of exercise at 65% of $\dot{V}O_{2max}$ is associated with an increase in $\dot{V}A/\dot{Q}$ inequality [33]. It seems that susceptible individuals can develop an increase in $\dot{V}A/\dot{Q}$ inequality with exercise, by exposure to short-term heavy exercise or by prolonged exercise at a lower intensity. The extent of the increased $\dot{V}A/\dot{Q}$ inequality is similar within individuals, regardless of which of these two type of exercise are used [33]. However, lung imaging after exercise is inconclusive; some studies demonstrate no change in lung water [56], and others show findings consistent with edema [57]. Thus conclusive proof of pulmonary edema occurring in humans or horses during sea level exercise is still awaited.

Exercise-induced pulmonary hemorrhage

The blood–gas barrier in lungs of mammals must fulfill two primary objectives. To allow pulmonary diffusion of oxygen and carbon dioxide, the blood–gas barrier of the lung must be very thin to allow the least possible resistance to pulmonary gas exchange.

At the same time, it must be able to withstand the high capillary wall stresses that develop during exercise when the capillary pressure rises [58]. The resistance to gas transport across the blood–gas barrier is proportional to its thickness; thus, conflicting forces potentially affect regulation of strength of the blood–gas barrier. As discussed previously, diffusion impairment of oxygen transport is in part responsible for the increase in $PAO_2 - PaO_2$ and the EIAH seen in many exercising humans and in horses. Therefore, an increase in mechanical strength of the blood–gas barrier by increasing thickness is undesirable, as diffusion equilibrium is expected to be compromised further. Therefore, it is not surprising that the structural integrity of the blood–gas barrier may be at risk during intense exercise.

Pulmonary capillary stress failure

For more than a decade, there has been increasing recognition that the blood–gas barrier of the lung is vulnerable to impairment in function induced by mechanical stress [59–64]. The nature of this stress (Fig. 3) relates to circumferential tension (a function of capillary transmural pressure and the radius of curvature of the capillary), longitudinal tension in the alveolar wall elements associated with the inflation of the lung, and surface tension of the alveolar lining layer. Since the original analyses by West of the mechanical forces placed on the lung [64], a great deal has been elucidated experimentally regarding the

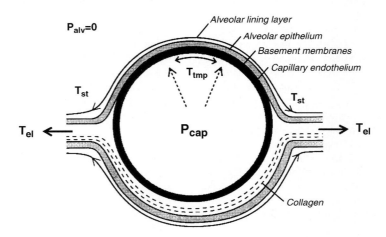

Fig. 3. Schematic representation of the three forces acting on the blood–gas barrier. T_{tmp} represents circumferential tension, a product of capillary transmural pressure ($P_{capillary} - P_{alveolar}$) × radius; T_{st} is the surface tension of the alveolar lining layer, which acts to support the capillary, and T_{el} is the longitudinal tension exerted by inflation of the lung. Exercise affects the forces placed on the pulmonary capillary by increasing T_{tmp} as capillary pressure rises and by increasing T_{el} as lung volumes increase with increased ventilation. (*From* West JB. Invited review: pulmonary capillary stress failure. J Appl Physiol 2000;89:2484; with permission.)

effects that extreme mechanical stresses have on the lung. The term, stress failure, is used to describe mechanically induced breaks in the blood–gas barrier. The vulnerability to pulmonary capillary stress failure is increased at high lung inflation [65] and varies between species. For example, dogs are more resistant to stress failure than rabbits. In experimental animal models of increased transmural pressure, ultrastructural changes in the blood–gas barrier are observed [66], consisting of discrete areas of structural damage to the blood–gas barrier, with rupture of the capillary endothelium, basement membrane, and the alveolar epithelium interspersed with large areas of structurally intact blood–gas barrier. Mechanical stress failure results in increased permeability of the blood–gas barrier to protein and red blood cells, but the blood–gas barrier retains sieving function for large molecular weight proteins [67]. Leukotriene B_4 is detected in the bronchoalveolar lavage fluid from these animals and likely represents activation of neutrophils or other white cells by exposed basement membrane [67].

Pulmonary capillary stress failure and exercise

Exercise, particularly in hypoxia, affects the mechanical forces placed on the pulmonary micro-

vasculature by increasing pulmonary arterial pressure, altering the pressure changes in the alveolus as expiration becomes active and by increasing lung inflation [58]. Thoroughbred racehorses almost universally develop EIPH [68–70]. Measurements of pulmonary artery (Fig. 4) and left atrial pressures in galloping racehorses show that these rise to extremely high levels, and capillary pressures are calculated at almost 100 mm Hg [71]. Electron micrographs of the lung taken from these animals after galloping show disruption of the capillary endothelium and the alveolar epithelium, and red cells and protein are observed in the alveolar space [69].

There is evidence that EIPH also occurs in some human athletes. Pulmonary capillary pressures as high as those observed in horses are not expected in humans during exercise, but using available data on pulmonary arterial and pulmonary arterial wedge pressures [51,72], it can be calculated that the capillary pressure near the base of the lung during heavy exercise in some humans exceeds 35 mm Hg [58]. Several studies report hemoptysis after exercise in human athletes. For example, after an ultramarathon, two athletes presented with shortness of breath, hemoptysis, and radiographic findings of pulmonary edema [73]. Similar findings were observed in military recruits who had excessive oral fluid intake before strenuous swimming exercise [74] and it is postulated that the combination of fluid overload combined with central vascular pooling and exercise may have raised pulmonary capillary pressure. EIPH was also described in an elite rugby player during exercise [75]. Bronchoscopy revealed frank bleeding from the lung periphery in this athlete. Also, increased concentrations of red blood cells, total protein, and leukotriene B_4 have been observed in bronchoalveolar lavage fluid of athletes who exercised at maximal levels for 6 to 8 minutes in a simulated race compared with sedentary controls [76]. These changes were not observed during exercise of lower intensity and longer duration [77], suggesting that the human lung is regulated to meet all but the highest demands.

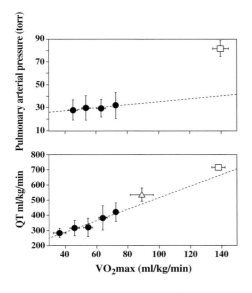

Fig. 4. Pulmonary arterial pressure versus $\dot{V}O_{2max}$ in humans and horses. Pulmonary arterial pressure is markedly elevated in horses compared with humans. Mass-specific cardiac output in humans, ponies, and horses. Cardiac output is higher in ponies and horses than expected from the human data.

Summary

Highly aerobic human athletes resemble their equine counterparts in many ways. Evidence suggests that both experience EIAH. Despite its much higher mass-specific $\dot{V}O_{2max}$, horses have only slightly greater gas exchange inefficiency than highly trained human athletes. The extent of diffusion limitation in horses likely is greater than in humans, but the extent of $\dot{V}A/\dot{Q}$ inequality is less. Horses hypoventilate markedly during exercise, however, and humans, although hyperventilation may be inadequate, do not experience frank hypoventilation. In humans and horses, the evidence for the development of interstitial edema during exercise is incomplete, but humans may be more vulnerable. Evidence suggests that some human athletes and virtually all Thoroughbred horses in training experience EIPH. As humans train harder for physical performance, pulmonary limitations during exercise may become even more evident.

References

[1] Academy of Achievement. Interview: Sir Roger Bannister. Available at: http://www.achievement.org/autodoc/page/banOint-3. Accessed July 6, 2005.

[2] Bryant J. 3:59.4 the quest to break the four minute mile. London: Arrow Books, LTD; 2005.

[3] An introduction to a general stud-book; containing (with few exceptions) the pedigree of every horse, mare & c. of note, that has appeared on the turf for the last fifty years with many of an earlier date. London: J. Weatherby; 1791.

[4] Taylor CR, Karas RH, Weibel ER, et al. Adaptive variation in the mammalian respiratory system in relation to energetic demand. Respir Physiol 1987;69: 1–127.

[5] Rose RJ, Evans DL. Cardiovascular and respiratory function in the athletic horse. In: Gillespie JR, Robinson NE, editors. Equine exercise physiology 2. Davis (CA): ICEEP Publications; 1987. p. 1–25.

[6] Bayly WM, Schultz DA, Hodgson DR, et al. Ventilatory responses of the horse to exercise: effect of gas collection systems. J Appl Physiol 1987;63:1210–7.

[7] Couetil LL, Rosenthal FS, Simpson CM. Forced expiration: a test for airflow obstruction in horses. J Appl Physiol 2000;88:1870–9.

[8] Bebout DE, Storey D, Roca J, et al. Effects of altitude acclimatization on pulmonary gas exchange during exercise. J Appl Physiol 1989;67:2286–95.

[9] Hopkins SR, Belzberg AS, Wiggs BR, et al. Pulmonary transit time and diffusion limitation during heavy exercise in athletes. Respir Physiol 1996;103:67–73.

[10] Hopkins SR, McKenzie DC, Schoene RB, et al. Pulmonary gas exchange during exercise in athletes I: ventilation-perfusion mismatch and diffusion limitation. J Appl Physiol 1994;77:912–7.

[11] Pluim BM, Zwinderman AH, van der Laarse A, et al. The athlete's heart: a meta-analysis of cardiac structure and function. Circulation 2000;101:336–44.

[12] Coltrain R, Kumar V, Robbins C. Diseases of the white cells, lymph nodes and spleen. In: Coltrain R, Kumar V, Robbins C, editors. Robbins pathological basis of disease. Philadelphia: Saunders; 1989. p. 173–320.

[13] Dempsey JA, Wagner PD. Exercise-induced arterial hypoxemia. J Appl Physiol 1999;87:1997–2006.

[14] Powers SK, Lawler J, Dempsey JA, et al. Effects of incomplete pulmonary gas exchange on VO_2 max. J Appl Physiol 1989;66:2491–5.

[15] Harms CA, McClaran SR, Nickele GA, et al. Effect of exercise-induced arterial O2 desaturation on VO2max in women. Med Sci Sports Exerc 2000;32:1101–8.

[16] Hopkins SR, Harms CA. Gender and pulmonary gas exchange during exercise. Exerc Sport Sci Rev 2004; 32:50–6.

[17] Bayly WM, Schulz D, Hodgson D, et al. Ventilatory response to exercise in horses with exercise-induced hypoxemia. In: Gillespie JR, Robinson NE, editors. Equine exercise physiology 2. Davis (CA): ICEEP Publications; 1987. p. 172–82.

[18] Wagner PD, Gillespie JR, Landgren GL, et al. Mechanism of exercise-induced hypoxemia in horses. J Appl Physiol 1989;66:1227–33.

[19] Parks CM, Manohar M. Blood-gas tensions and acid-base status in ponies during treadmill exercise. Am J Vet Res 1984;45:15–9.

[20] Dempsey JA, Hanson PG, Henderson KS. Exercised-induced arterial hypoxaemia in healthy human subjects at sea level. J Physiol (Lond) 1984;355:161–75.

[21] Powers SK, Dodd S, Lawler J, et al. Incidence of exercise-induced hypoxemia in elite endurance athletes at sea level. Eur J Appl Physiol 1988;58:298–302.

[22] Harms CA, McClaran SR, Nickele GA, et al. Exercise-induced arterial hypoxaemia in healthy young women. J Physiol (Lond) 1998;507(pt. 2):619–28.

[23] Hopkins SR, Barker RC, Brutsaert TD, et al. Pulmonary gas exchange during exercise in women: effects of exercise type and work increment. J Appl Physiol 2000;89:721–30.

[24] Gavin TP, Stager JM. The effects of exercise modality on exercise-induced hypoxemia. Respir Physiol 1999; 115:317–23.

[25] Mead J. Dysanapsis in normal lungs assessed by the relationship between maximal flow, static recoil, and vital capacity. Am Rev Respir Dis 1980;121:339–42.

[26] Thurlbeck WM. Postnatal human lung growth. Thorax 1982;37:564–71.

[27] Schwartz JD, Katz SA, Fegley RW, et al. Analysis of spirometric data from a national sample of healthy 6- to 24-year-olds (NHANES II). Am Rev Respir Dis 1988;138:1405–14.

[28] Hopkins SR, Bayly WM, Slocombe RF, et al. Effect of prolonged heavy exercise on pulmonary gas exchange in horses. J Appl Physiol 1998;84:1723–30.

[29] Wagner PD, Gillespie JR, Landgren GL, et al. Mechanism of exercise-induced hypoxemia in horses. J Appl Physiol 1989;66:1227–33.

[30] Rice AJ, Thornton AT, Gore CJ, et al. Pulmonary gas exchange during exercise in highly trained cyclists with arterial hypoxemia. J Appl Physiol 1999;87:1802–12.

[31] Piiper J, Scheid P. Gas transport efficacy of gills, lungs and skin: theory and experimental data. Respir Physiol 1975;23:209–21.

[32] Piiper J, Scheid P. Models for a comparative functional analysis of gas exchange organs in vertebrates. J Appl Physiol 1982;53:1321–9.

[33] Hopkins SR, Gavin TP, Siafakas NM, et al. Effect of prolonged, heavy exercise on pulmonary gas exchange in athletes. J Appl Physiol 1998;85:1523–32.

[34] Torre-Bueno JR, Wagner PD, Saltzman HA, et al. Diffusion limitation in normal humans during exercise at sea level and simulated altitude. J Appl Physiol 1985;58:989–95.

[35] Hammond MD, Gale GE, Kapitan KS, et al. Pulmonary gas exchange in humans during exercise at sea level. J Appl Physiol 1986;60:1590–8.

[36] McClaran SR, Harms CA, Pegelow DF, et al. Smaller lungs in women affect exercise hyperpnea. J Appl Physiol 1998;84:1872–81.

[37] Powers SK, Martin D, Cicale M, et al. Exercise-induced hypoxemia in athletes: role of inadequate hyperventilation. Eur J Appl Physiol 1992;65:37–42.

[38] Harms CA, Stager JM. Low chemoresponsiveness and inadequate hyperventilation contribute to exercise-induced hypoxemia. J Appl Physiol 1995;79:575–80.

[39] Franklin SH, Naylor JR, Lane JG. Effect of dorsal displacement of the soft palate on ventilation and airflow during high-intensity exercise. Equine Vet J Suppl 2002;379–83.

[40] Attenburrow DP. Time relationship between the respiratory cycle and limb cycle in the horse. Equine Vet J 1982;14:69–72.

[41] Bonsignore MR, Morici G, Abate P, et al. Ventilation and entrainment of breathing during cycling and running in triathletes. Med Sci Sports Exerc 1998; 30(2):239–45.

[42] Lafortuna CL, Saibene F, Albertini M, et al. The regulation of respiratory resistance in exercising horses. Eur J Appl Physiol 2003;90:396–404.

[43] Bayly W, Schott II H, Slocombe R. Ventilatory responses of horses to prolonged submaximal exercise. Equine Vet J Suppl 1995;18:23–8.

[44] Johnson BD, Saupe KW, Dempsey JA. Mechanical constraints on exercise hyperpnea in endurance athletes. J Appl Physiol 1992;73:874–86.

[45] Rasmussen BS, Hanel B, Jensen K, et al. Decrease in pulmonary diffusion capacity after maximal exercise. J Sports Sci 1984;4:185–8.

[46] Hanel B, Teunissen I, Rabol A, et al. Restricted postexercise pulmonary diffusion capacity and central blood volume depletion. J Appl Physiol 1997;83:11–7.

[47] Schaffartzik W, Poole DC, Derion T, et al. VA/Q distribution during heavy exercise and recovery in humans: implications for pulmonary edema. J Appl Physiol 1992;72:1657–67.

[48] Podolsky A, Eldridge MW, Richardson RS, et al. Exercise-induced VA/Q inequality in subjects with prior high-altitude pulmonary edema. J Appl Physiol 1996;81:922–32.

[49] Schaffartzik W, Arcos J, Tsukimoto K, et al. Pulmonary interstitial edema in the pig after heavy exercise. J Appl Physiol 1993;75:2535–40.

[50] Gale GE, Torre BJ, Moon RE, et al. Ventilation-perfusion inequality in normal humans during exercise at sea level and simulated altitude. J Appl Physiol 1985;58:978–88.

[51] Wagner PD, Sutton JR, Reeves JT, et al. Operation Everest II: pulmonary gas exchange during a simulated ascent of Mt. Everest. J Appl Physiol 1987;63: 2348–59.

[52] Hultgren HN. Pulmonary hypertension and pulmonary edema. In: Loeppsky JA, Reidsel ML, editors. Oxygen transport to human tissues. New York: Elsevier/North Holland; 1982. p. 243–54.

[53] Tsukimoto K, Arcos JP, Schaffartzik W, et al. Effect of common dead space on VA/Q distribution in the dog. J Appl Physiol 1990;68:2488–93.

[54] Wilkins PA, Gleed RD, Krivitski NM, et al. Extravascular lung water in the exercising horse. J Appl Physiol 2001;91:2442–50.

[55] Sosa Leon L, Hodgson DR, Evans DL, et al. Hyperhydration prior to moderate-intensity exercise causes arterial hypoxaemia. Equine Vet J Suppl 2002;34:425–9.

[56] Manier G, Duclos M, Arsac L, et al. Distribution of lung density after strenuous, prolonged exercise. J Appl Physiol 1999;87:83–9.

[57] Anholm JD, Milne EN, Stark P, et al. Radiographic evidence of interstitial pulmonary edema after exercise at altitude. J Appl Physiol 1999;86:503–9.

[58] West JB, Tsukimoto K, Mathieu-Costello O, et al. Stress failure in pulmonary capillaries. J Appl Physiol 1991;70:1731–42.

[59] West JB, Wagner PD. Pulmonary gas exchange. In: West JB, editor. Bioengineering aspects of the lung. New York: Marcel Dekker; 1977. p. 361–457.

[60] West JB, Mathieu-Costello O. Strength of the pulmonary blood-gas barrier. Respir Physiol 1992;88:141–8.

[61] West JB, Mathieu-Costello O. Stress failure of pulmonary capillaries in the intensive care setting. Schweiz Med Wochenschr 1992;122:751–7.

[62] West JB, Mathieu-Costello O. Stress failure of pulmonary capillaries: role in lung and heart disease. Lancet 1992;340:762–7.

[63] West JB, Mathieu CO. Vulnerability of pulmonary capillaries in heart disease. Circulation 1995;92:622–31.

[64] West JB. Invited review: pulmonary capillary stress failure. J Appl Physiol 2000;89:2483–9.

[65] Fu Z, Costello ML, Tsukimoto K, et al. High lung volume increases stress failure in pulmonary capillaries. J Appl Physiol 1992;73:123–33.

[66] Tsukimoto K, Mathieu-Costello O, Prediletto R, et al. Ultrastructural appearances of pulmonary capillaries at high transmural pressures. J Appl Physiol 1991; 71:573–82.

[67] Tsukimoto K, Yoshimura N, Ichioka M, et al. Protein, cell, and LTB4 concentrations of lung edema fluid produced by high capillary pressures in rabbit. J Appl Physiol 1994;76:321–7.

[68] Sweeney CR, Humber KA, Roby KA. Cytologic findings of tracheobronchial aspirates from 66 thoroughbred racehorses. Am J Vet Res 1992;53:1172–5.

[69] West JB, Mathieu CO, Jones JH, et al. Stress failure of pulmonary capillaries in racehorses with exercise-induced pulmonary hemorrhage. J Appl Physiol 1993; 75:1097–109.

[70] O'Callaghan MW, Pascoe JR, Tyler WS, et al. Exercise-induced pulmonary hemorrhage in the horse: Results of a detailed clinical, post mortem and imaging study. VIII. Conclusions and implications. Equine Vet J 1987;19:428–34.

[71] Jones JH, Smith BL, Birks EK, et al. Left atrial and pulmonary arterial pressures in exercising horses [abstract]. FASEB J 1992;6:A2020.

[72] Reeves JT, Groves BM, Cymerman A, et al. Operation Everest II: cardiac filling pressures during cycle exercise at sea level. Respir Physiol 1990;80: 147–54.

[73] McKechnie JK, Leary WP, Noakes TD, et al. Acute pulmonary oedema in two athletes during a 90-km running race. S Afr Med J 1979;56:261–5.

[74] Weiler RD, Shupak A, Goldenberg I, et al. Pulmonary oedema and haemoptysis induced by strenuous swimming. BMJ 1995;311:361–2.

[75] West JB, Mathieu-Costello O, Geddes DM. Intra-pulmonary hemorrhage caused by stress failure of pulmonary capillaries during exercise [abstract]. Am Rev Respir Dis 1991;143:A569.

[76] Hopkins SR, Schoene RB, Henderson WR, et al. Intense exercise impairs the integrity of the pulmonary blood-gas barrier in elite athletes. Am J Respir Crit Care Med 1997;155:1090–4.

[77] Hopkins SR, Schoene RB, Henderson WR, et al. Sustained submaximal exercise does not alter the integrity of the lung blood-gas barrier in elite athletes. J Appl Physiol 1998;84:1185–9.

ELSEVIER
SAUNDERS

Clin Chest Med 26 (2005) 469 – 484

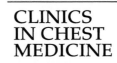

CLINICS
IN CHEST
MEDICINE

Aging of the Respiratory System: Impact on Pulmonary Function Tests and Adaptation to Exertion

Jean-Paul Janssens, MD

Outpatient Section of the Division of Pulmonary Diseases, Geneva University Hospital, 1211 Geneva 14, Switzerland

Life expectancy has risen sharply during the past century and is expected to continue to rise in virtually all populations throughout the world. In the United States population, life expectancy has risen from 47 years in 1900 to 77 in 2001 (74.4 for the male and 79.8 for the female population) [1]. The proportion of the population over 65 years of age currently is more than 15% in most developed countries and is expected to reach 20% by the year 2020. Healthy life expectancy, at the age of 60, is at present 15.3 years for the male population and 17.9 years for the female population [2]. These demographic changes have a major impact on health care, financially and clinically. Awareness of the basic changes in respiratory physiology associated with aging and their clinical implication is important for clinicians. Indeed, age-associated alterations of the respiratory system tend to diminish subjects' reserve in cases of common clinical diseases, such as lower respiratory tract infection or heart failure [3,4].

This review explores age-related physiologic changes in the respiratory system and their consequences in respiratory mechanics, gas exchange, and respiratory adaptation to exertion.

Structural changes in the respiratory system related to aging

Most of the age-related functional changes in the respiratory system result from three physiologic events: progressive decrease in compliance of the chest wall, in static elastic recoil of the lung (Fig. 1), and in strength of respiratory muscles.

Age-associated changes in the chest wall

Estenne and colleagues measured age-related changes in chest wall compliance in 50 healthy subjects ages 24 to 75: aging was associated with a significant decrease (-31%) in chest wall compliance, involving rib cage (upper thorax) compliance and compliance of the diaphragm-abdomen compartment (lower thorax) [5]. Calcifications of the costal cartilages and chondrosternal junctions and degenerative joint disease of the dorsal spine are common radiologic observations in older subjects and contribute to chest wall stiffening [6]. Changes in the shape of the thorax modify chest wall mechanics; age-related osteoporosis results in partial (wedge) or complete (crush) vertebral fractures, leading to increased dorsal kyphosis and anteroposteriordiameter (barrel chest). Indeed, prevalence of vertebral fractures in the elderly population is high and increases with age; in Europe, in female subjects over 60, the prevalence of vertebral fractures is 16.8% in the 60 to 64 age group, increasing to 34.8% in the 75 to 79 age group [7]. Men also show an increase in vertebral fractures with age, but rates are approximately half those of the female population [8]. A study of 100 chest radiographs of subjects ages 75 to 93 years, without cardiac or pulmonary disorders, illustrates the frequency of dorsal kyphosis in this age group: 25% had severe kyphosis as a consequence of vertebral wedge or crush fractures ($>50°$), 43% had moderate kyphosis ($35°-50°$), and only 23% had a normal curvature of the spine [6].

E-mail address: Jean-Paul.Janssens@hcuge.ch

0272-5231/05/$ – see front matter © 2005 Elsevier Inc. All rights reserved.
doi:10.1016/j.ccm.2005.05.004

chestmed.theclinics.com

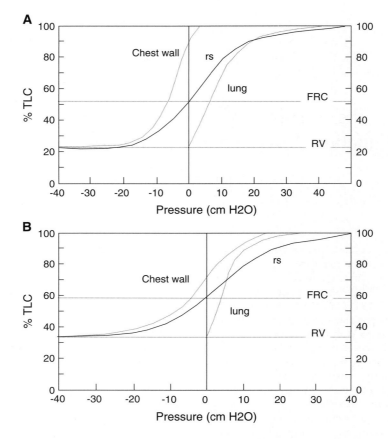

Fig. 1. Static pressure-volume curves showing changes in the compliance of the chest wall, the lung, and the respiratory system between an "ideal" 20-year-old (*A*) and a 60-year-old subject (*B*). Note increase in RV and FRC and decrease in slope of pressure-volume curve for the respiratory system (rs) in the older subject, illustrating decreased compliance of the respiratory system. (*Data from* Turner J, Mead J, Wohl M. Elasticity of human lungs in relation to age. J Appl Physiol 1968;25:664–71.)

Respiratory muscle function

Respiratory muscle performance is impaired concomitantly by the age-related geometric modifications of the rib cage, decreased chest-wall compliance, and increase in functional residual capacity (FRC) resulting from decreased elastic recoil of the lung (Fig. 2) [9]. The kyphotic curvature of the spine and the anteroposterior diameter of the chest increase with aging, thereby decreasing the curvature of the diaphragm and thus its force-generating capacity [6]. Changes in chest wall compliance lead to a greater contribution to breathing from the diaphragm and abdominal muscles and a lesser contribution from thoracic muscles. The age-related reduction in chest-wall compliance is somewhat greater than the increase in lung compliance; thus, compliance of the respiratory system is 20% less in a 60-year-old subject compared with a 20-year-old (see

Fig. 1) [9]. As such, during normal resting tidal breathing, the increase in breathing-related energy expenditure (elastic work) in a 60-year-old man is estimated at 20% compared with that of a 20-year-old, placing an additional burden on the respiratory muscles [8].

Respiratory muscle strength decreases with age (Table 1). Polkey and colleagues report a significant, although modest, decrease in the strength of the diaphragm in elderly subjects (n = 15; mean age 73, range 67–81 years) compared with a younger control group (n = 15; mean age 29, range 21–40 years): −13% for transdiaphragmatic pressure during a maximal sniff (sniff transdiaphragmatic pressure [Pdi]: 119 versus 136 cm H_2O) and −23% during cervical magnetic stimulation (twitch Pdi: 26.8 versus 35.2 cm H_2O) [10]. There was, however, a considerable overlap between groups, and the magnitude of the difference in this study was relatively small.

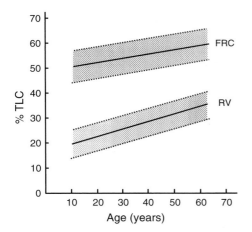

Fig. 2. Progressive and linear increase in RVand FRC between the ages of 20 and 60 years. Gray zones represent ± 1 SD. (*Data from* Turner J, Mead J, Wohl M. Elasticity of human lungs in relation to age. J Appl Physiol 1968;25: 664–71.)

Similarly, Tolep and coworkers report maximal Pdi values in healthy elderly subjects (n = 10; ages 65–75, 128 ± 9 cm H_2O), which were 25% lower than values obtained in young adults (n = 9; ages 19–28, 171 ± 8 cm H_2O) [11]. Although one cross-sectional study fails to demonstrate any relationship between age and maximal static respiratory pressures in 104 subjects over 55 [12], larger studies—also based on noninvasive measurements (maximal inspiratory and expiratory pressures [MIP and MEP] at the mouth and sniff nasal inspiratory pressure [SNIP])—document an age-related decrease in respiratory muscle performance [13–16].

Respiratory muscle strength is related to nutritional status, often deficient in the elderly. Enright and colleagues demonstrate significant correlations between MIP or MEP pressures and lean body mass (measured by bioelectric impedance), body weight, or body mass index [14]. Arora and Rochester show the deleterious impact of undernourishment on respiratory muscle strength or maximal voluntary ventilation: the decrease in respiratory muscle strength and maximal voluntary ventilation was highly significant in undernourished subjects (71 ± 6% of ideal body weight) compared with control subjects (104 ± 10% of ideal body weight) [17]. Necropsy studies confirm the correlation between body weight and diaphragm muscle mass further [18].

Age-associated alterations in skeletal muscles also affect respiratory muscle function [19]. MIP and MEP in elderly subjects are correlated strongly and independently with peripheral muscle strength (hand-grip) [13]. Peripheral muscle strength declines with aging. Bassey and Harries report a 2% annual decrease in handgrip strength in 620 healthy subjects over age 65 [20]. Decrease in muscle strength results from a decrease in cross-sectional muscle fiber area (process referred to as sarcopenia), a decrease in the number of muscle fibers (especially type II fast-twitch fibers and motor units), alterations in neuromuscular junctions, and loss of peripheral motor neurons with selective denervation of type II muscle fibers [21–26]. Other proposed mechanisms of age-related muscular dysfunction include impairment of the sarcoplasmic reticulum Ca^{++} pump resulting from uncoupling of ATP hydrolysis from Ca^{++} transport (which may reduce maximal shortening velocity and relaxation), loss of muscle proteins resulting from decreased synthesis (ie, decreased "repair" ability and protein turnover), and a decline in mitochondrial oxidative capacity [27–31].

Respiratory muscle function also is dependent on energy availability (ie, blood flow, oxygen content, and carbohydrate or lipid levels) [32]. Decreased respiratory muscle strength is described in patients who have chronic heart failure (CHF). Mancini and colleagues show that CHF has a highly significant impact on respiratory muscle strength and on the tension-time index [33]. The tension-time index describes the relationship between force of contraction (Pdi/Pdi$_{max}$) and duration of contraction (ratio of inspiratory time to total respiratory cycle duration [TI/TTOT]) and is related inversely to respiratory muscle endurance. In elderly subjects who have heart

Table 1
Maximal inspiratory and expiratory pressures measured at the mouth in older subjects, by age group and sex

Age group (y)	MIP (cm H_2O) n = 5201	MEP (cm H_2O) n = 756
Women		
65–69	59	125
70–74	56	121
75–79	49	102
80–84	45	84
>85	40	94
Men		
65–69	84	188
70–74	81	179
75–79	74	161
80–84	64	142
>85	56	131

Data from Enright PL, Kronmal RA, Manolio TA, et al. Respiratory muscle strength in the elderly: correlates and reference values. Am J Respir Crit Care Med 1994;149: 430–8.

failure, the tension-time index increases, primarily because of an increase in Pdi/Pdi_{max} and, during exercise, approaches values shown to generate fatigue [34]. Evans and coworkers show a significant correlation between cardiac index and sniff Pdi [35]. Nishimura and coworkers make a similar observation in subjects who have CHF, showing significant correlations between MIP and cardiac index or maximal oxygen consumption (VO_{2max}) per body weight, as an index of cardiovascular performance [36].

Other frequent clinical situations that produce diminished respiratory muscle function in the elderly include Parkinson's disease and sequelae of cerebral vascular disease [37,38]. Myasthenia gravis is another cause of respiratory muscle weakness, although encountered less commonly.

Changes in the lung parenchyma and peripheral airways

The human respiratory system is exposed continuously to air and a variety of inhaled pollutants. This creates a challenge for physiologists and clinicians, namely to differentiate—in studies of human lungs—the true impact of normal aging (ie, physiologic aging) from that of environmental exposure. Environmental tobacco smoke and particulate air pollution have measurable and well-documented effects on respiratory symptoms and disease in the elderly [39–41]. Appropriate animal models, therefore, are needed to study pathologic changes that occur with aging per se. Senescence-accelerated mice (SAM; a murine model of accelerated senescence) is proposed as such a model, permitting investigation of the differences between the aging lung and cigarette smoke–related airspace enlargement [42,43]. Morphometric studies of SAM show a notable homogeneous enlargement of alveolar duct size with aging. Cellular infiltrates in the alveoli rarely are seen, suggesting that the airspace enlargement does not result from inflammation, as opposed to what is seen in emphysema. The ratio of lung weight to body weight does not decrease with aging, suggesting little or no lung destruction [42]. Elastic fibers of the lung in SAM have a reduced recoil pressure, causing distention of the alveolar spaces and increased lung volume [43]. Age-related changes in the pressure-volume curves show a shift leftwards and upwards (ie, loss of elastic recoil of the lung) (see Fig. 1). These changes are similar to those described in senile hyperinflation of the lung in humans [9,44].

As noted in SAM during the course of aging, alveolar ducts in humans increase in diameter and alveoli become wider and shallower [45]. This enlargement is remarkably homogeneous as opposed to the irregular distribution of airspace enlargement in emphysema. Morphometric studies consistently find an increase in the average distance between airspace walls (mean linear intercept) and a decrease in the surface area of airspace wall per unit of lung volume beginning in the third decade of life. The decrease in surface area of airspace wall per unit of lung volume approximately is linear and continues throughout life, resulting in a 25% to 30% decrease in nonagenarians [46,47]. Although these changes are histologically different from emphysema (no destruction of alveolar walls), they result in similar changes in lung compliance. Thus, as described by Turner coworkers in subjects ages 20 to 60, static elastic recoil pressure of the lung decreases as a part of normal aging ($0.1-0.2$ cm $H_2O \cdot year^{-1}$), and the static pressure-volume curve for the lung is shifted to the left and has a steeper slope [9,48]. Verbeken and coworkers propose that the changes in structural and functional characteristics caused by isolated airspace enlargement that are seen in the elderly be differentiated from emphysema by the absence of alveolar wall destruction and inflammation and designated as senile lung [45].

In a postmortem study, mean bronchiolar diameter also decreased significantly after age 40 [49]. Bronchiolar narrowing and increased resistance were independent of any emphysematous changes or of previous bronchiolar injury. This decline in small airway diameter may contribute to the decrement in expiratory flow noted with aging [49]. Reduction in supporting tissues around the airways further increases the tendency for the small airways (<2 mm) to collapse.

Pulmonary function tests

Specifics of pulmonary function testing in an older population

The application of conventional quality control standards to objective assessment of pulmonary function in older subjects may prove difficult because of mood alterations, fatigability, lack of cooperation, or cognitive impairment. Indeed, prevalence of dementia increases with aging, reaching 5.6% after age 75, 22% after age 80, and 30% as of age 90 [50]. The relationship between ability to perform spirometry and cognitive function in the elderly is reported by several investigators [51–54]. The feasibility of high-quality spirometry in elderly subjects who do not have cognitive impairment is confirmed in a large

Italian study of 1612 ambulatory subjects ages 65 and older who did nor did not have chronic airflow limitation: tests with at least three acceptable curves were obtained in 82% of normal subjects and in 84% of patients who have chronic airflow limitation [55]. Cognitive impairment, however, lower educational level, and shorter 6-minute walking distance levels were found to be independent predictors of a poor acceptability rate [55]. Pezzoli and colleagues performed spirometric testing in 715 subjects who had respiratory symptoms and reported a feasibility rate (according to ATS criteria) of 82%; low Mini−Mental State Examination and activities of daily living scores were associated with poor spirometric performance [56]. Lower feasibility rates for spirometry are reported in elderly patients who were institutionalized (41%) and hospitalized (50%), with a clear relationship between the degree of cognitive impairment and feasibility of testing [53,54]. The prevalence of delirium in older people on hospital admission ranges from 10% to 24%, whereas delirium develops in 5% to 32% of older patients after admission [57]. Underdiagnosis, therefore undertreatment, of chronic obstructive pulmonary disease (COPD) in older subjects may be related to difficulties encountered in performing spirometry adequately in this population.

Alternative tests for the measurment of COPD in the elderly have been explored to find methods that may be less cooperation dependent for test subjects. Measurement of airway resistance using the forced oscillation technique (FOT) is applied more easily than spirometry in older patients who have cognitive disorders [53,54]. In elderly patients who are hospitalized or institutionalized, measurement of airway resistance by FOT was successful in 74% to 76% of patients tested. The reported sensitivity and specificity for the detection of COPD in older subjects were 76% and 78%, respectively; thus, FOT is useful in this population [54]. Conversely, assessment of airway resistance using the interrupter technique, widely used in epidemiologic and pediatric studies, in spite of its attractive simplicity, performed poorly in the detection of COPD in older subjects compared with FOT or spirometry, with a higher coefficient of variation than FOT [58]. The negative expiratory pressure technique (NEP), which does not require a forced expiratory maneuver, is useful to detect flow limitation [59]. The test involves applying negative pressure at the mouth during a tidal expiration. When the NEP elicits an increase in flow throughout the expiration, patients are not flow limited. In contrast, when patients do not have an increase in flow during most or part of the tidal expiration on application of NEP, they are considered flow limited. This technique has significant limitations, as it underestimated the presence of COPD without resting flow limitation in a study of 26 adults ages 42 to 87 (mean 65 ± 10 years) and, therefore, cannot be considered a substitute for spirometric screening for COPD [59].

For assessment of respiratory muscle performance, SNIP and MIP and MEP are feasible in older subjects, although SNIP tends to be easier to perform and better tolerated than MIP; these tests show an important learning effect and must be repeated at least five (MIP and MEP) to 10 (SNIP) times [60,61]. Reported coefficients of variation for MIP and MEP in healthy elderly subjects are, respectively, 10.2% and 12.8% [62].

Plethysmographic measurement of lung volumes seldom is required in this age group and, to the author's knowledge, no specific reference values are available for subjects over age 70.

Lung volumes

The major determinants of static lung volumes are the elastic recoil of the chest wall and that of the lung parenchyma. Loss of elastic recoil of the lung parenchyma and, to a lesser degree, decrease in respiratory muscle performance result in an increase in residual volume (RV): RV increases (air-trapping) by approximately 50% between ages 20 and 70 (see Fig. 2). Conversely, there is a progressive decrease in vital capacity to approximately 75% of best values. Because of the increased stiffness of the chest wall, the age-related diminished elastic recoil of the lungs is counterbalanced by an increased elastic load from the chest wall; total lung capacity (TLC) thus remains fairly constant throughout life [63]. Increased elastic recoil of the chest wall and diminished elastic recoil of the lung parenchyma also explain the increase in FRC (ie, elderly subjects breathe at higher lung volumes than younger subjects) (see Figs. 1 and 2) [63].

The closing volume (ie, the volume at which small airways in dependent regions of the lung begin to close during expiration) increases with age. Premature closure of terminal airways is related to a loss of supporting tissues around the airways. The closing volume begins to exceed the supine FRC at approximately 44 years of age and to exceed the sitting FRC at approximately 65 years of age [64]. Closing volume may reach 55% to 60% of TLC and equal FRC; as such, normal tidal breathing may occur with a significant proportion of peripheral airways not contributing to gas exchange (low ventilation-perfusion ratio [V/Q] zones). Although this is suggested as an important mechanism for the age-related decrease in PaO_2, increase in alveolar-arterial difference in partial pressure of oxygen ($PAO_2 - PaO_2$), and decrease in carbon monoxide transfer, measurement of V/Q inequality using the multiple inert gas elimination technique (MIGET) fails to show a significant increase in low V/Q areas with aging in 64 subjects ages 18 to 71 [65].

Spirometry

Forced expiratory volumes increase with growth up to the age of approximately 18. According to European Community for Coal and Steel data, no significant changes occur in forced expiratory volume in 1 second (FEV_1) or forced vital capacity (FVC) between the ages of 18 and 25 [66]. After this plateau, FEV_1 and FVC start to decrease, although more recent studies excluding smokers suggest a later start of FEV_1 and FVC decline in nonsmokers [67]. Cross-sectional and longitudinal studies show an accelerated decline in FEV_1 and FVC with age; the rate of decline is greater in cross-sectional versus longitudinal studies and in men versus women and more rapid in patients who have increased airway reactivity [63]. The age-related decrease in FEV_1 and FVC initially was considered linear, but more recent studies—including subjects ages 18 to 74—suggest that the decline may be nonlinear and accelerates with aging [68–71].

Regression equations, based on extrapolations from groups of younger subjects, tend to overestimate predicted values for FEV_1, FVC, and FEV_1/FVC in elderly subjects [67]. Few studies report results obtained in large samples of elderly subjects. Ericsson and Irnell, for example, report measurements performed on 264 normal "elderly" subjects, none of whom was older than 71 years of age [72]. Fowler and colleagues studied 182 Londoners over age 60, but only 44 subjects were over age 75 and 23 were over 80 [73]. The three largest studies (all cross-sectional) reporting spirometric data from healthy elderly subjects were published by Milne and Williamson, Enright and colleagues, and DuWayne Schmidt and colleagues[52,74,75]. DuWayne Schmidt and colleagues included patients ages 20 to 94 and found that decline in FEV_1 and FVC with age was linear (-31 mL/year in men and -27 mL/year in women). Values for FEV_1/FVC were stable in young adults and decreased in women over age 55 and in men over age 60 to 70 to 75% range [75]. The study by Milne and Williamson includes a large number of active or former smokers, and 20% of subjects had regular cough and phlegm; thus, it is unreliable [52].

Enright and colleagues selected 777 healthy non-obese, never-smokers ages 65 to 85 who had no history of lung disease from 5201 ambulatory elderly participants of the Cardiovascular Health Study; estimation of annual decline for FEV_1 was 32 mL/year in women and 27 mL/year for men and, for FVC, 33 mL/year in women and 20 mL/year in men (Box 1) [13,74,108,113,117]. Regression equations suggest a linear relationship between age and decline in FEV_1 and FVC in this study [73]. In summary, the average yearly decline of FEV_1 and FVC is approximately 30 mL/year, although it may be overestimated by cross-sectional studies. Whether or not decline of forced expiratory volumes with age is linear remains controversial, and longitudinal studies of older nonsmoking subjects are required to clarify this issue.

According to published reference values for FEV_1/FVC, using a threshold value of FEV_1/FVC less than 70% for defining the presence of airway obstruction, as suggested by the Global Initiative for Chronic Lung Diseases (GOLD) Workshop Summary, may lead to overdiagnosis of COPD. This is illustrated by a Norwegian study of forced expiratory volumes in 71 asymptomatic never-smokers, ages 70 or older; according to GOLD criteria, 25% had stage I COPD and 10% stage II; for subjects older than 80, results were, respectively, 32% and 18% [76]. Using the regression equations published by Enright and colleagues, normal values for FEV_1/FVC are less than 70% for men ages 80 and older and women ages 92 and older (see Box 1) [74].

Flow-volume curves and peak expiratory flow

Fowler and colleagues report characteristic modifications in the expiratory flow-volume curve with aging (Fig. 3) [73]. The changes in expiratory flow-volume suggested alterations in the small peripheral airways, with an obstructive pattern present even in lifetime nonsmokers, suggesting that this pattern may be normal in old age. Similar results are reported by Babb and Rodarte, who compared expiratory flow rates in 17 younger adults (ages 35–45) with those of 19 older adults (ages 65–75); in this study, decline in peak expiratory flow (PEF) in the older group is proportional to loss of lung elastic recoil [77]. Changes in peripheral airways and loss of supporting tissue around the airways ("senile lung") (discussed previously) are plausible explanations for these findings.

Although PEF rates tend to decrease with age, the variability in predicted peak flow values is large, and prediction equations are, therefore, not reliable [78,79]. PEF lability (maximal difference in PEF

Box 1. Regression equations for pulmonary function test variables in older subjects

Spirometry: men

FEV_1 (liters) = $(0.0378 \times height_{cm}) - (0.0271 \times age_{years}) - 1.73$; LLN = -0.84
FVC = $(0.0567 \times height_{cm}) - (0.0206 \times age_{years}) - 4.37$; LLN = -1.12
$FEV_1/FVC\%$ = $(-0.294 \times age_{years}) + 93.8$; LLN = -11.7

Spirometry: women

FEV_1 (liters) = $(0.0281 \times height_{cm}) - (0.0325 \times age_{years}) - 0.09$; LLN = -0.48
FVC = $(0.0365 \times height_{cm}) - (0.0330 \times age_{years}) - 0.70$; LLN = -0.64
$FEV_1/FVC\%$ = $(-0.242 \times age_{years}) + 92.3$; LLN = -9.3

Maximal mouth inspiratory and maximal mouth expiratory pressures: men

MIP (cm H_2O) = $(0.131 \times weight_{lb}) - (1.27 \times age_{years}) + 153$; LLN = -41
MEP (cm H_2O) = $(0.25 \times weight_{lb}) - (2.95 \times age_{years}) + 347$; LLN = -71

Maximal mouth inspiratory and maximal mouth expiratory pressures: women

MIP (cm H_2O) = $(0.133 \times weight_{lb}) - (0.805 \times age_{years}) + 96$; LLN = -32
MIP (cm H_2O) = $(0.344 \times weight_{lb}) - (2.12 \times age_{years}) + 219$; LLN = -52

6-minute walk test: men (n = 117; ages 40 to 80)

$6MWD_{meters}$ = $(7.57 \times height_{cm}) - (5.02 \times age_{years}) - 309$ m; LLN = -153 m

6-minute walk test: women (n = 173, ages 40 to 80)

$6MWD_{meters}$ = $(2.11 \times height_{cm}) - (2.29 \times weight_{kg}) - (5.78 \times age_{years}) + 667$ m;
LLN = -139 m

Maximal heart rate (n = 18712)

Maximal heart rate = $208 - (0.7 \times age)$

Maximal oxygen consumption (n = 100; ages 15 to 71)

VO_{2max} (L/min) = $(0.046 \times height_{cm}) - (0.021 \times age_{years}) - 0.62$ (0: male; 1: female) $- 4.31$ L;
LLN = $-.89$ L

Abbreviations: LLN, lower limit of normal (mean $- 1.96$ SD); 6MWD, distance walked during a 6-minute test.

per mean PEF) is shown to correlate with a diagnosis of asthma in younger subjects. Although middle-aged and older persons seem to be successful in providing a measure of PEF reliably at home, older age per se was a factor of increased variability in longitudinal monitoring of ambulatory PEF (independent predictor of higher PEF lability) [80]. In a study of 1223 subjects (mean age 66, range 43–80), Enright and colleagues report an upper limit of normal of 16% for PEF lability in older patients [80]. Another study

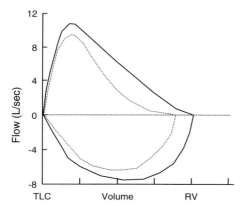

Fig. 3. Changes in the expiratory flow-volume curve with aging, suggesting obstruction to airflow. Curves from an older (*dashed line*) and a younger subject (*solid line*), normalized to percentage of vital capacity. (*Data from* Babb TG, Rodarte JR. Mechanism of reduced maximal expiratory flow with aging. J Appl Physiol 2000;89:505–11; and Fowler RW, Pluck RA, Hetzel MR. Maximal expiratory flow-volume curves in Londeners aged 60 years and over. Thorax 1987;42:173–82.)

by the same group, based on a larger community sample of 4581 persons ages 65 and older, reports an upper limit of normal of 29% for PEF lability. A cut-off value of 30% for PEF lability, therefore, is recommended in older subjects for the diagnosis of asthma [78].

No specific changes are noted regarding the inspiratory flow curves, although maximal inspiratory flow values decrease with aging. Because lung deposition of inhaled drugs is flow dependent with available powder-inhaling devices, determination of maximal inspiratory flow in older subjects may be relevant when considering topical bronchodilator or anti-inflammatory treatment with a powder inhaler [81,82]. Some powder-inhaling devices require minimal inspiratory flows (through the device) of up to $60 \ L \cdot min^{-1}$ and these values may not be attained in very elderly patients. With the Turbuhaler, for instance, lung deposition at an inspirator flow of $30 \ L \cdot min^{-1}$ is approximately half that obtained at $60 \ L \cdot min^{-1}$, although equivalent to that obtained with a metered-dose inhaler [82].

Airway resistance and conductance

When adjusted for lung volume, age has no significant effect on airway resistance. Peripheral airways contribute marginally to the total resistance of the airways and, therefore, changes in the peripheral airways are not reflected by changes in airway re-

sistance [63]. Using the FOT, Pasker and colleagues find a weak impact of age on resistance and reactance, with opposite effects according to sex; the investigators consider the relationship between FOT measurements and age clinically irrelevant [83].

Respiratory muscle testing

Respiratory muscle weakness may lead to shortness of breath, reduced exercise tolerance, and, in more severe cases, alveolar hypoventilation and respiratory failure. The overall strength of respiratory muscles can be measured noninvasively by recording MIP and MEP or by measuring SNIP [61,84]. These measurements can be performed easily at bedside [61,84]. Inspiratory pressures are measured at FRC or at RV. Expiratory pressures usually are measured at TLC. As discussed previously, the learning effect for MIP, MEP, and SNIP measurements is important, with significant increases over at least five consecutive maneuvers [13,61]. Values greater than or equal to 80 cm H_2O (in men) or 70 cm H_2O (in women) for MIP or greater than or equal to 70 cm H_2O in men and 60 cm H_2O in women for SNIP exclude clinically relevant respiratory muscle weakness [85].

Available reference values for these measurements show a decrease with age of respiratory muscle strength (see Table 1 and Box 1) [13–16]. Enright and colleagues measured MIP and MEP in ambulatory subjects ages greater than or equal to 65; normal values for women ages greater than or equal to 65 and males ages greater than or equal to 75 are below the aforementioned threshold for clinically relevant respiratory muscle dysfunction [13]. Nutritional status (body weight, bioelectric impedance, and body mass index) and peripheral muscle strength (handgrip) correlate significantly with MIP and MEP values [13]. Other investigators find values in the same range for MIP, MEP, or SNIP [15,16,86]. The decrease in respiratory muscle strength likely is relevant in elderly patients in clinical situations where an additional load is placed on the respiratory muscles, such as pneumonia or left ventricular failure [35,36]. The effects of poor nutritional status and CHF on respiratory muscle strength are discussed previously.

Gas exchange

Changes in arterial oxygen tension and ventilation-perfusion relationships

Wagner and coworkers, using the MIGET, report an increase, with aging, in V/Q imbalance, with a rise in units with a high V/Q (wasted ventilation or physiologic dead space) and in units with a low V/Q (shunt or venous admixture) [87,88]. The decrease in PaO₂ with age is described a consequence of this increased heterogeneity of V/Q and, in particular, of the increase in units with a low V/Q (dependent parts of the lung, poorly ventilated during tidal breathing, as reflected by an increased closing volume) [87]. These conclusions are based, however, on a small number of observations. More recently, Cardus and coworkers described the age-related changes in V/Q distribution in 64 healthy subjects ages 18 to 71 [65]. Although there was a slight increase in V/Q mismatch in older patients, shunt and low V/Q areas did not exceed 3% of total cardiac output, and decrease in PaO₂ with age was minimal (6 mm Hg). Most of the variance of V/Q mismatch was not a result of aging and remained unexplained; the role of an increase in closing volume with aging was not supported by these data. This elegant study included, unfortunately, a small number of older patients (only 4 were older than 60) and may not reflect changes in V/Q distribution occurring in the very old. Indeed, closing volume increases with age but may equal FRC only when subjects reach approximately 65 years of age (according to Leblanc and coworkers [89], FRC − closing volume = 1.95 − [0.03 × age]).

Regressions proposed for the computing of PaO₂ as a function of age vary widely, mainly in relation to the coefficient attributed to age [90]. Indeed, for an 82-year-old man, predicted values for PaO₂ range from 8.4 to 11.3 kPa (63–84 mm Hg). Delclaux and colleagues measured arterial blood gases in 274 subjects ages 65 to 100 (mean 82 years) with and without airway obstruction; mean PaO₂ was 10 ± 1.4 kPa (75 ± 11 mm Hg) [90]. These investigators suggest accepting as normal a PaO₂ of 10.6 to 11.3 kPa (80–85 mm Hg) for subjects 65 years of age and older [90]. Guenard and coworkers find no significant correlation between PaO₂ and age in 74 subjects ages 69 to 104; mean values reported were 11.2 ± 1.0 kPa (84 ± 7.5 mm Hg) [91]. Conversely, Sorbini and colleagues showed that there was a linear, but reciprocal, relationship between age and PaO₂ in nonsmoking healthy subjects, with the following regression equation: PaO₂ = 109 − (0.43 × age) (the fact that patients were supine during arterial sampling probably explains lower PaO₂ values obtained from this regression) [92]. More recently, Cerveri and coworkers suggest that the decrease in PaO₂ with aging is not linear [93]. In their study, arterial blood gas tests were analyzed in 194 nonsmoking subjects ages 40 to 90. Stratifying the results by 5-year age intervals, the investigators found a clear

decline in PaO₂ up to 70 to 74 years of age, followed by a slight rise in PaO₂ from ages 75 to 90. For healthy patients older than 75, PaO₂ was not correlated with age; mean values reported were 83 ± 9 mm Hg (11.1 ± 1.2 kPa), and fifth percentile was at 68.4 mm Hg (9.2 kPa) [93].

A modest increase in the PAO₂ − PaO₂ with age is expected because of the previously described increase in V/Q heterogeneity. According to Sorbini and coworkers [92], the highest normal value for the PAO₂ − PaO₂ at a certain age is given by the equation: PAO₂ − PaO₂ (mm Hg) ≤ 1.4 ± 0.43 × age (years). High values obtained by this equation (ie, 4.8 kPa [36 mm Hg] for 80 years of age) also may result from the supine position of subjects at time of sampling. More recent studies find no significant relationship between age and PAO₂ − PaO₂; however, values reported are well above normal values for younger adults (ie, 3.2 ± 1.4 kPa [24 ± 10 mm Hg] [90] and 4.4 ± 0.6 kPa [33 ± 4.5 mm Hg] [91]).

Carbon monoxide transfer factor

Flattening of the internal surface of the alveoli (ductectasia) in the elderly is associated with a reduction in alveolar surface (75 m² at the age of 30 years versus 60 m² at age 70 years, a reduction of 0.27 m² · year⁻¹) [63]. Because of loss of alveolar surface area, decreased density of lung capillaries, decline in pulmonary capillary blood volume, and increased V/Q heterogeneity, it is estimated that, even in healthy nonsmokers, there is a yearly decline in the diffusing capacity of the lung for carbon monoxide (DLCO) of 0.2 to 0.32 mL · min⁻¹ · mmHg⁻¹ from middle ages and onward in men and a decrease of 0.06 to 0.18 mL · min⁻¹ · mmHg⁻¹ in women [91,94]. Guénard and Marthan determined, in a population of 74 healthy subjects aged 69 to 104, the following regression equation for transfer capacity of the lung for carbon monoxide (TLCO) versus age (age explaining 29% of the variance of TLCO): TLCO (mL · min⁻¹ · kPa⁻¹) = 126 − 0.9 × age (years; r = 0.54, P < 0.001) [91].

Regulation of breathing

Aging and ventilatory responses

Aging is associated with a marked attenuation in ventilatory responses to hypoxia and hypercapnia [95–97]. Kronenberg and Drage compared the responses to hypercapnia and hypoxia in eight healthy young men (22–30 years old) with those of eight older men (64–73 years old) [95]. In the older subjects, ventilatory response to hypoxia was four times less than that of the younger group; response to hypercapnia was decreased by 58%. Mouth occlusion pressure ($P_{0.1}$), an index of respiratory drive, is the inspiratory pressure generated at the mouth when occluding the airway 0.1 second after the beginning of inspiration. Peterson and colleagues describe, in subjects ages 65 to 79, a 50% reduction in the response to isocapnic hypoxia and a 60% reduction in that to hyperoxic hypercapnia measured by $P_{0.1}$ compared with younger subjects [97]. More recently, however, two studies cast doubt on the age-related decrease in hypoxic ventilatory response. Smith and colleagues studied two groups of nonsmoking male subjects, ages 30 ± 7 and 73 ± 3, who were submitted to 20 minutes of acute isocapnic hypoxia; ventilatory responses and increment in neuromuscular drive were similar in both groups [98]. Similarly, Pokorski and Marczak compare the ventilatory response to isocapnic hypoxia in 19 women ages 71 ± 1 to 16 younger women and find no significant difference between groups in slopes of the ΔV_E (ventilation) to ΔSaO_2 (arterial oxygen saturation) ratio and $\Delta P_{0.1}/\Delta SaO_2$ [99].

The importance of the decrease in ventilatory response to hypercapnia in older subjects also is unsettled: as in the study by Kronenberg and Drage, Brischetto and colleagues report a reduction in the slope of the ventilatory response to hypercapnia in older subjects (−67%) versus a younger control group [95,96]. Rubin and coworkers, however, in a comparative study of ventilatory response and $P_{0.1}$ response to hypercapnia, fail to disclose significant differences between older (n = 10, ages over 60) versus younger adults (n = 18, ages under 30) [100].

Thus, although some studies suggest that there is an age-related decline in the ability to integrate information received from sensors (peripheral and central chemoreceptors and mechanoreceptors) and generate appropriate neural activity, further investigations are needed to clarify this issue.

Aging also is associated with a decreased perception of added resistive or elastic loads [57,101,102]. Older subjects have a lower perception of methacholine-induced bronchoconstriction than younger subjects. Although available evidence yields conflicting results, blunting of the response to hypoxia and hypercapnia and lower ability to perceive bronchoconstriction may represent a partial loss of important protective mechanisms (alarm signals).

During sleep

The prevalence of sleep-disordered breathing increases in elderly subjects. In middle-aged populations, the prevalence of the obstructive sleep apnea syndrome (OSAS), using an apnea/hypopnea index (AHI) of 15 events $\cdot$ h^{-1} as a cut-off value, is approximately 4% in women and 9% in men [103]. In older subjects, however, 13% to 62% of elderly subjects suffer from OSAS with an AHI greater than 10 events per hour [104]. Sleep-disordered breathing may be associated with impairment in cognitive function and is reported to be more frequent in Alzheimer's disease [105]. As discussed previously, aging is associated with a diminished perception of added resistive loads, such as that generated by bronchoconstriction or upper airway collapse. Indeed, respiratory effort in response to upper airway occlusion in elderly patients is decreased compared with younger subjects. Krieger and coworkers recorded esophageal pressure during sleep in 116 patients who had OSAS (AHI > 20) and showed that indexes of respiratory effort were reduced significantly in older compared with younger patients (inspiratory effort at end of apnea: maximal esophageal pressure 40 ± 2 versus 56 ± 3 cm H_2O) [106]. The lesser increase in respiratory effort in older patients may result from a decrease in respiratory drive and respiratory muscle performance. In spite of the fact that indexes of respiratory effort during apneic episodes were lower in older individuals, mean apnea duration was not prolonged significantly in older patients (28.3 ± 0.7 s versus 30.4 ± 0.9 s), and postapneic SaO_2 was higher in older individuals.

Ventilatory response to exercise

Performance during the 6-minute walk test

In subjects who do not have significant osteo-articular or neuromuscular limitation, the 6-minute walk test is a widely used standardized measurement for evaluating physical function; results of a 6-minute walk test are useful to quantify physical limitation and monitor progression of disease in chronic obstructive or restrictive disorders, CHF, or pulmonary vascular diseases; performance is correlated with health-related quality-of-life scores and predictive of morbidity and mortality in disorders, such as pulmonary hypertension or CHF [107]. There is a 15% learning effect when tests are performed on two successive days. Coefficient of variation is 8%. Enright and Sherrill established reference equations for the 6-minute walk test from results collected in 290 healthy subjects ages 40 to 80 (see Box 1) [108]. Predicted values for distance walked decrease linearly with age, with a difference of approximately 200 meters between the ages of 40 and 80 years. Mean baseline SaO_2 was stable at 96%. The 6-minute walk test is a submaximal exercise test (peak VO_{2max} during a 6-minute walk is approximately 80% of VO_{2max} during maximal exercise testing); thus, potentially it is less sensitive for the detection of cardiac or pulmonary disorders.

Maximal oxygen consumption and aging

The ability to perform physical tasks declines with advancing age. VO_{2max}, expressed in $L \cdot min^{-1}$, reaches a peak between 20 and 30 years of age. Longitudinal and cross-sectional studies thereafter show a decrease in VO_{2max} at an estimated rate of 9% to 10% per decade or -0.37 to -1.32 mL/kg/min/year (see Box 1) [109–114]. The ventilatory threshold also decreases with age, although less rapidly than VO_{2max} [115]. The decrease in VO_{2max} is more pronounced in sedentary subjects than in those remaining physically active [109]. In fact, loss in VO_{2max} is attenuated in fit elderly individuals and may not be significant clinically. VO_{2max} of older trained athletes is shown to be higher than that of middle-aged untrained men [116]. Thigh muscular mass also has a positive impact on VO_{2max} [113]. The Fick equation gives the relationship between cardiac output, peripheral oxygen extraction ($[Ca - Cv]O_2$), and oxygen consumption per unit time (VO_2): $VO_2 =$ cardiac output $\times [Ca - Cv]O_2$. Maximal heart rate (HR) in healthy adults decreases with age: Tanaka and colleagues, in a recent a meta-analysis compiling data from 18,712 subjects, show that maximal HR is independent of sex and level of physical activity and is predicted mainly by age alone; they computed the equation, maximal HR $= 208 - 0.7 \times$ age ($r = -0.90$ versus age), which gives slightly higher values than the commonly used predictive equation, maximal HR $= 220 -$ age [117]. Factors limiting VO_2 in older subjects are reduced maximal HR (resulting from a decrease in sensitivity of cardiac β-adrenergic receptors), decreased left ventricular ejection fraction, reduced maximal cardiac output, and reduced peripheral muscle mass. Fleg and Lakatta measured 24-hour urinary creatinine excretion, an index of muscle mass, in 184 healthy nonobese volunteers, aged 22 to 87, who performed a maximal treadmill exercise [118]. VO_{2max} showed a strong negative linear relationship with age. When VO_{2max} was normalized for creatinine excretion, a large portion of the age-associated decline in VO_{2max} was explained by the loss of muscle mass [118].

Ventilation and exercise

Ventilation during exercise in the elderly is associated with more abdominal contribution than in young adults and a concomitant change in respiratory pattern (higher rate and lower tidal volume), which may result from increased stiffness of the thoracic cage.

When compared with younger subjects, initial ventilatory (and circulatory) responses to exercise are slowed in the elderly. Although respiratory frequency increases rapidly, rise in tidal volume and total ventilation is delayed [119].

In contrast to the previously discussed decreased response to hypercapnia at rest, elderly subjects seem more responsive than younger subjects to carbon dioxide during exercise. Poulin and colleagues demonstrate, in a sample of 224 subjects aged 56 to 85, that, for a given carbon dioxide production (VCO_2), the ventilatory response (VE/VCO_2) increases with aging [120]. Similarly, Inbar and co-workers find a 14% increase in VE/VCO_2 and a 13% increase in VE/VO_2 between the ages of 20 and 70, in a large cross-sectional study of 1424 healthy subjects [114]. This also was reported by Brischetto and colleagues [95]. In both of these studies, this response was related neither to oxygen desaturation nor to increased metabolic acidosis; Prioux and colleagues, however, show that, above the anaerobic threshold, older subjects had, for a given carbon dioxide production, higher lactate concentrations [121]. A higher dead space–to–tidal volume ratio in elderly subjects most probably is contributive to the higher VE/VCO_2 ratio. In agreement with this hypothesis is the observation of a higher difference between end-tidal and arterial carbon dioxide tensions ($PaCO_2$) in older subjects and the increase in V/Q heterogeneity with aging (described previously) [65,114]. In itself, this may increase dyspnea for a given workload. Indeed, for a given VE, the oxygen cost of breathing is higher in elderly subjects.

Response to exercise training

Pulmonary rehabilitation programs are shown to improve exercise capacity in older patients who have COPD. A retrospective study by Couser and co-workers compares the impact of a 2-month rehabilitation program in 28 subjects ages 75 years and older versus 56 subjects aged less than 75. Improvement in 12-minute walking distance was significantly higher in the older patient group (+167 m; 38% increase) than in the younger group (+107 m; 23% increase) [122].

Aerobic training also is feasible in older healthy individuals and results in significant, although often modest, improvements in VO_2 peak in older subjects. For instance, Malbut and colleagues studied the effects of a 6-month aerobic training program on maximal aerobic power of 26 healthy elderly people (79 to 91 years) [123]. After training, VO_{2max} increased by 15% in women but not in men. Another study of 22 sedentary subjects (aged 80 to 92) shows, after 6 months of moderate-intensity aerobic exercise training, an improvement in exercise test duration (+33%) and peak VO_2 (+9%) [124]. Training programs of 4 to 12 months, in older individuals, show average increases in VO_{2max} of 8.5% to 25% [125–128].

Summary

Compliance of the chest wall and the respiratory system and lung elastic recoil decrease with aging, resulting in static air trapping (increased RV), increased FRC, and increased work of breathing. Respiratory muscle function also is affected by aging, either as a consequence of geometric changes in the rib cage, nutritional status (lean body mass, body weight), cardiac function, or through the age-related reduction in peripheral muscle mass and function, referred to as sarcopenia. In subjects 80 years of age and older, values of MIP may reach critically low values; this may result in alveolar hypoventilation or respiratory failure in clinical situations such as left-sided heart failure or pneumonia. Expiratory flow rates also decrease with aging, with characteristic changes in the flow-volume curves suggesting increased collapsibility of peripheral airways.

Gas exchange is remarkably well preserved at rest and during exertion in spite of a reduced alveolar surface area and increased ventilation-perfusion heterogeneity. In fact, in older athletes who have regular physical training, the respiratory system remains capable of adapting to high levels of exercise. In sedentary individuals, however, VO_{2max} decreases regularly with aging, whereas work of breathing, at a given level of ventilation, increases. Decreased sensitivity of respiratory centers to hypoxia or hypercapnia may result in a diminished ventilatory response in case of acute disease, such as heart failure, infection, or aggravated airway obstruction, although published data as to the ventilatory response to hypoxia in the elderly are inconclusive. Furthermore, blunted perception of added resistive loads (ie, bronchoconstriction) and diminished physical activity may result in a lesser awareness of respiratory disease and delay diagnosis.

References

[1] Arias E, Anderson R, Kung H, et al. National vital statistics reports. Hyattsville (MD): National Center for Health Statistics; 2003.

[2] World Health Organization. World health report 2004. Available at: http://www.who.int/whr/2004/annex/topic/en/annex_4_en.pdf.

[3] Janssens JP, Krause KH. Pneumonia in the very old. Lancet Infect Dis 2004;4:112–24.

[4] Janssens JP, Pache JC, Nicod LP. Physiological changes in respiratory function associated with ageing. Eur Respir J 1999;13:197–205.

[5] Estenne M, Yernault JC, De Troyer A. Rib cage and diaphragm-abdomen compliance in humans: effects of age and posture. J Appl Physiol 1985;59:1842–8.

[6] Edge JR, Millard FJ, Reid L, et al. The radiographic appearances of the chest in persons of advanced age. Br J Radiol 1964;37:769–74.

[7] Cummings SR, Melton LJ. Epidemiology and outcomes of osteoporotic fractures. Lancet 2002;359: 1761–7.

[8] Gunby MC, Morley JE. Epidemiology of bone loss with aging. Clin Geriatr Med 1994;10:557–71.

[9] Turner J, Mead J, Wohl M. Elasticity of human lungs in relation to age. J Appl Physiol 1968;25:664–71.

[10] Polkey MI, Harris ML, Hughes PD, et al. The contractile properties of the elderly human diaphragm. Am J Respir Crit Care Med 1997;155: 1560–4.

[11] Tolep K, Higgins N, Muza S, et al. Comparison of diaphragm strength between healthy adult elderly and young men. Am J Respir Crit Care Med 1995;152: 677–82.

[12] McElvaney G, Blackie S, Morrison NJ, et al. Maximal static respiratory pressures in the normal elderly. Am Rev Respir Dis 1989;139:277–81.

[13] Enright PL, Kronmal RA, Manolio TA, et al. Respiratory muscle strength in the elderly: correlates and reference values. Am J Respir Crit Care Med 1994;149:430–8.

[14] Enright PL, Adams AB, Boyle PJR, et al. Spirometry and maximal respiratory pressure references from healthy Minnesota 65 to 85 year old women and men. Chest 1995;108:663–9.

[15] Uldry C, Fitting J-W. Maximal values of sniff nasal inspiratory pressure in healthy subjects. Thorax 1995; 50:371–5.

[16] Black LF, Hyatt RE. Maximal respiratory pressures: normal values and relationship to age and sex. Am Rev Respir Dis 1969;99:696–702.

[17] Arora NS, Rochester DF. Respiratory muscle strength

and maximal voluntary ventilation in undernourished patients. Am Rev Respir Dis 1982;126:5–8.

[18] Arora NS, Rochester DF. Effect of body weight and muscularity on human diaphragm muscle mass, thickness, and area. J Appl Phsiol 1982;52:64–70.

[19] Tolep K, Kelsen S. Effect of aging on respiratory skeletal muscles. Clin Chest Med 1993;14:363–78.

[20] Bassey EJ, Harries UJ. Normal values for handgrip strength in 920 men and women aged over 65 years, and longitudinal changes over 4 years in 620 survivors. Clin Sci 1993;84:331–7.

[21] Evans WJ. What is sarcopenia? J Gerontol A Biol Sci Med Sci 1995;50(Spec no):5–8.

[22] Carmeli E, Reznick AZ. The physiology and biochemistry of skeletal muscle atrophy as a function of age. Proc Soc Exp Biol Med 1994;206:103–13.

[23] Carmeli E, Coleman R, Reznick AZ. The biochemistry of aging muscle. Exp Gerontol 2002;37:477–89.

[24] Booth FW, Weeden SH, Tseng BS. Effect of aging on human skeletal muscle and motor function. Med Sci Sports Exerc 1994;26:556–60.

[25] Baumgartner RN, Stauber PM, McHugh D, et al. Cross-sectional age differences in body composition in persons 60 + years of age. J Gerontol A Biol Sci Med Sci 1995;50:M307–16.

[26] Newman AB, Haggerty CL, Goodpaster B, et al. Strength and muscle quality in a well-functioning cohort of older adults: the Health, Aging and Body Composition Study. J Am Geriatr Soc 2003;51:323–30.

[27] Narayanan N, Jones D, Xu A, et al. Effects of aging on sarcoplasmic reticulum function and contraction duration in skeletal muscles of the rat. Am J Physiol 1996;271:1032–40.

[28] Balagopal P, Rooyackers O, Adey D, et al. Effects of aging on in vivo synthesis of skeletal muscle myosin heavy-chain and sarcoplasmic protein in humans. Am J Physiol 1997;273:790–800.

[29] Taylor D, Kemp G, Thompson C, et al. Ageing: effects on oxidative function of skeletal muscle in vivo. Moll Cell Biochem 1997;174:321–4.

[30] Trounce I, Byrne E, Marzuki S. Decline in skeletal muscle mitochondrial respiratory chain function: possible factor in ageing. Lancet 1989;1:637–9.

[31] Brierley E, Johnson M, James O, et al. Effects of physical activity and age on mitochondrial function. Q J Med 1996;89:251–8.

[32] Wilson DO, Rogers RM, Hoffman RM. Nutrition and chronic lung disease. Am Rev Respir Dis 1985;132:1347–65.

[33] Mancini D, Henson D, LaManca J, et al. Respiratory muscle function and dyspnoea in patients with chronic heart failure. Circulation 1992;86:909–18.

[34] Stassijns G, Lysens R, Decramer M. Peripheral and respiratory muscles in chronic heart failure. Eur Respir J 1996;9:2161–7.

[35] Evans S, Watson L, Hawkins M, et al. Respiratory muscle strength in chronic heart failure. Thorax 1995;50:625–8.

[36] Nishimura Y, Maeda H, Tanaka K, et al. Respiratory muscle strength and hemodynamics in chronic heart failure. Chest 1994;105:355–9.

[37] Brown LK. Respiratory dysfunction in Parkinson's disease. Clin Chest Med 1994;15:715–27.

[38] Vingerhoets F, Bogousslavsky J. Respiratory dysfunction in stroke. Clin Chest Med 1994;15:729–37.

[39] Anderson HR, Atkinson RW, Bremner SA, et al. Particulate air pollution and hospital admissions for cardiorespiratory diseases: are the elderly at greater risk? Eur Respir J Suppl 2003;40:39s–46s.

[40] Aga E, Samoli E, Touloumi G, et al. Short-term effects of ambient particles on mortality in the elderly: results from 28 cities in the APHEA2 project. Eur Respir J Suppl 2003;40:28s–33s.

[41] Jaakkola MS. Environmental tobacco smoke and health in the elderly. Eur Respir J 2002;19:172–81.

[42] Teramoto S, Fukuchi Y, Uejima Y, et al. A novel model of senile lung: senescence accelerated mouse (SAM). Am J Respir Crit Care Med 1994;150:238–44.

[43] Kurozumi M, Matsushita T, Hosokawa M, et al. Age-related changes in lung structure and function in the senescence-accelerated mouse (SAM): SAM-P/1 as a new murine model of senile hyperinflation of Lung. Am J Respir Crit Care Med 1994;149:776–82.

[44] Bode FR, Dosman J, Martin RR, et al. Age and sex differences in lung elasticity, and in closing capacity in nonsmokers. J Appl Physiol 1976;41:129–35.

[45] Verbeken E, Cauberghs M, Mertens I. The senile lung. Comparison with normal and emphysematous lungs. I: structural aspects. Chest 1992;101:793–9.

[46] Thurlbeck W. The internal surface area of nonemphysematous lungs. Am Rev Respir Dis 1967;95:765–73.

[47] Gillooly M, Lamb D. Airspace size in lungs of lifelong nonsmokers: effect of age and sex. Thorax 1993;48:39–43.

[48] Niewohner D, Kleinerman J, Liotta L. Elastic behaviour of post-mortem human lungs: effects of aging and mild emphysema. J Appl Physiol 1975;38:943–9.

[49] Niewoenner D, Kleinerman J. Morphologic basis of pulmonary resistance in human lung and effects of aging. J Appl Physiol 1974;36:412–8.

[50] Nussbaum RL, Ellis CE. Alzheimer's disease and Parkinson's disease. N Engl J Med 2003;348:1356–64.

[51] Sherman CB, Kern D, Richardson ER, et al. Cognitive function and spirometry performance in the elderly. Am Rev Respir Dis 1993;148:123–6.

[52] Milne JS, Williamson J. Respiratory function tests in older people. Clin Sci 1972;42:371–81.

[53] Carvalhaes-Neto N, Lorino H, Gallinari C, et al. Cognitive assessment of lung function in the elderly. Am J Respir Crit Care Med 1995;152:1611–5.

[54] Janssens JP, Nguyen M, Herrmann F, et al. Diagnostic value of respiratory impedance measurements in elderly subjects. Respir Med 2001;95:415–22.

[55] Bellia V, Pistelli R, Catalano F, et al. Quality control of spirometry in the elderly. The S.A.R.A. study. SAlute Respiration nell'Anziano = Respiratory

Health in the Elderly. Am J Respir Crit Care Med 2000;161(4 Pt 1):1094–100.

[56] Pezzoli L, Giardini G, Consonni S, et al. Quality of spirometric performance in older people. Age Ageing 2003;32(1):43–6.

[57] Manning H, Mahler D, Harver A. Dyspnea in the elderly. In: Mahler DA, editor. Pulmonary disease in the elderly patient. New York: Marcel Dekker; 1993. p. 81–111.

[58] Guo YF, Herrmann F, Ghezal S, et al. Comparison of airway resistance measurements by the forced oscillation technique and the interrupter technique for detecting obstructive lung disease in elderly patients. Swiss Med Wkly 2004;134(Suppl 139):S18.

[59] Koulouris NG, Valta P, Lavoie A, et al. A simple method to detect expiratory flow limitation during spontaneous breathing. Eur Respir J 1995;8:306–13.

[60] Larson JL, Covey MK, Vitalo CA, et al. Maximal inspiratory pressure. Learning effect and test-retest reliability in patients with chronic obstructive pulmonary disease. Chest 1993;104:448–53.

[61] Héritier F, Rahm F, Pasche P, et al. Sniff nasal inspiratory pressure: a noninvasive assessment of inspiratory muscle strength. Am J Respir Crit Care Med 1994;150:1678–83.

[62] McConnell AK, Copestake AJ. Maximum static respiratory pressures in healthy elderly men and women: issues of reproducibility and interpretation. Respiration (Herrlisheim) 1999;66:251–8.

[63] Crapo RO. The aging lung. In: Mahler DA, editor. Pulmonary disease in the elderly patient. New York: Marcel Dekker; 1993. p. 1–21.

[64] Tockman M. Aging of the respiratory system. In: Hazzard W, Bierman E, Blass J, et al, editors. Principles of geriatric medicine and gerontology. New York: McGraw-Hill; 1994. p. 555–64.

[65] Cardus J, Burgos F, Diaz O, et al. Increase in pulmonary ventilation-perfusion inequality with age in healthy individuals. Am J Respir Crit Care Med 1997;156(2 Pt 1):648–53.

[66] Quanjer P. Standardized lung function testing: report working party "Standardization of lung function tests". European Community for Coal and Steel, Luxembourg. Bull Eur Physiopathol Respir 1983; 19(Suppl 5):22–7.

[67] Kerstjens HA, Rijcken B, Schouten JP, et al. Decline of FEV_1 by age and smoking status: facts, figures, and fallacies. Thorax 1997;52:820–7.

[68] Dockery DW, Ware JH, Ferris Jr BG, et al. Distribution of forced expiratory volume in one second and forced vital capacity in healthy, white, adult never-smokers in six US cities. Am Rev Respir Dis 1985; 131:511–20.

[69] Glindmeyer HW, Lefante JJ, McColloster C, et al. Blue-collar normative spirometric values for Caucasian and African-American men and women aged 18 to 65. Am J Respir Crit Care Med 1995;151(2 Pt 1): 412–22.

[70] Brandli O, Schindler C, Kunzli N, et al. Lung function in healthy never smoking adults: reference values and lower limits of normal of a Swiss population. Thorax 1996;51:277–83.

[71] Burrows B, Lebowitz MD, Camilli AE, et al. Longitudinal changes in forced expiratory volume in one second in adults. Methodologic considerations and findings in healthy nonsmokers. Am Rev Respir Dis 1986;133:974–80.

[72] Ericcson P, Irnell L. Spirometric studies of ventilatory capacity in elderly people. Acta Med Scand 1969; 185:179–84.

[73] Fowler RW, Pluck RA, Hetzel MR. Maximal expiratory flow-volume curves in Londeners aged 60 years and over. Thorax 1987;42:173–82.

[74] Enright PL, Kronmal RA, Higgins M, et al. Spirometry reference values for women and men 65 to 85 years of age. Am Rev Respir Dis 1993;147: 125–33.

[75] DuWayne Schmidt C, Dickman ML, Gardner RM, et al. Spirometric standards for healthy elderly men and women: 532 subjects, ages 55 through 94 years. Am Rev Respir Dis 1973;108:933–9.

[76] Hardie JA, Buist AS, Vollmer WM, et al. Risk of over-diagnosis of COPD in asymptomatic elderly never-smokers. Eur Respir J 2002;20:1117–22.

[77] Babb TG, Rodarte JR. Mechanism of reduced maximal expiratory flow with aging. J Appl Physiol 2000;89:505–11.

[78] Enright PL, McClelland RL, Buist AS, et al. Correlates of peak expiratory flow lability in elderly persons. Chest 2001;120:1861–8.

[79] Bellia V, Pistelli F, Giannini D, et al. Questionnaires, spirometry and PEF monitoring in epidemiological studies on elderly respiratory patients. Eur Respir J Suppl 2003;40:21s–7s.

[80] Enright PL, Burchette R, Peters J, et al. Peak flow lability: association with asthma and spirometry in an older cohort. Chest 1997;112:895–901.

[81] Pauwels R, Newman S, Borgström L. Airway deposition and airway effects of antiasthma drugs delivered from metered-dose inhalers. Eur Respir J 1997;10:2127–38.

[82] Borgström L, Bondesson E, Morén F, et al. Lung deposition of budesonide inhaled via Turbuhaler®: a comparison with terbutaline sulphate in normal subjects. Eur Respir J 1994;7:69–73.

[83] Pasker H, Mertens I, Clement J, et al. Normal values of total respiratory input resistance and reactance for adult men and women. Eur Respir Rev 1994;4:134–7.

[84] Hamnegard C-H, Wragg S, Kyroussis D, et al. Portable measurement of maximum mouth pressures. Eur Respir J 1994;7:398–401.

[85] Polkey MI, Green M, Moxham J. Measurement of respiratory muscle strength. Thorax 1995;50:1131–5.

[86] Wijkstra PJ, Van der Mark TW, Boezen M, et al. Peak inspiratory mouth pressure in healthy subjects and in patients with COPD. Chest 1995;107:652–6.

[87] Wagner PD, Laravuso RB, Uhl RR, et al. Continuous distributions of ventilation-perfusion ratios in normal

subjects breathing air and 100 per cent O2. J Clin Invest 1974;54:54–68.

[88] Wagner PD, Saltzman HA, West JB. Measurement of continuous distributions of ventilation-perfusion ratios: theory. J Appl Physiol 1974;36:588–99.

[89] Leblanc P, Ruff F, Milic-Emili J. Effects of age and body position on "airway closure" in man. J Appl Physiol 1970;28:448–51.

[90] Delclaux B, Orcel B, Housset B, et al. Arterial blood gases in elderly persons with chronic obstructive pulmonary disease (COPD). Eur Respir J 1994;7:856–61.

[91] Guénard H, Marthan R. Pulmonary gas exchange in elderly subjects. Eur Respir J 1996;9:2573–7.

[92] Sorbini CA, Grassi V, Solinas E, et al. Arterial oxygen tension in relation to age in healthy subjects. Respiration (Herrlisheim) 1968;25:3–13.

[93] Cerveri I, Zoia MC, Fanfulla F, et al. Reference values of arterial oxygen tension in the middle-aged and elderly. Am J Respir Crit Care Med 1995;152:934–41.

[94] Butler C, Kleinerman J. Capillary density: alveolar diameter, a morphometric approach to ventilation and perfusion. Am Rev Respir Dis 1970;102:886–94.

[95] Brischetto M, Millman D, Peterson D, et al. Effect of aging on ventilatory response to exercise and CO2. J Appl Physiol 1984;56:1143–50.

[96] Kronenberg R, Drage G. Attenuation of the ventilatory and heart rate responses to hypoxia and hypercapnia with aging in normal man. J Clin Invest 1973; 52:1812–9.

[97] Peterson D, Pack A, Silage D, et al. Effects of aging on ventilatory and occlusion pressure responses to hypoxia and hypercapnia. Am Rev Respir Dis 1981; 124:387–91.

[98] Smith WD, Cunningham DA, Poulin MJ, et al. Ventilatory responses to isocapnic hypoxia in the eighth decade. Adv Exp Med Biol 1995;393:267–70.

[99] Pokorski M, Marczak M. Ventilatory response to hypoxia in elderly women. Ann Hum Biol 2003;30: 53–64.

[100] Rubin S, Tack M, Cherniack NS. Effect of aging on respiratory responses to CO2 and inspiratory resistive loads. J Gerontol 1982;37:306–12.

[101] Tack M, Altose M, Cherniack N. Effects of ageing on respiratory sensation produced by elastic loads. J Appl Physiol 1981;50:844–50.

[102] Tack M, Altose M, Cherniack N. Effect of aging on the perception of resistive ventilatory loads. Am Rev Respir Dis 1982;126:463–7.

[103] Young T, Palta M, Dempsey J, et al. The occurence of sleep-disordered breathing among middle-aged adults. N Engl J Med 1993;328:1230–5.

[104] Janssens JP, Pautex S, Hilleret H, et al. Sleep disordered breathing in the elderly. Aging Clin Exp Res 2000;12:417–29.

[105] Dealberto M, Pajot N, Courbon D, et al. Breathing disorders during sleep and cognitive performance in an older community sample: the EVA study. J Am Geriatr Soc 1996;44:1287–94.

[106] Krieger J, Sforza E, Boudewijns A, et al. Respiratory

effort during obstructive sleep apnea: role of age and sleep state. Chest 1997;112:875–84.

[107] American Thoracic Society. ATS statement: guidelines for the six-minute walk test. Am J Respir Crit Care Med 2002;166:111–7.

[108] Enright PL, Sherrill DL. Reference equations for the six-minute walk in healthy adults. Am J Respir Crit Care Med 1998;158(5 Pt 1):1384–7.

[109] Dehn MM, Bruce RA. Longitudinal variations in maximal oxygen intake with age and activity. J Appl Physiol 1972;33:805–7.

[110] Astrand I, Astrand PO, Hallback I, et al. Reduction in maximal oxygen uptake with age. J Appl Physiol 1973;35:649–54.

[111] Mahler DA, Cunningham LN, Curfman GD. Aging and exercise performance. Clin Geriatr Med 1986;2: 433–52.

[112] Robinson S, Dill DB, Tzankoff SP, et al. Longitudinal studies of aging in 37 men. J Appl Physiol 1975; 38:263–7.

[113] Jones NL, Makrides L, Hitchcock C, et al. Normal standards for an incremental progressive cycle ergometer test. Am Rev Respir Dis 1985;131:700–8.

[114] Inbar O, Oren A, Scheinowitz M, et al. Normal cardiopulmonary responses during incremental exercise in 20- to 70-yr-old men. Med Sci Sports Exerc 1994;26:538–46.

[115] Posner JD, Gorman KM, Klein HS, et al. Ventilatory threshold: measurement and variation with age. J Appl Physiol 1987;63:1519–25.

[116] Heath GW, Hagberg JM, Ehsani AA, et al. A physiological comparison of young and older endurance athletes. J Appl Physiol 1981;51:634–40.

[117] Tanaka H, Monahan KD, Seals DR. Age-predicted maximal heart rate revisited. J Am Coll Cardiol 2001; 37:153–6.

[118] Fleg JL, Lakatta EG. Role of muscle loss in the age-associated reduction in VO2 max. J Appl Physiol 1988;65:1147–51.

[119] Ishida K, Sato Y, Katayama K, et al. Initial ventilatory and circulatory responses to dynamic exercise are slowed in the elderly. J Appl Physiol 2000;89:1771–7.

[120] Poulin MJ, Cunningham DA, Paterson DH, et al. Ventilatory response to exercise in men and women 55 to 86 years of age. Am J Respir Crit Care Med 1994;149:408–15.

[121] Prioux J, Ramonatxo M, Hayot M, et al. Effect of ageing on the ventilatory response and lactate kinetics during incremental exercise in man. Eur J Appl Physiol 2000;81:100–7.

[122] Couser JI, Guthmann R, Abdulgany Hamadeh M, et al. Pulmonary rehabilitation improves exercise capacity in older elderly patients with COPD. Chest 1995;107:730–4.

[123] Malbut KE, Dinan S, Young A. Aerobic training in the 'oldest old': the effect of 24 weeks of training. Age Ageing 2002;31:255–60.

[124] Vaitkevicius PV, Ebersold C, Shah MS, et al. Effects of aerobic exercise training in community-based

subjects aged 80 and older: a pilot study. J Am Geriatr Soc 2002;50:2009–13.

[125] Yerg 2nd JE, Seals DR, Hagberg JM, et al. Effect of endurance exercise training on ventilatory function in older individuals. J Appl Physiol 1985;58:791–4.

[126] Vincent KR, Braith RW, Feldman RA, et al. Improved cardiorespiratory endurance following 6 months of resistance exercise in elderly men and women. Arch Intern Med 2002;162:673–8.

[127] Seals DR, Hurley BF, Schultz J, et al. Endurance training in older men and women II. Blood lactate response to submaximal exercise. J Appl Physiol 1984;57:1030–3.

[128] Posner JD, Gorman KM, Windsor-Landsberg L, et al. Low to moderate intensity endurance training in healthy older adults: physiological responses after four months. J Am Geriatr Soc 1992;40:1–7.

ELSEVIER
SAUNDERS

Clin Chest Med 26 (2005) 485 – 507

CLINICS
IN CHEST
MEDICINE

Pulmonary Function Testing and Extreme Environments

Thomas A. Dillard, MD[a,*], Seema Khosla, MD[a], Frank W. Ewald, Jr, MD[b],
M. Asif Kaleem, MBBS[a]

[a]Division of Pulmonary/Critical Care, Medical College of Georgia, BBR 5513, 1120 15th Street, Augusta, GA 30912-3135, USA
[b]Veteran's Administration Medical Center, 1 Freedom Way, Augusta, GA 30904, USA

Millions of people around the world engage in leisure or occupational activities in extreme environments [1]. These environments sometimes entail health risks even for normal subjects. The presence of lung disease, or other conditions, further predisposes to illness or injury. Patients who have known lung conditions should, but often do not, consult with their pulmonary clinicians before traveling [2]. Normal subjects, including elderly or deconditioned adults, may be referred to pulmonologists for evaluation of risk prior to exposure. Other patients may present for consultations after complications occur. In many instances, pulmonary function testing before or after exposure can assist physicians counseling patients about the likelihood of complications.

Extreme environments (Table 1) may be natural or manmade but differ from usual conditions in at least one of the following variables of the physical environment: (1) the breathing atmosphere, which consists of gas composition, barometric pressure, humidity, and temperature; (2) the body envelope, which includes anything in physical contact with the subject, such as ambient pressure, clothing, air or water temperature, and humidity; (3) kinematics, including velocity, acceleration, and gravity; and (4) radiation from energy sources, including heat, electromagnetic fields, or emissions, such as x-rays (see Table 1).

Biologic and nonbiologic variables may influence tolerance of extreme environments strongly. These

include: (1) psychomotor activity, such as exercise, posture, sleep/wake cycle, and emotional or mental state; (2) diet, including source of energy and hydration; (3) biohazards, such as biologic toxins, microbiologicpathogens, pollutants, and poisons; (4) the chronic state of health of the subject; and, finally, (5) unexpected threats, such as wildlife, failure of equipment or performance, and common illnesses that can increase the harshness of an otherwise mild environment and contribute to intolerance.

Extreme environments often involve more than one of these variables, which may compound each other. Mountain climbing, for example, entails moderate to heavy exertion (psychomotor activity) in a setting of reduced inspired PaO_2 and low ambient humidity (breathing atmosphere), cold ambient temperature and high winds (body envelope), and increased ultraviolet light exposure (radiation) [3].

Table 2 presents general levels of medical supervision of exposures to extreme environments. Specific guidelines for patient management with respect to extreme environments differ in various fields of interest, such as military medicine, emergency medicine, wilderness medicine, aerospace medicine, and pulmonary medicine. This article includes recent guidelines most likely to be of interest to chest physicians.

Because of the daunting task of trying to simulate exposures for millions of would-be travelers, however, the authors favor future studies that examine and validate measures of clinical value in day-to-day practice as predictors of outcomes of extreme exposures. Simulations, such as chamber exposures, may need to be applied for higher-risk subjects or settings and to develop predictors.

* Corresponding author.
E-mail address: tdillard@mail.mcg.edu (T.A. Dillard).

Table 1
Examples of extreme environments

Variable	Spectrum	Examples
Atmospheric pressure	Hypobaric	Mountain climbing; aviation (air travel)
	Hyperbaric	Diving
	Transients	Explosion blast wave; sound
Gravitational force	Zero G	Parabolic flight; space travel
	High G	Rocket launch; aviation; centrifuge
Electromagnetic radiation	Ultraviolet	Mountain climbing
	X-ray	Occupation
Temperature	Low	Polar exploration; mountain climbing
	High	Various

The scope of this article precludes a detailed review of all extreme environments. Several examples are considered with respect to selected lung diseases and common medical illnesses. Recommendations for pulmonary function testing are included, such as spirometry, exercise testing, bronchial challenge testing, hypoxic gas inhalation testing, and blood gas analysis or other evaluation along with recommendations for restrictions from participation. Readers are referred to earlier works [4].

Hyperbaric environments: diving

The different forms of diving include breath-hold diving; compressed gas diving with the familiar self-contained underwater breathing apparatus (scuba) and closed circuit systems; surface supplied gas diving using a life line to a diving helmet or suit; and saturation diving, where the divers typically stay in a habitat pressurized to the depth at which they are working [5]. This section briefly reviews effects of diving on lung function, common hazards of diving,

and specific recommendations for patients who have common conditions.

Hazards of diving

Diving presents major challenges to cardiovascular and respiratory systems. Drowning, myocardial infarction, and pulmonary barotrauma constitute the most common causes of death in divers [6]. Decompression sickness (DCS) and systemic arterial gas embolism (SAGE), sometimes jointly referred to as decompression illness (DCI), constitute common hazards of diving that often are preventable and respond to hyperbaric recompression therapy. Table 3 shows hazards of diving by likeliest phase of the dive for presentation. This information is useful to clinicians who may be called on to provide emergency care for amateur divers who sustain injuries.

DCS is a multiorgan system disorder that results from micro- or macroscopic nitrogen bubble formation when ambient pressure decreases on surfacing. Bubbles can cause injury by rupturing cell walls, accumulating in veins or arteries and impairing perfusion, activating coagulation or inflammation pathways, and other mechanisms. SAGE may result from a variety of mechanisms, including pulmonary overinflation injury (POI) with passage of air from the pulmonary interstitial space into pulmonary capillaries or veins and accumulation of bubbles in the pulmonary artery raising right heart pressure enough to create right-to-left shunting through a patent foramen ovale (PFO). Other mechanisms, such as passage of air bubbles directly through the pulmonary capillary bed [7] or through a pulmonary arteriovenous malformation, could contribute to the pathogenesis of SAGE. The effects of SAGE include occlusion of cranial, coronary, spinal, mesenteric, and renal arteries with severe consequences. Elevated serum creatinine phosphokinase, mostly of skeletal muscle origin, is proposed as a useful marker for recent SAGE [8].

Table 2
Levels of medical supervision of subjects exposed to extreme environments

Level	Subject	Supervision	Monitoring	Example
0	Normal	None	None	Trekking (N); skiing (N)
1	Ambulatory	Remote	Pre-exposure	Diving (N); air travel (P)
2	High-risk[a]	On-site	Symptomatic	Deep diving (N); medical spa (P)
3	Hospitalized	On-site	Intermittent	Air evacuation of mass casualties (P)
4	Critically ill	On-site	Continuous	Critical care air transport (P)

Abbreviations: N, normal subjects; P, patients.

[a] Indicates high-risk subject or high-risk activity warranting on-site medical assistance.

Table 3
Some common hazards of scuba diving by phase of dive

Hazard	Dive phase	Comment
Drowning	Any	
Squeeze injuries	Descent	Middle ear, sinuses, lung (uncommon)
Nitrogen narcosis	Descent	Narcotic effect of nitrogen (100–200 fsw)
High-pressure neurologic syndrome	Bottom	Heliox (500 fsw)
Hypercapnia	Bottom	Equipment failure
Hyperoxia	Bottom	Central nervous system or lung toxicity
POI	Ascent	Pneumomediastinum, pneumothorax
Carbon monoxide poisoning	Ascent	Contaminated air
SAGE	Ascent	Within 10 min after surfacing
Hypoxia	Ascent	Can occur in any phase
DCS	Postdive	10 min to 24 h after surfacing

POI typically occurs during ascent from scuba diving. Macklin and Macklin [9], Pierson [10], and others propose a sequence of events for the pathogenesis of POI. Alveolar rupture, particularly at the border of the alveolar connection to the bronchovascular sheath, can occur at transpulmonary pressures of 80 mm Hg or less [11,12]. A greater pressure change can occur with one body length of ascent in seawater with glottis closed. High transpulmonary pressures overdistend the lung and disrupt the continuity of the pulmonary epithelium. Air enters the interstitial space and dissects centrally to the hilum along the bronchovascular compartment. If the mediastinal pleura remains intact, then pneumomediastinum occurs without pneumothorax. Subcutaneous emphysema and pneumoperiotoneum or pneumoretroperitoneum can occur by dissection superiorly or inferiorly, respectively. Pneumothorax occurs if a defect in the pleura permits air to enter the pleural space. Dissection of air outwardly to the periphery of the lung to cause pneumothorax also is proposed [13]. This mechanism occurs with trauma to the chest wall and possibly other mechanisms.

Factors that increase the likelihood of POI include scuba divers holding their breath during ascent, ascending too rapidly, and having underlying obstructive lung disease, such as asthma, chronic obstructive pulmonary disease (COPD), or a focal anatomic ab-

normality. Such injuries also can occur in normal subjects who use safe diving practices. Table 4 shows a differential diagnosis of common signs and symptoms that may develop during dives.

Tetzlaff and colleagues [14] explored the link between pulmonary function abnormalities and diving illnesses. These investigators compared preinjury spirometry and chest radiograph findings with postinjury chest CT findings from 15 consecutive cases of diving-related barotrauama (pneumothorax, pneumomediastinum, or arterial gas embolism) to a group of 15 cases of DCS without barotrauma. There were 11 male and 4 female divers in both groups. Seven patients in the barotrauma group were current smokers versus nine in the DCS group. All patients had normal preinjury values for vital capacity and forced expiratory volume in 1 second (FEV_1) and group means exceeded mean predicted values.

Pulmonary barotrauma patients showed significantly lower forced expiratory flow rates at 50% and 25% of vital capacity ($P < 0.05$ and $P < 0.02$, respectively) compared to patients who had DCS. In a subgroup of 10 barotrauma patients, forced expiratory rate at 25% was below 80% of the predicted values, whereas only one patient who had DCS had a similarly reduced forced expiratory rate at 25%. Results of chest CT scans in 12 patients who had barotrauma revealed subpleural emphysematous blebs in five patients that were not detected in preinjury or postinjury chest radiographs. Presumably these were pre-existing lesions. Chest CT was negative in four patients who had DCS.

Table 4
Clinical manifestations of diving injuries and selected causes

Manifestation	Causes
Chest pain	Coronary thrombosis; SAGE; pneumomediastinum; pneumothorax; pulmonary oxygen toxicity
Dyspnea	Bronchospasm; pneumothorax; hypercapnia; anxiety
Hemoptysis	Pulmonary artery gas embolism; lung squeeze; pulmonary edema[a]; middle ear squeeze[a]; sinus squeeze[a]
Paralysis	Spinal DCS; cranial artery gas embolism
Seizures	Central nervous system oxygen toxicity; hypercapnia; high pressure neurologic syndrome; SAGE; DCS
Loss of consciousness	SAGE; hypoxia; hypercapnia; nitrogen narcosis; hyperoxia; vasovagal syncope
Paresthesias	Cutaneous DCS; spinal DCS

[a] Conditions that may mimic hemoptysis.

Table 5
Fitness for diving: selected contraindications

Condition	Absolute	Relative
Cardiovascular	Coronary ischemia	Post myocardial ischemia
	Arrhythmias	Angioplasty
	PFO, atrial septal defect, ventricular septal defect	Prior thoracic surgery
	Congestive heart failure	Hypertension
		Raynaud's phenomenon
Pulmonary	Active asthma	History of asthma
	Active pneumothorax	History of pneumothorax
	Active pulmonary infections	
	Cavitary lung disease	
	COPD	
	Bullous lung disease	
Ear, nose, and throat	Active upper respiratory infection	Allergic rhinitis
	Otitis media	Sinus obstruction
	Monomeric tympanic membrane	Cholesteatoma
	Active ruptured tympanic membrane	Ear atresia/stenosis
	Poststapedectomy	Chronic otitis externa
	Dental caries	Unilateral sensorineural hearing loss
	Meniere's disease	
	Tracheostomy	
Neurologic	Seizure disorders	Migraine headaches
	Other central nervous system disease	
Other	Prior arterial gas embolism	Previous DCS
	Late pregnancy	Early pregnancy
	Insulin-dependent diabetes mellitus	Other medications
	Osteomyelitis	Herniated nucleus pulposus
	Esophageal diverticulae	
	Sickle cell disease	

The study by Tetzlaff suggests that lung diseases causing abnormalities in pulmonary function or anatomy predispose to diving barotrauma. Accordingly, many common medical conditions represent absolute contraindications to diving, whereas other conditions are relative contraindications (Table 5). Pulmonary physicians should counsel patients who have known or suspected lung disease of any significance that they may risk death or serious impairment if they dive.

Effects of diving on pulmonary function

Diving poses many challenges to the respiratory system. Head out immersion reduces lung volume subdivisions and dynamic compliance and increases work of breathing [15–17]. Simply standing in the water with the head out reduces vital capacity by 5% to 10% as a result of the vertical gradient of water pressure (1 cm H_2O pressure per cm of depth). Immersion displaces blood from the limbs into the thorax, reducing lung volume and increasing elastance. Work of breathing increases as a result of a combination of increased gas density, increased hydrostatic pressure, and altered respiratory mechanics [3,18]. Scuba adds dead space and increases resistance to breathing. Work of breathing rises with increasing minute ventilation and higher flow rates needed to meet metabolic demands of exertion.

Regular divers in general have larger than predicted total lung capacities and reduced expiratory flow rates at low lung volumes, possibly reflecting obstructive disease [19,20] Scuba diving reduces spirometric volumes and diffusing capacity during the event followed by substantial recovery within 1 to 2 days [21–25]; however, cumulative effects, with gradual development of obstructive defects over time, are suggested [26]. Closed circuit oxygen scuba diving also reduces spirometric volumes acutely compared to air diving [27].

Saturation diving causes a decline in carbon monoxide diffusing capacity that returns toward predive values [28], although there may be cumulative decline. In several studies of saturation divers, Thorsen and coworkers attribute changes in lung function to hyperoxia, including cummulative hyperoxia, and bubble emboli [29–32]. The potential effects of diving have direct implications for initial and serial testing of divers (discussed later).

Routine evaluation of diving candidates

Most professional dives have prearranged medical supervision. In other situations, medical evaluation, including spirometry, is recommended for all dive candidates. The history should include current respiratory symptoms and history of lung disease, pneumothorax, trauma or surgery to the chest, and lung disease (including childhood asthma). Respiratory system examination and spirometry should be performed. For patients who have no medical history of lung disease, FEV_1, forced vital capacity (FVC), and peak expiratory flow rate (PEF) normally should be greater than 80% of predicted and the FEV_1/FVC ratio greater than 70%. Variations from these values should lead to further evaluation (discussed later). Whether or not pulse oximetry adds to the evaluation is unknown.

The potential for change in lung function as a result of recurrent diving exposure remains a concern. Such changes may increase the difficulty in interpreting test results and distinguishing the onset of a new illness from expected change from diving alone. Professional and frequent amateur divers should have initial and serial annual testing of spirometry and diffusing capacity in order to identify cumulative chronic effects early. Testing should be deferred at least 2 to 7 days after the last dive to allow acute effects to resolve. Patients who have mild asthma, if approved to dive at all, require more frequent monitoring (discussed later).

The British Thoracic Society (BTS) guideline recommends chest radiograph examination for all dive instructors but omits chest radiograph examination for other divers who have normal examination and spirometry and no respiratory symptoms or history of chest trauma or lung disease [18]. Chest radiography is appropriate if there is a history of any significant respiratory symptoms, past illness, or abnormal finding on examination. History of pneumonia, pleurisy, recurrent bronchitis, sarcoidosis, chest surgery or trauma, allergic rhinitis, sinusitis, smoking, cough, dyspnea, asthma, pneumothorax, or other pulmonary diseases warrants further evaluation with chest radiograph or high-resolution CT scanning and complete lung volumes, diffusing capacity, or airway challenge testing based on individual concerns. Patients who have other anatomic defects should be excluded from diving with few exceptions. Selected topics are discussed later.

Aerobic fitness

Scuba divers should have strong swimming skills and aerobic capacity sufficient to permit at least moderately strenuous exertion. Divers may encounter strong currents or other unexpected events requiring increased exertion. Pulmonary function laboratories may be asked to assess exercise capacity of older or deconditioned normal subjects who want to begin scuba diving. Evaluation of cardiopulmonary fitness and exercise capacity may add additional insights and should receive further study as a predictor of tolerance or intolerance to diving.

Table 6 shows steady-state oxygen requirements for underwater swimming in comparison to running on land. Underwater swimming at a medium speed of 1 mile per hour (0.85 nautical miles per hour) typically requires steady-state oxygen consumption of 1.4 liters per minute (STPD [standard temperature and pressure, dry]) for United States Navy divers [33]. Because only approximately half of peak exercise capacity can be sustained, peak oxygen consumption should approach at least 2.8 L per minute for average-sized men to maintain underwater swimming at medium speed. Patients unable to complete stage 4 of the Bruce protocol (13 METS [metabolic equivalents]) may have insufficient cardiopulmonary reserves for diving [34]. This relatively high level of peak exertion equates to approximately 240 watts of incremental cycle exercise or running on level ground at a pace reaching 8 minutes per mile [35]. Subjects who have reduced aerobic fitness may have difficulty meeting these requirements.

Table 6
Oxygen consumption and ventilation requirements in liters per minute during steady-state land exercise and underwater swimming

Exercise	MPH[a]	Oxygen consumption	Exercise ventilation	Exertion
Walking	2	0.7	16	Light
Swimming	0.58	0.8	18	Light
Walking	4	1.2	27	Moderate
Swimming	0.98	1.4	30	Moderate
Running	8	2.0	50	Heavy
Swimming	1.15	1.8	40	Heavy
Swimming	1.38	2.5	60	Very heavy

Table assumes a healthy, conditioned subject performing steady-state exercise.

[a] Statute miles per hour; to convert to nautical miles, divide by 1.15.

Data from US Navy diving manual, volume 1. Air diving, revision 3. Publication no. 0994-LP-001-9010. US Navy Sea Systems Command; 1993. p. 3–10.

Asthma

Scuba diving entails exposure to factors, such as cold air, dry air, and exercise, known to provoke bronchoconstriction in susceptible nondivers [36,37]. Compressed air released from scuba tanks typically has a lower relative humidity and temperature than air at the surface. In addition, accidental aspiration of hypotonic fresh water or hypertonic seawater through the glottis into the tracheobronchial tree could trigger laryngospasm or bronchospasm in susceptible persons. Aerosolized sea water also is proposed as a risk of diving [38] because of the known potency of nebulized hypertonic saline to induce bronchospasm [39,40]. Emotional stress also can trigger bronchial constriction in some patients. Shortness of breath and panic at depth may result in an uncontrolled ascent.

Investigators recommend disqualification of divers who have asthma precipitated by exercise, cold, or emotion and divers who have moderate or severe persistent asthma [41]. United States Army medical fitness standards for initial selection for marine dive training reject candidates who have a history of asthma at any age, abnormal spirometry, or positive bronchial challenge test [42].

Whether or not all asthma, including well-controlled allergic asthma of mild degree, should be considered a relative or absolute contraindication remains controversial. Some investigators believe that the risk of barotrauma in asthmatics is increased only slightly provided spirometry is normal [43]. At a minimum, established divers who have mild asthma should monitor their peak flow twice daily and refrain from diving if they have (1) active bronchospasm, as evident by wheezing on physical examination or airflow obstruction on spirometry; (2) history of rescue use of β-agonist inhaler within 48 hours; or (3) reduced PEF below 90% of personal best (BTS) or PEF variation of greater than 20% within day [41]. Divers who have clinical exacerbations should remain disqualified until FEV_1 is stable above 80% of predicted for 2 weeks. The authors recommend airway hyper-responsiveness (AHR) testing, on contoller therapy without rescue β-agonist use, before considering a request for temporary medical clearance to dive during a defined interval. Positive responses to cold air or exercise challenge indicate an absolute contraindication to diving. Detailed counseling also is recommended.

Smoking

Tobacco smoke causes nonspecific AHR in smokers. The Lung Health Study finds that approxi-

mately 12% of male and 35% of female smokers, ages 35 to 59, who have normal FEV_1 exhibited pronounced AHR to methacholine, 5 mg/mL or less; 44% and 76% of men and women, respectively, responded to methacholine, 25 mg/mL or less [44]. The apparent gender difference in methacholine sensitivity results from smaller size of airways in women [45]. Other studies also show AHR in smokers. This tendency may place smokers who have AHR at equal or greater risk than patients who have asthma when diving. Smokers who have AHR risk acute bronchial constriction in the diving environment, with potential for further consequences, such as barotrauma, SAGE, or DCS [46,47].

Buch and coworkers analyzed data from 4350 adverse event reports submitted by individual divers (36% smokers) to the Diver's Alert Network between 1986 and 1997 [48]. After adjusting for variables known to contribute to DCI, the investigators found significantly higher severity of DCI in the smokers (>5 pack years) compared to nonsmokers. Because the database did not include smoking history from uneventful dives or fatal accidents, their results extend only to the severity of nonfatal DCI and do not address the risk of smoking on the incidence of DCI or death. Further confirmation of smoking risk to divers would be helpful.

The history of smoking and risk of DCI in divers warrants further study. In the meantime, the authors favor counseling divers to refrain from smoking. Consideration of spirometry or airway challenge testing should be considered in some predive settings. This becomes a high priority with any airway symptoms. Complete pulmonary function testing and high-resolution CT scanning may be helpful in selected cases [49].

Pneumothorax

Whether or not previous pneumothorax should be considered a relative or absolute contraindication remains controversial. Some authorities consider a single primary spontaneous pneumothorax, even if treated surgically, to be a permanent disqualification from diving because of the potential for ipsilateral or contralateral recurrence. Selection for marine diving training in the United States Army requires complete recovery, normal lung function, and a 3-year period without recurrence after a single spontaneous pneumothorax. The presence of residual spirometric or anatomic abnormalities should disqualify. (See previous discussion of risks of diving.)

Cardiovascular disease

Symptomatic coronary artery disease, including stable angina pectoris on medications, is a contraindication to safe diving. Older divers and those who have significant risk factors for coronary artery disease should have regular medical evaluations and a treadmill EKG test, at a minimum, before diving. Caruso recommends treadmill stress testing with EKG monitoring before diving for selected patients, including older subjects, patients who have significant coronary disease risk factors, and patients 6 to 12 months after coronary bypass or angioplasty [6]. Active chest pain, arrhythmias, or EKG changes should be disqualifying. Divers also should have adequate aerobic fitness (discussed previously).

Uncontrolled hypertension may cause acute pulmonary edema during diving; however, divers who have demonstrated adequate control of blood pressure and have no significant decrease in performance in the water because of the side effects of drugs should be able to dive safely [50]. Other cardiovascular diseases, such as peripheral vascular diseases, disqualify if exercise capacity is limited.

Patent foramen ovale

As many as one third of the population may have patent foramen ovale. Those individuals who dive are at increased risk for right-to-left shunting of air bubbles causing SAGE and DCS in some divers [51]. A study by Schwerzmann and colleagues, using transesophageal contrast echocardiograms and MRI of the brain found that divers who have PFO have 4.5-fold greater risk for decompression events and a twofold greater risk for ischemic brain lesions than divers who do not have PFO [52]. Accordingly, diving is contraindicated in patients who have a patent foramen ovale. If positive, transcutaneous bubble contrast echocardiography should be sufficient to raise this as a concern. It seems appropriate to test for PFO in diving candidates who have any cardiac symptoms or findings on examination, such as a murmur.

Prior decompression illness

In divers who have sustained an injury, such as DCS, SAGE, or barotrauma, thorough evaluation with pulmonary function tests, high-resolution CT scanning of the lung parenchyma, and bubble contrast echocardiography detect the cause of many injuries. Transesophageal contrast echocardiography and MRI of the brain are appropriate in selected cases.

Pulmonary function testing should include lung volumes, diffusing capacity, and spirometry with bronchodilator testing and bronchial challenge testing if spirometry is normal.

Medical clearance to return to diving after DCS should not be granted if residual symptoms or signs persist, or if divers adhered correctly to decompression guidelines [53]. The latter circumstance implies future risk even with proper dive procedures. Engaging in air travel after diving increases the risk for DCS. Most experts advise waiting at least 12 hours after no-decompression dives and 24 hours after decompression stop dives or multiple dives.

Hypobaric exposures: altitude

Hypobaric hypoxia occurs to varying degrees in passenger air travel, mountain sojourning, and aviation. Although hypoxia is a risk for all three exposure settings, other risks differ. The following sections address acute or short-term hypobaric hypoxia for these exposure scenarios. The scope of this article excludes long-term hypobaric exposure, as in permanent residence at high altitude.

Although the fraction of inspired oxygen (FIO_2) remains constant at 20.9% as altitude increases, the PaO_2 declines in proportion to barometric pressure [54]. Acute manifestations of hypoxia begin in normal subjects when dry inspired PaO_2 declines below 0.14 ata (equivalent to 14% oxygen at sea level). Tachycardia, increased systemic blood pressure, tachypnea, and cyanosis typically occur. Other manifestations include inability to concentrate on task, loss of coordination, loss of color vision, drowsiness, generalized weakness, incapacitation (0.11 ata oxygen), loss of consciousness (below 0.10 ata oxygen), and death [33].

Tolerance of hypoxia depends on the rapidity of onset, duration, and magnitude of exposure. Even moderate hypoxia for several hours in patients could cause clinical manifestations even if well tolerated for a shorter duration. The nadir of PaO_2 during acute hypobaric hypoxia, such as with air travel, occurs during the first hours of exposure, as soon as mass equilibration of gases in the lungs and body occurs. Mass equilibration may require a longer time in some patients who have delayed washout [55–57]. Increased ventilation in response to hypoxia then lowers $PaCO_2$ and raises PaO_2, but this compensation is modulated by the respiratory depressant effect of alkalosis. Full respiratory compensation depends on metabolic correction of respiratory alkalosis over time.

Aerospace exposures

Environmental factors that may contribute to acute adverse outcomes in flight crew members include sudden decompression, acceleration forces (+Gz) and anti-G maneuvers, breathing pure oxygen by mask, dry cabin air, ozone and smoke in the cockpit [58]. Other environmental factors associated with chronic occupational illnesses, space travel and adaptations to chronic weightlessness are beyond the scope of this article.

Exposures

Sudden decompression can occur after a breach in the fuselage of a pressurized aircraft, failure of cabin air compression systems, or an unrestrained ascent in various situations. Acute hypoxemia rapidly ensues as a result of reduced PaO_2. This limits subjects to the "time of useful consciousness," a matter of seconds to minutes, to remedy the situation before hypoxic syncope ensues [59]. The practical remedies consist of breathing oxygen from a contained source and rapid descent to lower altitude and higher barometric pressure. Commercial aircraft keep a temporary supply of oxygen that typically cannot be accessed for a single individual for this contingency.

Altitude DCS and SAGE are two forms of dysbarism that can occur during flight ascent. SAGE usually is associated with underlying lung disease and its occurrence should prompt an evaluation. The risk for altitude DCS increases with the rate of change and magnitude of hypobaric exposure [60], duration of exposure, and exercise. The risk decreases with the nitrogen depletion by pre-exposure oxygen treatment [61]. The threshold for DCS is described as 18,000 feet (5487 m) to 25,000 feet (7620 m) above sea level. Webb and colleagues report that DCS developed in 55% of subjects without prior depletion of oxygen at 22,500 feet [62].

Altitude DCS typically occurs during the early phases of a flight. Treatment with oxygen and return to sea level succeeds in the majority of patients. Some patients require hyperbaric oxygen as treatment for DCS after diving. Clearance can be granted to return to flight duty 72 hours after symptoms resolve. Engaging in air travel after diving increases the risk for DCS. Most experts advise waiting at least 12 hours after no-decompression dives and 24 hours after decompression stop dives or multiple dives before flying.

G-induced loss of consciousness (G-LOC) can afflict pilots of high performance aircraft, typically military fighter jets, in situations that require tactical maneuvering for evasion. The presumptive mechanism consists of reduced cerebral perfusion. G-forces occur not only with rapid ascent but also with turning at high speeds. Countermeasures for G-LOC include positive pressure breathing.

Fitness for flight duty

Clinicians who are not flight surgeons should be aware that many common self-limited conditions, such as rhinitis, sinusitis, and otitis, and most prescription medications have implications for temporary suspension of flight duty status. Flight organizations may have a list of approved medications, but even these usually require notification of the organization flight surgeon to continue on flight duty.

Medical illnesses that can cause sudden loss of consciousness or incapacitation in pilots create the greatest concerns for pilot and passenger safety. Conditions, such as cardiac arrhythmias and other cardiac diseases, syncope, seizure disorders, and diabetes mellitus, requiring hypoglycemic agents call for immediate suspension of flight status for medical evaluation.

Cardiovascular disease exceeds all other medical causes of premature termination for civilian airline pilots. Selvester and colleagues have proposed a four-step screening algorithm to detect asymptomatic coronary artery disease in flight school candidates, cadets, and rated flyers of the Unites States Air Force [63]. Risk factors for coronary disease, such as adequately treated hypertension, usually are not disqualifying [64,65].

Two common pulmonary disorders, acute bronchial asthma and spontaneous pneumothorax, frequently have implications for entry or continuation on flight duty status. In 1997, the Aeromedical Center of the Israeli Air Force published an algorithm for evaluating respiratory disorders in military candidates for flight training [66]. The algorithm presents decision logic and disqualification criteria based on history, physical examination, spirometry, postbronchodilator and postexercise spirometry, methacholine challenge testing, lung volumes, diffusing capacity, radiograph, and CT scanning in the evaluation of fitness for military flight duty.

Asthma

According to the Israeli algorithm, a personal history of asthma with an attack-free period greater than 5 years does not disqualify from flight training if further testing is normal. A negative personal history of asthma with a positive family history of either asthma or atopy, especially among first-order relatives, requires further testing. Wheezing on unforced exhalation indicates asthma or, less commonly, localized airway obstruction, both of which are disqualifying factors. Prolonged exhalation without wheezing during quiet breathing requires further investigation. A recent respiratory infection should delay screening by at least 6 weeks.

Some investigators favor routine testing for non-specific bronchial hyperresponsiveness, with an agent, such as methacholine, as a prerequisite for initial entry on military flight duty status in circumstances where uncompromised lung function under all environmental conditions is considered essential. Alternatively, a study of United States Army Reserve Officers' Training Corps cadets raises concerns over false-positive tests when higher concentrations of methacholine provocation are considered positive results [67].

Pneumothorax

According to the Israeli algorithm, a history of spontaneous pneumothorax may qualify for a medical waiver if: (1) 5 years have passed since the last episode; (2) chest CT gives no hint of subpleural blebs, localized overinflation, or generalized over-inflation; and (3) pulmonary function testing reveals no airways obstruction. In borderline cases, the candidate may be evaluated further by monitored hypobaric chamber exposure. Traumatic pneumothorax may qualify for a medical waiver after 1 year without recurrence if residual lung damage is minimal or absent.

United States Army regulations differ somewhat from the Israeli recommendations [42]. A single spontaneous pneumothorax disqualifies a candidate for selection to begin United States Army pilot training. Before pilots or crewmembers already on flight status can return to aviation duties after a spontaneous pneumothorax, a 2-month waiting period and clinical evaluation that shows complete recovery, full expansion of the lung, normal lung function, and no additional lung pathology are recommended.

After a recurrent spontaneous pneumothorax, pilots and crewmembers should not continue on flight duty status. Waiver of this restriction may be requested after effective treatment by pleurodesis or pleurectomy with complete recovery and successful completion of an altitude chamber exposure to 18,000 feet. Selection for free fall parachute training or marine diving training in the United States Army requires complete recovery, normal lung function, and a 3-year period without recurrence after a single spontaneous pneumothorax.

Mass screening of all flight duty applicants with chest radiographs may not be cost effective. Keesling and colleagues reviewed results of 3500 screening chest radiographs performed for flight duty to determine the rate of detection of significant abnormalities. Of 107 abnormal chest radiographs (3%), 55 were found to be false positive. Only two medically significant conditions were found in the screening population [68].

Other defects

Martin and colleagues compared echocardiograms from military pilots (n = 46) who had flown at least 1000 hours in high-performance aircraft to nonpilots (n = 201) in a retrospective study [69]. Martin and colleagues found a greater incidence of pulmonic insufficiency and tricuspid regurgitation in the pilots. Possible explanations offered by the investigators include transient increase in right ventricular pressure as a result of acceleration forces or straining maneuvers used to prevent or postpone +Gz-induced G-LOC.

Air travel

It was estimated 30 years ago that approximately 5% of passengers on commercial aircraft were ambulatory patients who had common ailments [70]. As the average age of Western populations rises, so does the likelihood that airline passengers have a chronic medical condition. In addition, flights are getting longer and aircraft bigger. The new Airbus 380, for example, carries approximately 600 passengers for 20 hour flights and longer [71].

Commercial jet aircraft routinely expose passengers to conditions equivalent to 6,000 to 8,000 feet above sea level [72]. Because of difficulties predicting cabin altitude for a given flight, clinicians can assume exposure to 8,000 feet (2438 m) as a realistic worst-case scenario for most airline travel. This exposure presents little risk to normal subjects but can cause severe hypoxemia in patients who have lung diseases even if oxygen is not required at sea level [73].

Patients who have lung diseases often undertake airline travel without prior medical supervision. In one study, 38% of patients took at least one airline trip within a 2-year period [2]. A minority of patients (27.3%) consulted a physician beforehand, but a significant number of patients (18.2%) reported clinical signs and symptoms during or after air travel, such as dyspnea, wheezing, chest pain, cyanosis, and right heart failure, leading to urgent requests for oxygen during flights. Even light physical exertion during flight can increase the risk for an exacerbation of symptoms [74].

Although death resulting from a purely respiratory cause rarely occurs during flight, the frequency of less morbid events, including worsening symptoms after exiting the plane, may be underreported to airlines and physicians. In one survey, 17% of respiratory in-flight emergencies resulted in diversion of the aircraft, the third most common cause of diversions [75]; however, hypoxia could have contributed to diversions in cardiac, neurologic, and obstetric patients, amounting to 97% of diversions and 55% of all reported emergencies. The number of passengers who have air travel hypoxemia contributing to cardiac arrest, stroke, seizure, or pulmonary embolism during flight is unknown but deserves further study.

Clinical strategy

Most investigators recommend maintenance of PaO_2 greater than 50 mm Hg during air travel [76,77]. The pathophysiologic basis for maintaining this level of oxygenation involves the likelihood of pulmonary vasoconstriction, right heart failure, and preserving oxygen delivery. Resting pulmonary artery pressure rises rapidly in patients who have lung diseases even during moderate altitude exposures [78]. An even higher PaO_2 during flight may be preferable in some high-risk patients. Outcome data establishing a safe threshold are needed [79].

For high-risk patients, maintenance of PaO_2 at altitude equal to PaO_2 at baseline ground level is desirable. This category includes compensated but "brittle" patients who have severe single organ impairments and those who have multiple defects in oxygen delivery, such as moderate lung disease along with comorbid conditions, such as chronic right heart failure, coronary artery disease, cerebrovascular disease, anemia, and other illnesses.

Preflight assessment

Patients who do not require home oxygen may not be aware of the potential risk for hypoxemia during air travel. Physicians can educate patients to seek evaluation for air travel hypoxemia. The preflight assessment should include the following steps in most cases: (1) estimate the expected degree of hypoxemia at altitude; (2) identify comorbid disease conditions; (3) prescribe oxygen if necessary; (4) counsel the patient; and (5) provide medical contact information in the event of emergency. Provid-

ing copies of recent clinic notes or lab results may be helpful.

Candidates for preflight evaluation (Box 1 and Table 7) include: (1) patients already on chronic oxygen for lung disease; (2) patients who have severe impairment of spirometry resulting from COPD or interstitial lung diseases even if not on oxygen at sea level; (3) patients who have conditions that may be affected by hypoxemia, such as coronary artery disease, congestive heart failure, arrhythmias, and other cardiac diseases; cerebrovascular disease; anemia; seizure disorders and other neurologic diseases; and pulmonary vascular disease, including pul-

---

Box 1. American Thoracic Society chronic obstructive pulmonary disease guideline: indications for hypoxia inhalation testing of patients who have chronic obstructive pulmonary disease

Comorbid disease that may be affected by hypoxaemia

   Coronary artery disease
   Congestive heart failure
   Arrhythmias and other cardiac diseases
   Cerebrovascular disease
   Anemia
   Seizure disorders and other
      neurologic diseases
   Pulmonary vascular disease including
      pulmonary embolism

Symptoms manifested during prior air travel
   Recovery phase after acute exacerbation
   Tendency to hypoventilation with oxygen administration
   Prediction of altitude $PaO_2 = 50 + 3$ mm Hg by regression equation
   Reassurance before embarking on air travel

From Berg BW, Dillard TA, Celli BR. Management of stable COPD: air travel in standards for the diagnosis and treatment of patients with chronic obstructive pulmonary disease. Available at: http://www. thoracic.org/COPD. Accessed July 20, 2005. American Thoracic Society/European Thoracic Society, 2004; with permission.

Table 7
Indications for preflight assessment of adults

Condition	Evidence grade
Severe COPD or asthma	B
Severe restriction (including chest wall or neuromuscular disease), especially with hypoxemia or hypercapnia	C
Cystic fibrosis	C
History of air travel intolerance with respiratory symptoms (dyspnoea, chest pain, confusion, or syncope)	C
Comorbid conditions exacerbated by hypoxemia (cerebrovascular disease, coronary artery disease, heart failure)	C
Pulmonary tuberculosis or other potentially contagious infection	C
Within 6 wk of hospital discharge for acute respiratory illness	C
Recent pneumothorax	B
Risk for, or history of, venous thromboembolism	B
Pre-existing requirement for oxygen or ventilator support	C

Modified from British Thoracic Society Standards of Care Committee. Managing passengers with respiratory disease planning air travel: British Thoracic Society recommendations Thorax 2002;57:290. Reproduced with permission from the BMJ Publishing Group.

monary embolism; (4) subjects who manifested symptoms previously during air travel; (5) patients recovering from pneumonia, heart attack, or acute exacerbations of COPD; (6) patients who have lung disease and are known to develop hypoventilation with oxygen administration; (7) patients who require additional reassurance before embarking on air travel; and (8) selected other patients. These recommendations were published recently by the American Thoracic Society (see Box 1).

The timing of preflight testing should be within 2 to 14 days of travel. Most airlines require at least 48 hours' notice. Assessments within a few hours of flight have greater accuracy but lack practicality. Test modalities to predict PaO_2 at altitude or assess tolerance to air travel include spirometry and arterial blood gas values at sea level; hypoxia inhalation testing (HIT); pulse oximetry; and exercise testing.

Regression estimates of PaO_2 during flight

Regression estimates based on ground level measures should be the first step in evaluation of

patients who have known or suspected lung impairment [80]. Regression estimates can achieve reasonable accuracy provided patients in question match the population from which the equation was derived [81]. The regression approach affords the opportunity to model the hypoxemic response to longer exposures in hypobaric conditions. As a practical matter, blood gas determination and spirometry obtained at sea level have more usefulness in day-to-day clinical management than blood gases obtained during HIT. Future studies to test existing regression models or develop new models for a mixed population, including patients who have interstitial lung disease and normal subjects, would be welcome.

PaO_2 at sea level, alone, as a predictor has limited usefulness: threshold values for PaO_2 at sea level, such as 68 to 72 mm Hg, as predictors of PaO_2 above 50 or 55 mm Hg at altitude, respectively, misclassify many patients. Also, neither the alveolar minus arterial (A-a) gradient for oxygen nor the PaO_2/FIO_2 ratio at sea level remain the same at altitude [82]. The A-a gradient and a/A ratio for oxygen at sea level did not improve accuracy of predicting the PaO_2 at altitude in one study [83]. Preferred regression equations use PaO_2 at sea level with additional variables to predict PaO_2 at altitude.

In patients who have stable COPD, the authors favor regression estimates that incorporate PaO_2 and FEV_1 at sea level as the initial step for estimating PaO_2 at altitude. Estimated values for PaO_2 at altitude close to 50 mm Hg (eg, ±3 mm Hg) may warrant HIT if available. Eq. 1 uses the FEV_1/FVC ratio and PaO_2 at sea level [80]. The study sample included male and female subjects and patients who had COPD:

$$PaO_2 \text{ at 8000 ft} = 0.238 \, [PaO_2 \text{ at sea level}]$$
$$+ 20.098 \, [FEV_1/FVC]$$
$$+ 22.258 \qquad (1)$$

After inserting mean subject values from the study of Naughton and colleagues [84] for the variables in the Eq. 1, the estimate from Eq. 1 (61.4 mm Hg) agrees within 0.3 mm Hg with the observed PaO_2 at 8000 feet of hypobaric exposure in their normal subjects (61.7 mm Hg). The estimate from Eq. 1 for patients who have COPD (48.3 mm Hg) agrees within 1.2 mm Hg with the hypobaric exposure to 8000 feet in patients who have COPD in the study by Naughton and colleagues (49.5 mm Hg). By this analysis, Eq. 1 has comparable accuracy to HIT testing by Naughton and colleagues within 2 hours of hypobaric exposure in patients who have COPD (Naughton average

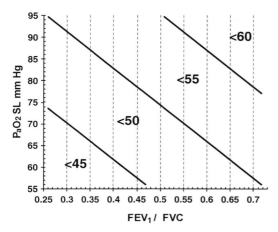

Fig. 1. Graph for estimating PaO$_2$ at 8000 feet based on PaO$_2$ at sea level and FEV$_1$/FVC ratio in patients who have COPD of varying degree. The diagonal lines represent PaO$_2$ values of 45, 50, and 55 mm Hg, respectively, at 8000 feet. To estimate PaO$_2$: (1) place a straight edge at the subject's value for FEV$_1$/FVC on the x-axis; (2) follow the straight edge directly upward, parallel to the y-axis and perpendicular to the x-axis, until reaching the subject's PaO$_2$ at sea level and mark that point; and (3) observe if that point falls above or below the line for PaO$_2$ at 8000 feet equal to 50 mm Hg. (*Data from* Dillard TA, Moores LK, Bilello KL, et al. The preflight evaluation: a comparison of the hypoxia inhalation test with hypobaric exposure. Chest 1995; 107(2):354.)

difference 1.1 mm Hg) and normal subjects (Naughton average difference −0.7 mm Hg).

Fig. 1 reveals a graphic method of estimating PaO$_2$ during air travel in patients who have COPD from PaO$_2$ at sea level and FEV$_1$/FVC based on Eq. 1. Users should trace perpendicular lines from each axis and read the estimate for PaO$_2$ at 8000 feet at the point of intersection.

Eq. 2 (COPD) is derived from a study sample of ambulatory men who had FEV$_1$ below 60% of predicted and did not require home oxygen.

PaO$_2$ at 8000 ft = 0.453 [PaO$_2$ at sea level]

$$+ 0.386 \text{ [FEV}_1\% \text{ predicted]}$$

$$+ 2.440 \qquad (2)$$

The authors have developed a 3-axis nomogram to estimate altitude oxygen tension using Eq. 2 [4].

The study by Naughton and colleagues comparing altitude chamber exposures with HIT and regression estimates shows better precision (lower SD of differences) compared to Schwartz and coworkers for each of three regression equations estimating PaO$_2$ at

8000 feet, although there is greater bias reported for some equations. Naughton did not report height, gender or actual FEV$_1$ in liters for the control subjects or COPD patients nor specify which equation from Dillard was studied.

Hypoxia inhalation test

The HIT permits assessment of symptoms and EKG tracings for individual patients and has been applied to mixed populations, including those who have interstitial lung disease. An early study by Schwartz and colleagues compared a normobaric HIT using 17.2% oxygen at sea level with a hypobaric altitude exposure of 1650 meters (5413 ft; barometric pressure, 623 mm Hg) in a small airplane 3 weeks to 4 months later in patients who had COPD [85]. The exposures in that study had nearly equivalent inspired PaO$_2$ (120 + 1 mm Hg, saturated with water vapor). Those investigators found an average difference in PaO$_2$ of 1.46 mm Hg (SD 6.46 mm Hg) with a maximum individual difference of 11 mm Hg between HIT and hyporbaric exposure.

The Naughton study reports that a 15.1% HIT by facemask done within 2 hours of an 8000-foot hypobaric exposure had higher accuracy than regression estimates (Fig. 2). The Naughton data raise the

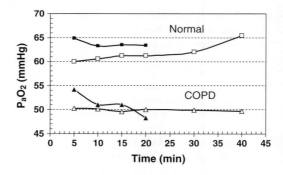

Fig. 2. Comparison of normobaric hypoxia (HIT) (*closed symbols*) with hypobaric chamber exposures (*open symbols*) between normal subjects (*squares*) and patients who have COPD (*triangles*). Data plotted at an altitude of 8000 feet. In normal subjects, HIT exceeded hypobaric exposure by 2 to 3 mm Hg at several time intervals. In patients who had COPD, HIT may not have reached nadir at full equilibration in the time shown. PaO$_2$ varied from 54 mm Hg at 5 minutes to 48 mm Hg at 20 minutes. Data were reported as not statistically significant. (*Data from* Naughton MT, Rochford PD, Pretto JJ, et al. Is normobaric simulation of hypobaric hypoxia accurate in chronic airflow limitation? Am J Respir Crit Care Med 1995;152:1959.)

Table 8
British Thoracic Society guideline for evaluating patients
before air travel with pulse oximetry

Saturation by pulse oximetry at sea level on room air	British Thoracic Society recommendation	Evidence grade
>95%	Oxygen not required	B
92%–95% without risk factor[a]	Oxygen not required	C
92%–95% with risk factor[a]	Perform hypoxic inhalation challenge with arterial or capillary measurements	B
<92%	Prescribe inflight oxygen	B
Chronic supplemental oxygen	Increase the flow while at cruising altitude	B

[a] Risk factors: hypercapnia; FEV_1 <50% predicted; lung
cancer; restrictive lung disease involving the parenchyma
(fibrosis), chest wall (kyphoscoliosis), or respiratory muscles; ventilator support; cerebrovascular or cardiac disease;
within 6 weeks of discharge for an exacerbation of chronic
lung or cardiac disease.
Modified from British Thoracic Society Standards of Care
Committee. Managing passengers with respiratory disease
planning air travel: British Thoracic Society recommendations. Thorax 2002;57:293. Reproduced with permission from
the BMJ Publishing Group.

question of potential lack of full equilibration of HIT
PaO_2 in the patients who had COPD (see Fig. 2) over
the 20-minute exposure. Also, the normal group HIT
values exceeded the hypobaric values (see Fig. 2).

Limitations of HIT include the following concerns. A 10- or 15-minute HIT may not allow sufficient time for inspired gas to reach mass equilibrium
in subjects who have COPD and may be too brief to
fully assess the physiologic effects of hypoxemia.
Patients seldom develop any symptoms or objective
findings during a HIT [86]. As a practical matter, a
2-hour turnaround time to perform a HIT before air
travel seems impractical for patient care.

The authors favor a 15- to 25-minute exposure
to 15.1% oxygen at sea level (simulating 8000 ft)
breathing from a reservoir through a mouthpiece with
nose clips in place for the HIT to approximate altitude
most closely. An appealing but possibly less accurate
alternative consists of facemask devices applied over
nasal cannulae to permit simultaneous hypoxia exposure and titration of oxygen [87]. This method requires further study. The primary endpoints for the
HIT consist of sampling arterial blood in the upright
position and EKG monitoring for ischemia and
arrhythmias. Patients who have PaO_2 during HIT
below 50 mm Hg require oxygen supplementation.

The criteria for use of pulse oximetry instead of
arterial blood gases during HIT testing remain to be
fully studied in relation to hypobaric exposure. A
pulse oximetry value during HIT of 85% is proposed
as a threshold for oxygen prescription [88] but this
may underestimate actual PaO_2 (discussed later).

Pulse oximetry

The oxyhemoglobin saturation as measured by
pulse oximetry (SpO_2) constitutes a convenient assessment of gas exchange but has limitations. At sea
level, the main weaknesses of SpO_2 are inaccuracy in
smokers and others exposed to carbon monoxide and
susceptibility to transient hyperventilation.

During acute brief hypoxia exposure, in the
absence of acclimatization, pulse oximetry overesti-
mates true arterial oxygen as a result of change in
oxyhemoglobin affinity with respiratory alkalosis
[89]. The clinical significance of a single measurement of SpO_2 in the acute altitude setting in the
absence of apparent illness is unclear [90]; however,
the authors favor maintenance of SpO_2 of 90% or
above in patients who have significant lung disease
during air travel. Higher levels may be appropriate for
high-risk patients.

The BTS incorporates resting pulse oximetry at
sea level into a guideline for evaluating patients
before air travel (Table 8) [91]. Some investigators
caution about use of resting pulse oximetry at sea
level to assess patients for air travel [92,93]. The BTS
guideline recommends inflight oxygen for patients
with room air SpO_2 below 92% at sea level and HIT
testing for patients with room air SpO_2 at sea level in
the range of 92% to 95%. Table 9 shows recom-

Table 9
Guideline for evaluating patients before air travel with
15.1% oxygen for 20 minutes

PaO_2 on 15.1%	Recommendation	Evidence grade
>55 mm Hg	Oxygen not required	B
50–55 mm Hg	Borderline; a walk test may be helpful	C
<50 mm Hg	Prescribe in-flight oxygen (2 L/min)	B

Modified from British Thoracic Society Standards of Care
Committee. Managing passengers with respiratory disease
planning air travel: British Thoracic Society recommendations. Thorax 2002;57:293. Reproduced with permission from
the BMJ Publishing Group.

mendations based on arterial blood samples during HIT from the BTS guideline. Overall, this guideline seems promising but should be validated in a variety of patient groups.

The criteria for use of pulse oximetry instead of arterial blood gases during HIT testing remain to be fully studied in relation to hypobaric exposure in adults. One article recommends oxygen at altitude for patients who have cystic fibrosis desaturated to 83% or below by pulse oximetry during HIT testing [93]. For now, pulse oximetry should not substitute for arterial blood gas measurement during HIT but does seem useful to titrate oxygen during a HIT [87].

In steady-state altitude settings, pulse oximetry is a more useful measure of changes in gas exchange. For example, Bendrick and colleagues successfully used a threshold of 90% pulse oximetry saturation to provide supplemental oxygen to air-transported patients who had ischemic heart disease exposed to a mean cabin altitude of 6900 feet (range 2500–8100 ft) without serious events [94]. In another study, Kramer and coworkers report a series of 19 of 21 of patients accompanied by physicians on flights of 4 to 21 hours to medical centers for evaluation for lung transplantation or pulmonary thromboembolectomy [95]. Saturation was maintained at values of 85% or above in most patients for the entire flight. In that study, three patients had hemodynamic instability and one patient died during flight. This series included patients who had diagnoses of emphysema, pulmonary fibrosis, cystic fibrosis, Eisenmenger's syndrome, primary pulmonary hypertension, dilated cardiomyopathy with amiodarone lung, and severe pulmonary hypertension resulting from thromboemboli.

In stable ambulatory patients, the authors favor maintenance of a minimum of 90% saturation by pulse oximetry during air travel in patients based on the two studies cited previously and other reasons. This should assure a PaO_2 above 50 mm Hg during flight. For high-risk patients, such as those in the two studies cited previously, maintenance of PaO_2 equal to ground level is the most desirable goal. This may require an SpO_2 above ground level during the early stages of exposure. Portable blood gas analyzers or other measures of oxygenation may become more useful in this setting [96].

In an era of inexpensive portable pulse oximeters, physicians should resist the temptation of having patients monitor their own pulse oximetry during flights without an oxygen prescription and a statement of intent to monitor pulse oximetry approved in advance by the airline medical director. Further study of this topic would be helpful.

Exercise testing

The text of the BTS guideline advocates a 50-meter or 6-minute walk at ground level to assess desaturation and functional status. Those who have desaturation or limited exercise capacity at sea level may warrant further medical decisions. Christensen and colleagues report that all patients who had aerobic capacity exceeding 12.1 mL/min/kg during cycle ergometry at sea level had PaO_2 values higher than 50 mm Hg at rest at 8000 feet (2438 m) [74]. In that study, exercise testing started at 20 watts and increased by 5 watts per minute until exhaustion.

Exercise testing during altitude simulation in patients who have lung disease has received less study than altitude assessment at rest. The BTS guideline suggests exercise testing (see Table 8), presumably during HIT, for patients who have PaO_2 between 50 and 55 mm Hg during HIT. Patients who desaturate would receive in-flight oxygen. Exercise testing with HIT testing warrants careful monitoring and emergency equipment.

Oxygen prescription

Berg and colleagues report that 28% oxygen (2438 m) via Venturi mask at altitude-corrected PaO_2 at 8000 feet to 90% of sea level values [97]. Oxygen, 4 L/min, via nasal prongs (equivalent to a 34% by mask) overcorrected PaO_2 at 8000 feet to values above the baseline sea level values. For most stable patients who have COPD who do not receive long-term oxygen therapy, 2 liters of oxygen by nasal cannulae nearly completely restores the PaO_2 lost at 8000 feet compared to sea level.

Patients receiving continuous oxygen at home require more supplemental oxygen during flight. The treatment of such patients would benefit from further study. In general, the maximum oxygen flow should not be applied below the cruising altitude to avoid hyperoxic suppression of ventilatory drive in some patients [91]. If the elevation at the destination is significantly greater than at home, patients also require additional oxygen supplementation on the ground. Stable patients who have COPD and do not require home oxygen, who do not have comorbid diseases, who recently have traveled safely by air without oxygen, and who have been clinically stable since their previous air travel can make an informed decision to travel without oxygen.

Airlines generally do not permit patients to bring their own oxygen aboard but provide oxygen on receipt of a prescription from a physician at least

48 hours before the intended flight. In one review, 7 of 11 United States–based air carriers and 18 of 22 international carriers allow oxygen supplementation [98]. Air carriers typically provide oxygen from nasal cannulae at discrete flow rates typically ranging from 2 to 8 L per minute. An oxygen prescription may be required for each segment of the travel itinerary (see Stoller for more details [99]).

Laboratory confirmation of correction of hypoxia with nasal cannulae would be useful during HIT testing to avoid overcorrection. Vohra and Klocke [87] used a Venturi mask powered with nitrogen flow to entrain room air, thereby creating normobaric hypoxia. After hypoxia exposure with the mask, they added oxygen by nasal cannulae titration with continuation of hypoxia. The Venturi mask method of hypoxia challenge warrants further study with blood gases and modifications to allow more precise settings of FIO_2 and, therefore, altitude, equivalence.

Deep venous thrombosis and pulmonary embolism

Several studies report that airline travel predisposes to deep venous thrombosis and pulmonary embolism: "the economy class syndrome" [100]. In a study of illness upon arrival in Paris, Lapostolle and coworkers report that flight distance greater than 3000 miles (5000 km) contributes significantly greater risk for massive pulmonary embolism [101]. In another study, 10% of healthy passengers passengers not wearing elastic compression stockings had symptomless calf vein thrombosis after lengthy trips (median duration 24 hours) [102]. A study of high-risk flights with mean flight duration of 12.4 hours reports deep vein thrombosis in 4.5% compared with 0.24% of controls treated with below-the-knee stockings [103].

The risk for deep venous thrombosis from short, domestic flights presumably should be lower than international or transoceanic flights. Patients who have cor pulmonale or a sedentary lifestyle before travel presumably have higher risk for thrombosis than the general population. Patients who do not have symptoms initially could develop pulmonary embolism hours or days after deplaning [104]. Such events after deplaning likely are unreported to airlines.

Interventions to prevent thrombosis seem justified in many patients. Guidelines of the Aerospace Medical Association identify low-, moderate-, and high-risk patients for prevention of thrombosis with physical means, aspirin, and low molecular weight heparin, respectively, in addition to support tights or compression stockings [105].

Pneumothorax

Pneumothoraces occur during air travel but relatively rarely considering the large number of people who travel by air each year. Expansion of a preexisting subclinical pneumothorax during air travel also could occur and lead to symptoms during flight. Under such circumstances, a pneumothorax could expand by up to 34.5% of its initial volume when going from sea level to 8000 feet (2438 m). In patients who have pre-existing lung impairment, this expansion could critically jeopardize ventilatory reserves. Postoperative patients should delay air travel until a pneumothorax resolves.

Terrestrial altitude

Mountain trekking, snow skiing, and sight seeing are popular forms of recreation throughout the world that involve hypobaric exposure, often in the remotest areas of underdeveloped countries. In one year, for example, more than 27,000 people visited Sagarmatha National Park in Nepal where Mount Everest is found. Of these, 12,000 trekked beyond Namche Bazaar to Thame (elevation 12,304 ft), 5000 traveled to Goyko (17,575 ft) to view Mount Everest, and a similar number went to Mount Everest base camp (17,600 ft) [106]. Millions of travelers visit more accessible venues, such as ski resorts and national parks.

Terrestrial altitude exposures, such as mountain climbing, usually involve slower rate of change of barometric pressure than air travel. Slower ascent permits gradual acclimatization to lower PaO_2. Mountain venues usually entail longer hypoxia exposures and more exercise at altitude than air travel. Subjects may seek medical supervision to accelerate acclimatization by pharmacologic means or to anticipate treatment of altitude sickness if it develops. Combination exposures, such as air travel to a mountain venue, may make the management plan more complex. No single test excludes all risks; however, exercise testing while monitoring vital signs and pulse oximetry, without or with hypoxia challenge, could provide sufficient grounds for oxygen prescription during travel for many conditions.

The risks for terrestrial altitude exposure include AMS, high-altitude pulmonary edema (HAPE), and high-altitude cerebral edema (HACE) [107]. In general, patients who have lung impairments have greater risk for these events resulting from greater hypoxia at any altitude. Patients needing oxygen at sea level because of lung disease require an increase in flow rate or FIO_2 at a higher elevation. The needed FIO_2 can be estimated from change in alveolar oxygen tension. The following section addresses lung function changes at altitude that theoretically could influence the degree of hypoxia adversely or favorably.

Pulmonary function at altitude

Changes in lung function induced by altitude could worsen the severity of hypoxemia beyond that anticipated and reduce the ventilatory reserves available for exercise or further predispose to altitude illnesses. In an earlier review of studies pertaining to change in lung function at moderately high altitude [4], the authors conclude that FEV_1 and TLC change little. Decline in FVC can be detected at approximately 2500 meters but may not be detectable at milder exposures [108]. FVC declines further at higher altitude. PEF increases modestly at altitude in normal subjects but not in patients who have COPD. Correlation of spirometric changes with gas exchange variables or maximum ventilation do not seem to be consistent or significant. Increasing residual volume mirrors decreasing FVC. Terrestrial field studies have greater potential than hypobaric chamber studies for confounding factors to alter pulmonary function tests [109,110].

The pulmonary function changes with altitude exposure involve interesting questions of pathophysiology. Plausible mechanisms for changes in pulmonary function include pulmonary interstitial edema [111–114], pulmonary vasoconstriction with redistribution of pulmonary blood volume [115], and regional changes in lung elastic recoil, among others [116]. Mechanisms for reduced vital capacity, such as distention of abdominal gas [47] and reduced peak respiratory muscle strength, have less credibility at the present time [117].

Disorders of respiratory drive

A variety of disorders that can interfere with respiratory drive or neuromuscular function may predispose to illnesses at altitude [3]. Reduced respiratory drive may result from dysfunction of peripheral or central chemoreceptors. Hackett [3] includes the following defects in this category: stroke, CNS trauma, neuromuscular disease, primary alveolar hypoventilation, obesity hypoventilation syndrome, and COPD. Medications or illicit drugs and hypothyroidism also reduce respiratory drive. Hypoxia inhalation testing of these patients may reveal

oxygenation that is worse than expected resulting from inhibition of ventilation.

Periodic breathing during sleep

Periodic breathing during sleep occurs commonly at high altitude even in normal climbers and also can become manifest at moderate altitude. Zielinski studied nine nonsmoking healthy men (mean age 20 years) with full polysomnography at 760 meters and at 3200 meters [118]. Periodic breathing appeared at altitude mostly during non–rapid-eye-movement sleep, ranging from 0.1% to 24% of total sleep time in different individuals. In addition, the number of arousals and awakenings doubled at high altitude; episodes of central and obstructive apneas also increased ($P < 0.001$). Mean pulse oximetry saturation was lower during the study nights at high altitude. Some ventilatory acclimatization was suggested by greater saturation during the sixth night compared with the first night at altitude ($P < 0.001$).

Sleep-disordered breathing

This category of illness can include obstructive sleep apnea/hypopnea syndrome and other disorders of respiratory control, such as central hypoventilation. Sleep-disordered breathing (SDB) can worsen air travel hypoxia in patients who fall asleep on an airplane; however, SDB more often is a concern for terrestrial altitude situations. Patients who have SDB at sea level risk more severe hypoxemia while at high altitudes with attendant risks for cardiac dysrhythmia and pulmonary hypertension. SDB at high altitudes is implicated in the pathogenesis of AMS and HAPE. Patients on continuous positive airway pressure or bilevel positive airway pressure treatment at sea level should not discontinue treatment at high altitudes. Pressure adjustments should be made to higher settings because of decreased delivered pressure at high altitude from the continuous positive airway pressure generator [3]. Ideally, the new settings are verified by direct pressure measurement. More study of this topic would be helpful.

Chronic obstructive pulmonary disease

The findings of Graham and Houston [119] represent typical results of exposure in patients who have moderate to severe COPD in the setting of terrestrial altitude. They report a cohort of eight ambulatory patients who had COPD (PaO_2 66 mm Hg at 50 m elevation; FEV_1 1.27 L, 42% predicted) before and after ground transport to an altitude of 6300 feet (1920 m) for 4 days. Patients had a mean PaO_2 after 3 hours at altitude of 51.5 mm Hg at rest measured. PaO_2 rose to 54.5 by day 4 of the study because of ventilatory compensation for hypoxia. Some patients had symptoms, including headache and dyspnea on exertion, but no major complications. This study supports a contention that PaO_2 above 50 mm Hg can be tolerated at least temporarily in uncomplicated COPD, albeit with some symptomatology. Nevertheless, oxygen administration reduced the cardiovascular stress of altitude in patients who have COPD [120]. Use of a high carbohydrate diet [121] to combat hypoxia cannot be recommended for hypercapnic patients who have COPD at this time because of risk for worsening hypercapnia from increased carbon dioxide production.

Cystic fibrosis

Travel should be considered very carefully in patients who have cystic fibrosis. Exacerbation of infection in a remote location should be a major concern, especially in those who have severe obstruction on spirometry or frequent exacerbations. Drying of secretions can be anticipated because of reduced ambient water vapor pressure. Patients who have cystic fibrosis with mild obstruction and without hypoxia at sea level tolerate mild to moderate altitude exposures well [122]. Some investigators maintain that younger patients who have cystic fibrosis may tolerate moderate hypoxemia better than older patients who have severe COPD [123]. Speechly-Dick and colleagues [124] report that a hypoxic challenge with 15% FIO_2 is a better predictor of arterial oxygen saturation at altitude than spirometry and baseline oxygen saturation. These investigators also report that measurements obtained at rest underestimate FIO_2 requirements during sleep and exertion in the altitude setting. The authors favor maintenance of PaO_2 above 50 mm Hg during air travel and above 55 mm Hg during longer exposures in patients who have cystic fibrosis.

Asthma

Convincing evidence is lacking that lower air density at altitude conveys much advantage in patients who have COPD and asthma. Stable asthmatics who do not have hypoxemia at sea level have little added risk at altitude other than remote location in the event of bronchospasm. Reduced exposure to allergens and pollutants in mountain areas may reduce the likelihood of exacerbation, although com-

plete absence of these triggers cannot be assumed. Exercise in cold, dry air theoretically could provoke some asthmatics, although Matsuda and coworkers [125] report no changes from sea level in FEV_1, exercise time, oxygen consumption, or heart rate in children who have exercise-induced asthma exposed in a hypobaric chamber. Nonspecific airway challenge testing on current asthma therapy before travel may provide some reassurance.

Asthmatics may opt to monitor spirometry in field settings. Jensen and colleagues tested several devices by mechanical means in an altitude chamber and found that portable flow meters underestimate PEF as a function of increasing altitude and increasing target peak flow [126]. Pedersen and colleagues address similar issues and advocate carefully developed correction factors for meaningful use of selected instruments in settings of variable barometric pressure [127].

Cardiovascular diseases

Systemic circulatory changes on ascent to altitude include increase in resting and exercise heart rate, systemic blood pressure, systemic vascular resistance, and cardiac output [128]. The combination of exercise and hypoxia in susceptible patients predisposes to cardiac ischemia to a greater extent than either stimulus alone. In addition, cold ambient temperature may add to cardiovascular stress. These changes, which are associated with increased catecholamine release on exposure to hypoxia, lead to increased myocardial oxygen consumption and cardiac work in the first 7 to 14 days of exposure and then diminish thereafter [129]. Ventricular ectopy also increases in some individuals [130]. Pulmonary vasoconstriction, triggered directly by alveolar hypoxia, persists throughout the stay at altitude. Pulmonary hypertension plays a role in the development of HAPE.

Coronary artery disease

When allowed to fully acclimate over days to weeks, normal subjects can tolerate severe hypoxemia ($PaO_2 < 30$ mm Hg) without cardiac ischemia. Alternatively, Halhuber and colleagues caution that the risk for sudden death increases significantly in unacclimated, sedentary men who have subclinical coronary artery disease and who perform strenuous exercise, such as skiing or hiking at altitude above 2500 meters. The greatest risk occurs in the first few days after exposure before adaptations occur. Levine and colleagues [130] note that the double product needed to induce 1 mm ST segment depression decreases by approximately 5% at altitude compared to sea level but that after 5 days of acclimatization, this level returns to baseline.

Many investigators recommend that patients who have angina should reduce their activity at higher altitude to avoid chest pain. Hultgren [131] recommends exercise testing prior to ascent for men over 50 years of age who have risk factors for ischemic heart disease. Patients of any age who have known cardiac disease should be considered for stress testing before ascent. Self-monitoring of cardiac frequency and blood pressure during exercise at altitude could allow patients to titrate exertion to remain below 95% of the ischemia inducing double product at sea level. Some investigators [132] suggest that initiating an exercise program at sea level prior to exercising at altitude may reduce the risk for sudden death.

A two-stage testing procedure, with exercise testing on room air followed by exercise testing with hypoxia inhalation, may prove helpful to evaluate patients. Patients who desaturate on exercise at sea level should be considered for supplemental oxygen during altitude exposure. For stable angina patients who do not desaturate on room air at sea level, use of hypoxia inhalation with monitored exercise testing may define a double product at altitude that induces ischemia by EKG.

Hypertension

Both systolic and diastolic blood pressure at rest and exercise increase at moderate altitude compared to sea level in patients who have pre-existing systemic hypertension. Worsening of hypertension can occur in patients under control at sea level [131]. Patients who have pre-existing systemic hypertension may manifest a greater pulmonary pressor response to hypoxia and this predisposes to HAPE. Physicians should counsel patients to monitor blood pressure after arrival at altitude and that increased medication may be required for blood pressure control. Undiagnosed hypertension may be unmasked by altitude exposure.

Congestive heart failure

Patients who have congestive heart failure run the risk for decompensation at altitude. Contributing mechanisms include increased fluid retention and those mechanisms (discussed previously) for the systemic and pulmonary circulations. Exercise testing to exclude desaturation on room air with continuation of exercise with added hypoxia inhalation may aid in clinical decision making as to whether or not to prescribe oxygen for patients who have congestive

heart failure at altitude. Patients also may need to increase their diuretic use and monitor their weight and edema. Preventive measures for altitude illnesses should be considered.

Other cardiac defects

Patients who have uncorrected atrial and ventricular septal defects may experience worsening of right-to-left shunt at altitude [133,134]. The extent of shunting and desaturation depends on the degree of hypoxia-induced pulmonary vasconstriction. Pulmonary vasoconstriction at altitude may exacerbate pre-existing pulmonary hypertension of any cause. Patients who have primary pulmonary hypertension may vary in susceptibility to hypoxic vasoconstriction. Patients who have pulmonary hypertension who must travel may benefit from low-flow oxygen in addition to vasodilator therapy. Exercise testing before and after hypoxic gas breathing can be used to assess patients' likely response to altitude hypoxia. Desaturation justifies oxygen prescription.

Neurologic disorders

Many mechanisms may contribute to neurologic events at altitude, including hypoxia, hypocapnia, alkalosis, and circulatory changes. Adverse clinical events seem more likely if patients have comorbid heart or lung disease contributing to hypoxia before exposure, which may justify hypoxia inhalation testing. The symptoms of acute mountain sickness and HACE overlap significantly with symptoms of focal neurologic disorders. This overlap can contribute to diagnostic uncertainty in altitude settings.

Neurologic symptoms, including vertigo, seizures, headache, and syncope, constitute common causes of airline diversions [75]. Syncope occurs commonly at high altitude [135]. The possible contribution of exercise desaturation to syncope should be kept in mind. The authors recommend evaluation to exclude an underlying hypoxic pulmonary or cardiac disorder in patients who manifest neurologic symptoms at altitude.

Seizures occur at altitude in susceptible patients, presumably as a result of hypoxia, alkalosis, or hyperventilation. Seizures seem more likely to occur in susceptible patients not receiving effective antiepileptic therapy and rarely occur in healthy climbers. Ascent to altitude can trigger migraine headaches [136]. Supplemental oxygen, descent, or increased pharmacotherapy can ameliorate these events. Strokes occur rarely in healthy sojourners but may occur unpredictably in patients who have cerebrovascular disease traveling to high altitude. The risk for stroke during altitude exposure in susceptible individuals relative to baseline elevation is undetermined. The role of pre-exposure hypoxia inhalation testing in the management of patients who have seizures, migraine headaches, or stroke remains to be studied fully.

Long airplane flights or terrestrial altitude exposures reportedly can precipitate cerebral venous thrombosis [137]. This disorder has clinical manifestations similar to HACE. Cerebral venous thrombosis can be suspected if no improvement occurs after descent from altitude, as should occur with HACE. Case reports note apparent unmasking of intracranial disease processes, such as arteriovenous malformation, aneurysm, or brain tumor [138].

Other medical conditions

Hypobaric hypoxia may alter organ function adversely in a number of medical conditions. Pre-exposure hypoxia inhalation testing can be considered in patients who have comorbid lung disease or otherwise in selected cases. Patients who have significant desaturation because of lung disease may be considered for oxygen therapy at altitude; however, evidence-based outcome data need further development.

Patients who have anemia of any cause have reduced exercise performance at altitude [139]. Hypoxia promotes sickling of red blood cells containing hemoglobin S [140].Up to 20% of patients who have sickle cell anemia as a result of hemoglobin SS, hemoglobin SC, and sickle-thalessemia may have sickling events during airline travel [141]. For travelers who have sickle cell anemia, oxygen prescription to prevent a sickle crisis should be considered. In one controlled study of healthy aviators who had sickle cell trait, there was little if any risk for clinical events after altitude chamber exposures from 5000 to 25,000 feet [142]. Radial keratotomy predisposes to hyperopia at altitude in contrast to photorefractive keratectomy, which does not [143]. Corrective lenses can compensate hypoxia-induced visual changes in patients who have had radial keratotomy. Retinal hemorrhages occur in AMS and HAPE. Patients who have significant visual impairments because of retinal hemorrhages, as with diabetes mellitus or hypertension, may warrant hypoxia inhalation testing and oxygen therapy if they desaturate sharply because of comorbid lung disease.

Women who have normal pregnancies tolerate moderate altitude well, although travel should be curtailed during the third trimester. Women who have higher-risk pregnancies because of underlying maternal lung or heart disease should travel only with greatest reluctance. Such cases may warrant hypoxia inhalation testing before travel to monitor oxygenation of the mother and cardiac effects on the fetus during hypoxia. Outcome data on this issue are lacking.

This article reviews some effects of extreme environments and approaches to evaluation and management using pulmonary function and other clinical testing. In view of the large number of subjects at risk and the impracticality of simulation testing for all subjects, the authors favor development of a clinical strategy that employs readily available clinical tests and functional assessments performed in the usual clinical environment to screen the growing population of subjects before exposure. Specific simulations remain necessary for some populations and settings.

References

[1] Backer H. Travel-related emergencies: limitations to wilderness travel. Emerg Med Clin North Am 1997; 15:17–41.

[2] Dillard TA, Beninati WA, Berg BW. Air travel in patients with chronic obstructive pulmonary disease. Arch Intern Med 1991;151:1793–5.

[3] Hackett PH. High altitude and common medical conditions. In: Hornbein TF, Schoene RB, editors. High altitude: an exploration of human adaptation. New York: Marcel-Dekker; 2001. p. 839–85.

[4] Dillard TA, Ewald FW. The use of pulmonary function testing in piloting, air travel, mountain climbing and diving. Clin Chest Med 2001;22:795–816.

[5] Dillard TA, Grathwohl KW. Near-drowning and diving accidents. In: Baum GL, Crapo JD, Celli BR, et al, editors. Textbook of pulmonary diseases. 6th edition. Philadelphia: Lippincott-Raven Publishers; 1998. p. 901–17.

[6] Caruso JL. Cardiovascular fitness and diving. Alert diver (July/August 1999). Available at: http://www.diversalertnetwork.org/medical/articles/article.asp?articleid=11. Accessed August 20, 2001.

[7] Butler BD, Hills BA. Transpulmonary passage of venous air emboli. J Appl Physiol 1985;59(2):543–7.

[8] Smith RM, Neuman TS. Elevation of serum creatine kinase in divers with arterial gas embolization. N Engl J Med 1994;330:19–24.

[9] Macklin MT, Macklin CC. Malignant interstitial emphysema of the lungs and mediastinum as an important occult complication in many respiratory diseases and other conditions. Medicine 1944;23:281–354.

[10] Pierson DJ. Pneumomediastinum. In: Murray JF, Nadel JA, editors. Textbook of respiratory medicine.

2nd edition. Philadelphia: WB Saunders; 1994. p. 2250–65.

[11] Schaeffer KE, Nutly WP, Carey C, et al. Mechanisms in development of interstitial emphysema and air embolism on decompression from depth. J Appl Physiol 1958;13:15–29.

[12] Malhotra MC, Wright HC. The effect of raised intrapleural pressure on the lungs of fresh unchilled cadavers. J Pathol Bacteriol 1961;82:198–202.

[13] Newton NI, Adams AP. Excessive airway pressure during anesthesia: hazards, effects and prevention. Anaesthesia 1978;33:689–99.

[14] Tetzlaff K, Reuter M, Leplow B, et al. Risk factors for pulmonary barotrauma in divers. Chest 1997;112: 654–9.

[15] Thorsen E, Skogstad M, Reed JW. Subacute effects of inspiratory resistive loading and head-out water immersion on pulmonary function. Undersea Hyperb Med 1999;26:137–41.

[16] Morrison JB, Taylor NA. Measurement of static and dynamic pulmonary work during pressure breathing. Undersea Biomed Res 1990;17:453–67.

[17] Baer R, Dahlback GO, Balldin UI. Pulmonary mechanics and atelectasis during immersion in oxygen-breathing subjects. Undersea Biomed Res 1987; 14:229–40.

[18] British Thoracic Society Fitness to Dive Group. British Thoracic Society guidelines on respiratory aspects of fitness for diving. Thorax 2003;58:3–13.

[19] Thorsen E, Segadal K, Myrseth E, et al. Pulmonary mechanical function and diffusion capacity after deep saturation dives. Br J Ind Med 1990;47:242–7.

[20] Thorsen E, Segadal K, Kambestad BK. Mechanisms of reduced pulmonary function after a saturation dive. Eur Respir J 1994;7:4–10.

[21] Skogstad M, Thorsen E, Haldorsen T, et al. Divers' pulmonary function after open-sea bounce dives to 10 and 50 meters. Undersea Hyperb Med 1996;23:71–5.

[22] Dujic Z, Eterovic D, Denoble P, et al. Effect of a single air dive on pulmonary diffusing capacity in professional divers. J Appl Physiol 1993;74:55–61.

[23] Catron PW, Bertoncini J, Layton RP, et al. Respiratory mechanics in men following a deep air dive. J Appl Physiol 1986;61:734–40.

[24] Dougherty Jr JH. Use of H2 as an inert gas during diving: pulmonary function during H2- O2 breathing at 7.06 ATA. Aviat Space Environ Med 1976;47: 618–26.

[25] Thorsen E, Risberg J, Segadal K, et al. Effects of venous gas microemboli on pulmonary gas transfer function. Undersea Hyperb Med 1995;22:347–53.

[26] Skogstad M, Thorsen E, Haldorsen T. Lung function over the first 3 years of a professional career. Occup Environ Med 2000;57:390–5.

[27] Neubauer B, Tetzlaff K. Prospective lung function determination using an electronic miniature spirometer for detection of acute obstructive respiratory changes in diving students during occupational diving training. Pneumologie 1999;53:219–25.

[28] Eckenhoff RG, Dougherty Jr JH, Messier AA, et al. Progression of and recovery from pulmonary oxygen toxicity in humans exposed to 5 ATA air. Aviat Space Environ Med 1987;58:658–67.

[29] Thorsen E, Kambestad BK. Persistent small-airways dysfunction after exposure to hyperoxia. J Appl Physiol 1995;78:1421–4.

[30] Thorsen E, Segadal K, Reed JW, et al. Contribution of hyperoxia to reduced pulmonary function after deep saturation dives. J Appl Physiol 1993;75: 657–62.

[31] Thorsen E, Segadal K, Kambestad BK, et al. Pulmonary function one and four years after a deep saturation dive. Scand J Work Environ Health 1993;19:115–20.

[32] Smith RM, Hong SK, Dressendorfer RH, et al. Hana Kai II: a 17-day dry saturation dive at 18.6 ATA. IV. Cardiopulmonary functions. Undersea Biomed Res 1977;4:267–81.

[33] US Navy diving manual, volume 1. Air diving, revision 3. Publication no. 0994-LP-001-9010. US Navy Sea Systems Command; 1993. p. 1-1–8-72 [appendices A-1 to O-1].

[34] Caruso JL. Cardiovascular fitness and diving. Alert diver (July/August 1999). Available at: http://www. diversalertnetwork.org/medical/articles/article.asp? articleid=11. Accessed August 20, 2001.

[35] Janicki JS, Weber KT. Equipment and protocols to evaluate exercise response. In: Cariopulmonary exercise testing. Philadelphia: WB Saunders; 1986. p. 138–50.

[36] Deal EC, Wasserman SI, Soter NA, et al. Evaluation of the role played by mediators of immediate hypersensitivity in exercise-induced asthma. J Clin Invest 1980;65:659–65.

[37] Strauss RH, McFadden ER, Ingram RH, et al. Enhancement of exercise-induced asthma by cold air. N Engl J Med 1977;297:743–6.

[38] Van Hoesen KB, Neuman TS. Asthma and scuba diving. Immunol Allergy Clin North Am 1996;16: 917–28.

[39] Smith CM, Anderson SD. Inhalation provocation tests using non-isotonic aerosols. J Allergy Clin Immunol 1989;84:781–90.

[40] Smith CM, Anderson SD. Inhalational challenge using hypertonic saline in asthmatic subjects: a comparison with responses to hyperpnea, methacholine and water. Eur Respir J 1990;3:144–51.

[41] Tezlaff K, Muth CM, Waldhauser LK. A review of asthma and SCUBA diving. J Asthma 2002;39: 557–66.

[42] Army regulation 40-501. Standards of medical fitness. Unclassified US GPO 1995-387-857:20005. Washington (DC): Department of the Army; 1995. p. 24–33.

[43] Neuman TS, Bove AA, O'Connor RD, et al. Asthma and diving. Am Allergy 1994;73:344–50.

[44] Tashkin DP, Altose MD, Bleecker ER, et al. The lung health study: airway responsiveness to in-

haled methacholine in smokers with mild to moderate airflow limitation. The Lung Health Study Research Group. Am Rev Respir Dis 1992;145(2 Pt 1): 301–10.

[45] Kanner RE, Connett JE, Altose MD, et al. Gender difference in airway hyperresponsiveness in smokers with mild COPD. The Lung Health Study. Am J Respir Crit Care Med 1994;150:956–61.

[46] Tetzlaff K, Reuter M, Leplow B, et al. Risk factors for pulmonary barotrauma in divers. Chest 1997;112: 654–9.

[47] Wilmshurst P, Davidson C, O'Connell G, et al. Role of cardiorespiratory abnormalities, smoking and dive characteristics in the manifestations of neurological decompression illness. Clin Sci (Lond) 1994;86: 297–303.

[48] Buch DA, El Moalem H, Dovenbarger JA, et al. Cigarette smoking and decompression illness severity: a retrospective study in recreational divers. Aviat Space Environ Med 2003;74:1271–4.

[49] Reuter M, Tetzlaff, Warninghoff V, et al. Computed tomography of the chest in diving related pulmonary barotrauma. Br J Radiol 1997;70:440–5.

[50] Moon RE. Treatment of diving emergencies. Crit Care Clin 1999;15:429–56.

[51] Moon RE, Camporesi EM, Kisslo JA. Patent foramen ovale and decompression sickness in divers. Lancet 1989;1:513–4.

[52] Schwerzmann M, Seiler C, Lipp E, et al. Relation between directly detected patent foramen ovale and ischemic brain lesions in sport divers. Ann Intern Med 2001;134:21–4.

[53] Strauss MB, Borer RC. Diving medicine: contemporary topics and their controversies. Am J Emerg Med 2001;19:232–8.

[54] Virtual Naval Hospital. US Naval flight surgeon manual. 3rd edition, 1991. Available at: http://www.vnh.org.FSManual/01/01Atmosphere.html. Accessed July 1, 2001.

[55] Howe JP, Alpert JS, Rickman FD, et al. Return of arterial PO2 values to baseline after supplemental oxygen in patients with cardiac disease. Chest 1975; 67:256–8.

[56] Sherter CB, Jablour SM, Kovnat DM, et al. Prolonged rate of decay of arterial PO2 following oxygen breathing in chronic airways obstruction. Chest 1975;67:259–61.

[57] Cugell DW. How long should you wait [editorial]? Chest 1975;67:254.

[58] Hartmann CM, Steinhoff-Lankes D, Maya-Pelzer P. Lung function requirements in flying duty: the problem of bronchial hyperresponsiveness in military aircrew. Eur J Med Res 1999;4:375–8.

[59] Yoneda I, Tomoda M, Tokumaru O, et al. Time of useful consciousness determination in aircrew members with reference to prior altitude chamber experience and age. Aviat Space Environ Med 2000;71: 72–6.

[60] Kannan N, Raychaudhuri A, Pilmanis AA. A log-

logistic model for altitude decompression sickness. Aviat Space Environ Med 1998;69:965–70.

[61] Pilmanis AA, Olson RM, Fischer MD, et al. Exercise-induced altitude decompression sickness. Aviat Space Environ Med 1999;70:22–9.

[62] Webb JT, Pilmanis AA, O'Connor RB. An abrupt zero-preoxygenation altitude threshold for decompression sickness symptoms. Aviat Space Environ Med 1998;69:335–40.

[63] Selvester RH, Ahmed J, Tolan GD. Asymptomatic coronary artery disease detection: update 1996. A screening protocol using 16-lead high-resolution ECG, ultrafast CT, exercise testing, and radionuclear imaging. J Electrocardiol 1996;29(Suppl):135–44.

[64] McCall NJ, Wick Jr RL, Brawley WL, et al. A survey of blood lipid levels of airline pilot applicants. Aviat Space Environ Med 1992;63:533–7.

[65] Booze Jr CF, Simcox LS. Blood pressure levels of active pilots compared with those of air traffic controllers. Aviat Space Environ Med 1985;56:1092–6.

[66] Schwarz YA, Erel J, Davidson B, et al. An algorithm for pulmonary screening of military pilots in Israel. Chest 1997;111:916–21.

[67] Roth BR, Hammers LM, Dillard TA. Methacholine challenge testing in reserve officer training corps cadets. Chest 2001;19:701–7.

[68] Keesling CA, Johnson CE, Grayson DE, et al. The utility of screening chest radiographs for flight physicals. Milit Med 2000;165:667–9.

[69] Martin DS, D'Aunno DS, Wood ML, et al. Repetitive high G exposure is associated with increased occurrence of cardiac valvular regurgitation. Aviat Space Environ Med 1999;70:1197–200.

[70] Iglesias R, Cortes MDCG, Almanza C. Facing air passengers' medical problems while on board. Aerosp Med 1974;45:204–6.

[71] Coker RK, Partridge MR. Flying with respiratory disease: what happens to patients with respiratory disease when they fly? Thorax 2004;59:919–20.

[72] Cottrell JJ. Altitude exposures during aircraft flight: flying higher. Chest 1988;92:81–4.

[73] Dillard TA, Berg BW, Rajagopal KR, et al. Hypoxemia during air travel in patients with chronic obstructive pulmonary disease. Ann Intern Med 1989;111:362–7.

[74] Christensen CC, Ryg M, Refvem OK, et al. Development of severe hypoxaemia in chronic obstructive pulmonary disease patients at 2438 m (8000 ft) altitude. Eur Respir J 2000;15:635–9.

[75] Sirven JI, Claypool DW, Sahs KL, et al. Is there a neurologist on this flight? Neurology 2002;58: 1739–44.

[76] AMA Commission on Emergency Medical Services. Medical aspects of transportation aboard commercial aircraft. JAMA 1982;247:1007–11.

[77] ATS/ERS Task Force. Standards for the diagnosis and treatment of patients with COPD: a summary of the ATS/ERS position paper. Eur Respir J 2004;23: 932–46.

[78] Matthys J, Volz H, Ernst H. [Kardiopulmonale belanstung von flugpassagieren mit obsrruktiven ventilationsstorungen]. Schweiz Med Wochenschr 1975;104:1786–9 [in German].

[79] Pierson DJ. Controversies in home respiratory care: conference summary. Respir Care 1994;39(4):294–308.

[80] Dillard TA, Moores LK, Bilello KL, et al. The preflight evaluation: a comparison of the hypoxia inhalation test with hypobaric exposure. Chest 1995; 107:352–7.

[81] Muhm JM. Predicted arterial oxygenation at commercial aircraft cabin altitudes. Aviat Space Environ Med 2004;75:905–12.

[82] Chi-Lem G, Rerez-Padilla R. Gas exchange at rest during simulated altitude in patients with chronic lung disease. Arch Med Res (Mexico) 1998;29:57–62.

[83] Dillard TA, Piantadosi S. Arterial hypoxemia at altitude and the arterial-to-alveolar oxygen ratio. Ann Intern Med 1990;112:147–8.

[84] Naughton MT, Rochford PD, Pretto JJ, et al. Is normobaric simulation of hypobaric hypoxia accurate in chronic airflow limitation? Am J Respir Crit Care Med 1995;152:1956–60.

[85] Schwartz JS, Bencowitz HZ, Moser KM. Air travel hypoxemia with chronic obstructive pulmonary disease. Ann Intern Med 1984;100:473–7.

[86] Gong H, Tashkin DP, Lee EY, et al. Hypoxia-altitude simulation test. Am Rev Respir Dis 1984;130:980–6.

[87] Vohra KP, Klocke RA. Detection and correction of hypoxemia associated with air travel. Am Rev Respir Dis 1993;148:1215–9.

[88] Cramer D, Ward S, Geddes D. Assessment of oxygen supplementation during air travel. Thorax 1996;51: 202–3.

[89] Mehm WJ, Dillard TA, Berg BW, et al. Accuracy of oxyhemoglobin saturation monitors during simulated altitude exposure of men with chronic obstructive pulmonary disease. Aviat Space Environ Med 1991;62:418–21.

[90] Cottrell JJ, Lebovitz BL, Fennell RG, et al. In-flight arterial saturation: continuous monitoring by pulse oximetry. Aviat Space Environ Med 1995;66: 126–30.

[91] British Thoracic Society Standards of Care Committee. Managing passengers with respiratory disease planning air travel: British Thoracic Society recommendations. Thorax 2002;57:1–15.

[92] Seccombe LM, Kelly PT, Wong CK, et al. Effect of simulated commercial flight on oxygenation in patients with interstitial lung disease and chronic obstructive pulmonary disease. Thorax 2004;59:966–70.

[93] Oades PJ, Buchdhal RM, Bush A. Prediction of hypoxaemia at high altitude in children with cystic fibrosis. BMJ 1994;308(6920):15–8.

[94] Bendrick GA, Nicolas DK, Krause BA, et al. In-flight oxygen saturation decrements in aeromedical evacuation patients. Aviat Space Environ Med 1995; 66:40–4.

[95] Kramer MR, Jakobson DJ, Springer C, et al. The safety of air transportation of patients with advanced lung disease: experience with 21 patients requiring lung transplantation or pulmonary thromboendarterectomy. Chest 1995;108:1292–6.

[96] Maillard D, Ferracci F, Marotte H, et al. Testing of the AVL OPTI 1 portable blood gas analyzer during inflight conditions. Aviat Space Environ Med 1999; 70:346–50.

[97] Berg BW, Dillard TA, Rajagopal KR, et al. Oxygen supplementation during air travel in patients with chronic obstructive lung disease. Chest 1992;101: 638–41.

[98] Stoller JK, Hoisington E, Auger G. A comparative analysis of arranging in-flight oxygen aboard commercial air carriers. Chest 1999;115:991–5.

[99] Stoller JE. Oxygen and air travel. Respiratory Care 2000;45:214–22.

[100] Cruickshank JM, Gorlin R, Jennet B. Air travel and thrombotic episodes: the economy class syndrome. Lancet 1988;2:497–8.

[101] Lapostolle F, Surget V, Borron SW, et al. Severe pulmonary embolism associated with air travel. N Engl J Med 2001;345:779–83.

[102] Scurr JH, Machin SJ, Bailey-King S, et al. Frequency and prevention of symptomless deep-vein thrombosis in long-haul flights: a randomised trial. Lancet 2001; 357:1485–9.

[103] Belcaro G, Geroulakos G, Nicolaides AN, et al. Venous thromboembolism from air travel: the LONFLIT study. Angiology 2001;52:369–74.

[104] Rege KP, Bevan DH, Chitolie A, et al. Risk factors and thrombosis after airline flight. Thromb Haemost 1999;81:995–6.

[105] Aerospace Medical Association, Medical Guidelines Task Force. Medical guidelines for airline travel. 2nd edition. Aviat Environ Med 2003;74(5 section II):A1–19.

[106] National Geographic Society. Everest 50. National Geographic [map insert]. March 2003.

[107] Hackett PH, Yarnell PR, Hill R, et al. High-altitude cerebral edema evaluated with magnetic resonance imaging: clinical correlation and pathophysiology. JAMA 1998;280:1920–5.

[108] Dillard TA, Rajagopal KR, Slivka WA, et al. Lung function during moderate hypobaric hypoxia in normal subjects and patients with chronic obstructive pulmonary disease. Aviat Space Environ Med 1998; 69:979–85.

[109] Pollard AJ, Barry PW, Mason NP, et al. Hypoxia, hypocapnia and spirometry at altitude. Clin Sci 1997; 92:593–8 [erratum: Clin Sci (Colch) 1997;93:611].

[110] Mason NP, Barry PW, Pollard AJ, et al. Serial changes in spirometry during an ascent to 5,300 m in the Nepalese Himalayas. High Alt Med Biol 2000; 1:185–95.

[111] Welsh CH, Wagner PD, Reeves JT, et al. Operation Everest II: spirometric and radiographic changes in acclimatized humans at simulated high altitudes. Am Rev Respir Dis 1993;147:1239–44.

[112] Levine BD, Kubo K, Kobayashi T, et al. Role of

barometric pressure in pulmonary fluid balance and oxygen transport. J Appl Physiol 1988;64:419–28.

[113] Houston CS, Sutton JR, Cymmerman A, et al. Operation Everest II: man at extreme altitude. J Appl Physiol 1987;63:531–9.

[114] Vock P, Fretz C, Franciolli M, et al. High altitude pulmonary edema: findings at high altitude chest radiography and physical examination. Radiology 1989;170:661–6.

[115] Gray G, Coates G, Powles P. Lung volume changes during acute hypobaric hypoxia. J Appl Physiol 1986; 61:1599.

[116] Gautier H, Peslin R, Grassino A, et al. Mechanical properties of the lungs during acclimatization to altitudes. J Appl Physiol 1982;52:1407–15.

[117] Forte Jr VA, Leith DE, Muza SR, et al. Ventilatory capacities at sea level and high altitude. Aviat Space Environ Med 1997;68:488–93.

[118] Zielinski J, Koziej M, Mankowski M, et al. The quality of sleep and periodic breathing in healthy subjects at an altitude of 3,200 m. High Alt Med Biol 2000;1:331–6.

[119] Graham WG, Houston CS. Short-term adaptation to moderate altitude. Patients with chronic obstructive pulmonary disease. JAMA 1978;240:1491–4.

[120] Berg BW, Dillard TA, Derderian SS, et al. Hemodynamic effects of altitude exposure and oxygen administration in chronic obstructive pulmonary disease. Am J Med 1993;94:407–12.

[121] Hansen JE. Diet and flight hypoxemia [letter]. Ann Intern Med 1989;111:859–60.

[122] Blau H, Mussaffi-Georgy H, Fink G, et al. Effects of an intensive 4-week summer camp on cystic fibrosis: pulmonary function, exercise tolerance, and nutrition. Chest 2002;121:1117–22.

[123] Rose DM, Fleck B, Thews O, et al. Blood gas-analyses in patients with cystic fibrosis to estimate hypoxemia during exposure to high altitudes in a hypobaric-chamber. Eur J Med Res 2000;5:9–12.

[124] Speechly-Dick M, Rimmer S, Hodson M. Exacerbations of cystic fibrosis after holidays at high altitude—a cautionary tale. Respir Med 1992;86: 55–6.

[125] Matsuda S, Onda T, Iikura Y. Bronchial responsiveness of asthmatic patients in an atmosphere-changing chamber. Int Arch Allergy Immunol 1995;107:402–5.

[126] Jensen RL, Crapo RO, Berlin SL. Effect of altitude on hand-held peak flowmeters. Chest 1996;109:475–9.

[127] Pedersen OF, Miller MR, Sigsgaard T, et al. Portable peak flow meters: physical characteristics, influence of temperature, altitude, and humidity. Eur Respir J 1994;7:991–7.

[128] Palatini P, Businaro R, Berton G, et al. Effects of low altitude exposure on 24-hour blood pressure and adrenergic activity. Am J Cardiol 1989;64:1379–82.

[129] Halhuber M, Humpeler E, Inama K, et al. Does altitude cause exhaustion of the heart and circulatory system? Med Sport Sci 1985;19:192–202.

[130] Levine B, Zuckerman J, deFilippi C. Effect of high altitude exposure in the elderly: the 10th Mountain Division Study. Circulation 1997;96:1224–32.

[131] Hultgren H. Coronary heart disease and trekking. J Wilderness Med 1990;1:154–60.

[132] Burtsher M, Philadelphy M, Likar R. Sudden cardiac death during mountain hiking and downhill skiing. N Engl J Med 1993;329:1738–9.

[133] Levine BD, Grayburn PA, Voyles WF, et al. Intracardiac shunting across a patent foramen ovale may exacerbate hypoxemia in high altitude pulmonary edema. Ann Intern Med 1991;114:569–70.

[134] Dalen J, Bruce R, Cobb L. Interaction of chronic hypoxia of moderate altitude on pulmonary hypertension complicating defect of the atrial septum. N Engl J Med 1962;266:272–7.

[135] Nicholas R, O'Meara P. High-altitude syncope: history repeats itself. JAMA 1993;269:587.

[136] Jenzer G, Bartsch P. Migraine with aura at high altitude: case report. J Wilderness Med 1993;4:412–5.

[137] Pflauser B, Volbert H, Bosch S, et al. Cerebral venous thrombosis-a new diagnosis in travel medicine? J Travel Med 1996;3:165–7.

[138] Shlim DR, Meijer H. Sudden symptomatic brain tumors at altitude. Ann Emerg Med 1991;20:315–6.

[139] Beard JL, Haas JD, Tufts DA, et al. Iron deficiency anemia and steady-state work performance at high altitude. J Appl Physiol 1988;64:1878–84.

[140] Green RL, Huntsman RG, Serjeant GRl. The sickle-cell and altitude. BMJ 1971;4:593–5.

[141] Mahoney BS, Githens H. Sickling crisis and altitude: occurrence in the Colorado patient population. Clin Pediatr 1979;18:431–4.

[142] Dillard TA, Kark JA, Rajagopal KR, et al. Pulmonary function in men with sickle cell trait. Ann Intern Med 1987;106:191–6.

[143] Mader TH, Blanton CL, Gilbert BN, et al. Refractive changes during 72-hour exposure to high altitude after refractive surgery. Ophthalmology 1996;103(8): 1188–95.

Clin Chest Med 26 (2005) 509–515

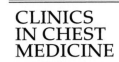

Index

Note: Page numbers of article titles are in **boldface** type.

A

Acute high-altitude pulmonary illness
  in sojourners, 396–397

Acute mountain sickness
  features of, 397

Aerobic fitness
  in divers, 489

Aerosol(s)
  inhaled
    in microgravity studies, 432

Aerospace exposures
  pulmonary function effects of, 492–493

Aging
  effects on respiratory system, **469–483.** See also
    Respiratory system, aging effects on.

Air travel
  pulmonary function effects of, 493–499

Airway(s)
  extra-thoracic
    limitations of
      respiratory response to exercise and,
        446–447
  intra-thoracic
    limitations of
      respiratory system response to exercise
        and, 447–453
  limitations of
    exercise and, 453–454
  peripheral
    age-associated changes in, 472

Airway resistance and conductance
  in older persons, 476

Altitude
  high
    drive to breathe at, 406
    respiration at
      limits of, **405–414.** See also *High-
      altitude environment.*
    pulmonary effects of, 491
  terrestrial
    pulmonary function effects of, 499–503

Alveolar ventilation
  EIAH and, 463

Apnea diving
  cardiovascular effects of, 389–391
  changes in partial pressure of breathing gases
    during descent and ascent, 385–387
  decompression sickness due to, 387–389
  described, 381–382
  excessive hyperventilation during, 387
  nitrogen narcosis due to, 387–389
  physiological and clinical aspects of, **381–394**

Asthma
  at terrestrial altitude, 501
  exercise effects on, 447–450
  in divers, 490

B

Barotrauma
  pulmonary
    diving while breathing compressed gas and,
      358–363

Breath-hold diving. See *Apnea diving.*

Breathing
  at depth, **355–380.** See also *Diving, while
    breathing compressed gas.*
  regulation of
    in older persons, 477–478
  sleep-disordered
    at terrestrial altitude, 500
  work of
    at high altitude, 407–410
    during exercise
      minimization of
        in healthy untrained normal
          subjects, 440

0272-5231/05/$ – see front matter © 2005 Elsevier Inc. All rights reserved.
doi:10.1016/S0272-5231(05)00085-7

chestmed.theclinics.com

Breathing gases
  partial pressure of
    changes in
      during apnea diving, 385–387

C
Carbon monoxide transfer factor
  in older persons, 477
Cardiac output
  in microgravity studies, 423–424
  increased
    in healthy untrained normal subjects, 441
Cardiovascular disease
  at terrestrial altitude, 501–502
  in divers, 491
Cardiovascular system
  apnea diving effects on, 389–391
Chest wall
  age-associated changes in, 469
  shape and movement of
    in microgravity studies, 420
Chest wall mechanics
  lung volumes and, 417–420
CHF. See *Congestive heart failure (CHF)*.
Chronic mountain sickness, 396
Chronic obstructive pulmonary disease (COPD)
  at terrestrial altitude, 500–501
Compressed gas
  diving while breathing, **355–380.** See also
    Diving, while breathing compressed gas.
Congestive heart failure (CHF)
  at terrestrial altitude, 502
COPD. See *Chronic obstructive pulmonary
  disease (COPD)*.
Coronary artery disease
  at terrestrial altitude, 501–502
Cystic fibrosis
  at terrestrial altitude, 501

D
Decompression illness
  diving while breathing compressed gas and,
    363–368
  prior
    in divers, 491
Decompression sickness
  apnea diving and, 387–389

Decompression stress
  effects on lung function during diving, 357
Deep venous thrombosis
  at high altitude, 499
Diffusing capacity
  lung water and
    in microgravity studies, 425
Diffusion limitation
  EIAH and, 462
Dive(s)
  single
    respiratory effects of, 358
Diving
  aerobic fitness in, 489
  apnea
    physiological and clinical aspects of, **381–394**
  asthma and, 490
  breath-hold. See *Apnea diving.*
  cardiovascular disease and, 491
  depth of
    theoretic limits of, 382–385
  fitness for
    concomitant respiratory diseases and,
      369–372
    respiratory assessment of, 371–372
  hazards of, 486–488
  lung function during
    decompression stress and, 357
    diving exposure and, 356
    gas density and, 357–358
    hyperoxia and, 356–357
    physical and physiological factors affecting,
      356–358
    respiratory heat and water loss and, 358
    respiratory mechanical loading and, 357–358
  methods of, 355–356
  patent foramen ovale and, 491
  pneumothorax and, 490
  prior decompression illness and, 491
  pulmonary function effects of, 486–491
    described, 488–489
    long-term, 372–373
  routine evaluation of candidates for, 489
  smoking and, 490
  while breathing compressed gas, **355–380**
    clinical problems related to, 358–369
    decompression illness due to, 363–368
    fitness to dive effects on concomitant
      respiratory diseases, 369–372
    pulmonary barotrauma due to, 358–363
    pulmonary edema due to, 368–369
  with respiratory diseases, 370–371

E

Edema
  pulmonary
    diving while breathing compressed gas and,
        368–369
    interstitial, 463–464

EIAH. See *Exercise-induced arterial
  hypoxemia (EIAH)*.

Energetic(s)
  in high-altitude environment, 407–410

Environment(s)
  extreme
    pulmonary function in, **485–507.** See also
        *Pulmonary function, extreme environments
        effects on.*
  high-altitude. See *High-altitude environment*.
  hyperbaric
    pulmonary function effects of, 486–491
  hypobaric
    pulmonary function effects of, 491
  space, 415–417

Exercise
  effects on asthma, 447–450
  extra-thoracic obstruction due to, 446–447
  in high-altitude pulmonary edema–prone persons
    pulmonary vascular response to, 445–446
  in microgravity studies, 429
  in persons with intrapulmonary arteriovenous
    shunting, 444–445
  maximal
    lung at, **459–468**
  pulmonary capillary stress failure due to, 465
  respiratory system response to, **439–457**
    asthma, 447–450
    extra-thoracic airway limitations of, 446–447
    in healthy untrained normal subjects, 439–441
      exercise hyperventilation, 439–440
      increased cardiac output, 441
      maximizing gas exchange efficiency,
        440–441
      minimization of work of breathing, 440
      shunting, 441–444
    intra-thoracic airway limitations, 447–453
    pulmonary vascular and airway limitations,
      453–454
    pulmonary vascular limitations, 441–446
  responses to
    pulmonary function and, 460
  ventilation and
    in older persons, 478
  ventilatory response to
    in older persons, 478–480

Exercise hyperventilation
  in healthy untrained normal subjects, 439–440

Exercise testing
  at high altitude, 498

Exercise training
  response to
    in older persons, 478

Exercise-induced arterial hypoxemia (EIAH),
    460–463
  alveolar ventilation and, 463
  described, 460–462
  diffusion limitation and, 462
  mechanisms of, 462
  shunts and, 462
  ventilation-perfusion ratio inequality and, 462

Exercise-induced pulmonary hemorrhage, 464–465

Extra-thoracic airway
  limitations of
    respiratory system response to exercise and,
        446–447

Extravehicular activity
  in microgravity studies, 433–434

Extreme environments
  pulmonary function effects of
    aerospace exposures, 492–493
    air travel, 493–499
    altitude, 491
    hyperbaric, 486–491. See also *Diving*.
    hypobaric, 491
    terrestrial altitude, 499–503

F

Flow-volume curves
  in older persons, 474–476

Functional residual capacity
  in microgravity studies, 417–418

G

Gas(es)
  breathing
    changes in partial pressure of
        during apnea diving, 385–387
    compressed
      diving while breathing, **355–380.** See also
          Diving, while breathing compressed gas.

Gas density
  effects on lung function during diving, 357–358

Gas exchange
  in lung
    in high-altitude environment
      limitations of, 410–413
  in older persons, 476–477

Genetic(s)
  in high-altitude–related pulmonary disease,
    399–401

H

Hemorrhage
  pulmonary
    exercise-induced, 464–465

High-altitude environment, **405–414**
  described, 405–406
  drive to breathe in, 406
  energetics in, 407–410
  gas exchange in lung in
    limitations of, 410–413
  ventilatory demand at, 406–407
  work of breathing at, 407–410

High-altitude pulmonary edema–prone persons
  exercise in
    pulmonary vascular response to, 445–446

High-altitude–related pulmonary disease, **395–404**
  demographics of, 396, 398
  described, 395
  epidemiology of, 396–398
  genetics in, 399–401
  in inbred populations, 400
  risk factors for, 398–401

High-altitude–related pulmonary edema
  features of, 397–398

Hyperbaric environments
  pulmonary function effects of, 486–491

Hyperoxia
  effects on lung function during diving, 356–357

Hypertension
  at terrestrial altitude, 502
  pulmonary. See *Pulmonary hypertension.*

Hyperventilation
  excessive
    apnea diving and, 387
  exercise
    in healthy untrained normal subjects, 439–440

Hypobaric exposures
  pulmonary function effects of, 491

Hypoxemia
  arterial
    exercise-induced, 460–463. See also *Exercise-induced arterial hypoxemia (EIAH).*

Hypoxia
  chronic
    high-altitude pulmonary illness due to, 396

Hypoxia inhalation test
  at high altitude, 496–497

Hypoxic pulmonary hypertension
  altered
    animal models of, 401
  animal models of, 401

I

Inhaled aerosols
  in microgravity studies, 432

International Space Station, 416

Interstitial pulmonary edema, 463–464

Intrapulmonary arteriovenous shunting
  exercise tolerance in persons with, 444–445

Intra-thoracic airway
  limitations of
    respiratory system response to exercise and,
    447–453

L

Lung(s)
  at maximal exercise, **459–468**
  diving effects on
    long-term, 372–373
  gas exchange in
    in high-altitude environment
      limitations of, 410–413
  in space, **415–438**

Lung function
  during diving
    physical and physiological factors affecting,
    356–358

Lung parenchyma
  age-associated changes in, 472

Lung volumes
  chest wall mechanics and, 417–420
  in older persons, 473–474

Lung water
  diffusing capacity and
    in microgravity studies, 425

M

Maximal oxygen consumption
  in older persons, 479

Maximizing gas exchange efficiency
  during exercise
    in healthy untrained normal subjects, 440–441

Maximum expiratory flows
  in microgravity studies, 419–420

Microgravity
  analogs of, 417
  making measurements in, 415–416
  studies in, 417–434
    cardiac output, 423–424
    diffusing capacity and lung water, 425
    exercise, 429
    extravehicular activity, 433–434
    functional residual capacity, 417–418
    inhaled aerosols, 432
    lung volumes and chest wall mechanics, 417–420
    maximum expiratory flows, 419–420
    pulmonary gas exchange, 427–428
    pulmonary perfusion, 425–427
    pulmonary ventilation, 420–423
    residual volume, 418–419
    shape and movement of chest wall, 420
    sleep, 431–432
    ventilation-perfusion ratio, 427–428
    ventilatory control, 429–431
    vital capacity, 417–418

Mountain sickness
  acute, 397
  chronic, 396
  subacute, 396

N

Neurologic disorders
  at terrestrial altitude, 502–503

Nitrogen narcosis
  apnea diving and, 387–389

O

Oxygen consumption
  maximal
    in older persons, 479

Oxygen prescription
  at high altitude, 498–499

P

Parenchyma
  lung
    age-associated changes in, 472

Patent foramen ovale
  in divers, 491

Peak expiratory flow
  in older persons, 474–476

Periodic breathing during sleep
  at terrestrial altitude, 500

Peripheral airways
  age-associated changes in, 472

Pneumothorax
  at high altitude, 499
  in divers, 490

Pulmonary capillary stress failure, 464–465
  exercise and, 465

Pulmonary disease
  high-altitude–related, **395–404.** See also
    High-altitude–related pulmonary disease.

Pulmonary edema
  diving while breathing compressed gas and, 368–369
  interstitial, 463–464

Pulmonary embolism
  at high altitude, 499

Pulmonary function
  at altitude, 500
  exercise responses to, 460
  extreme environments effects on, **485–507**

Pulmonary function tests
  in older persons, 472–476
    airway resistance and conductance, 476
    flow-volume curves, 474–476
    lung volumes, 473–474
    peak expiratory flow, 474–476
    respiratory muscle testing, 476
    spirometry, 474

Pulmonary gas exchange
  in microgravity studies, 427–428

Pulmonary hemorrhage
  exercise-induced, 464–465

Pulmonary hypertension
  hypoxic
    altered
      animal models of, 401
    animal models of, 401
    in high-altitude residents, 396

Pulmonary perfusion
  in microgravity studies, 425–427

Pulmonary vascular limitations
  during exercise, 441–446

Pulmonary vascular response
  to exercise in high-altitude pulmonary edema–
    prone persons, 445–446

Pulmonary vascular system
  limitations of
    exercise and, 453–454

Pulmonary ventilation
  in microgravity studies, 420–423

Pulse oximetry
  at high altitude, 497–498

R

Residual volume
  in microgravity studies, 418–419

Respiration
  at high altitude
    limits of, **405–414.** See also *High-
      altitude environment.*

Respiratory diseases
  diving with, 370–371

Respiratory drive
  disorders of
    at terrestrial altitude, 500

Respiratory heat and water loss
  effects on lung function during diving, 358

Respiratory mechanical loading
  effects on lung function during diving, 357–358

Respiratory muscle function
  age-associated changes in, 470–472

Respiratory muscle testing
  in older persons, 476

Respiratory system
  aging effects on, **469–483**
    carbon monoxide transfer factor, 477
    chest wall changes, 469
    gas exchange, 476–477
    lung parenchyma, 472
    maximal oxygen consumption, 479
    peripheral airways, 472
    pulmonary function tests related to, 472–476
    regulation of breathing, 477–478

respiratory muscle function, 470–472
structural changes, 469–472
ventilatory response to exercise, 478–480

S

Shunt(s)
  EIAH and, 462

Shunting
  in healthy untrained normal subjects, 441–444

Sleep
  in microgravity studies, 431–432
  periodic breathing during
    at terrestrial altitude, 500

Sleep-disordered breathing
  at terrestrial altitude, 500

Smoking
  in divers, 490

Space
  lung in, **415–438**

Space environment, 415–417

Space flight
  early, 417

Space Shuttle, 416

Spirometry
  in older persons, 474

Stress
  decompression
    effects on lung function during diving, 357

Subacute mountain sickness, 396

T

Terrestrial altitude
  pulmonary function effects of, 499–503

Travel
  air
    pulmonary function effects of, 493–499

V

Venous thrombosis
  deep
    at high altitude, 499

Ventilation
  alveolar
    EIAH and, 463

exercise and
   in older persons, 478
pulmonary
   in microgravity studies, 420–423

Ventilation-perfusion ratio
  in microgravity studies, 427–428

Ventilation-perfusion ratio inequality
  EIAH and, 462

Ventilatory control
  in microgravity studies, 429–431

Ventilatory demand
  at high altitude, 406–407

Ventilatory response to exercise
  in older persons, 478–480

Vital capacity
  in microgravity studies, 417–418

Changing Your Address?

Make sure your subscription changes too! When you notify us of your new address, you can help make our job easier by including an exact copy of your Clinics label number with your old address (see illustration below.) This number identifies you to our computer system and will speed the processing of your address change. Please be sure this label number accompanies your old address and your corrected address—you can send an old Clinics label with your number on it or just copy it exactly and send it to the address listed below.

We appreciate your help in our attempt to give you continuous coverage. Thank you.

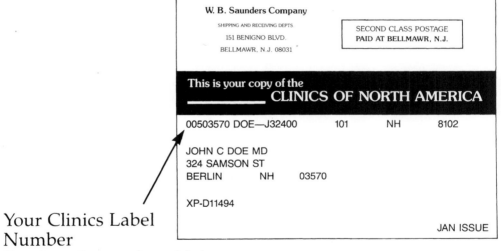

W. B. Saunders Company

SHIPPING AND RECEIVING DEPTS.
151 BENIGNO BLVD.
BELLMAWR, N.J. 08031

SECOND CLASS POSTAGE
PAID AT BELLMAWR, N.J.

This is your copy of the
CLINICS OF NORTH AMERICA

00503570 DOE—J32400   101   NH   8102

JOHN C DOE MD
324 SAMSON ST
BERLIN   NH   03570

XP-D11494

JAN ISSUE

Your Clinics Label Number
Copy it exactly or send your label
along with your address to:
W.B. Saunders Company, Customer Service
Orlando, FL 32887-4800
Call Toll Free 1-800-654-2452

Please allow four to six weeks for delivery of new subscriptions and for processing address changes.